D1240241

CURING CANCER
with
IMMUNOTHERAPY

*How it happened a century ago,
what we learned as we attempted it,
and why it is possible today.*

RENE CHEE, PhD and EDWARD CHEE, MS

FOUNDRYSOFT PRESS
SAN DIEGO

This book is intended to supplement, not replace the advice of trained oncology professionals. The authors and publisher specifically disclaim any liability, loss or risk, personal or otherwise, incurred as a consequence, directly or indirectly, of the use and application of any contents in this book.

Foundrysoft LLC
11835 Carmel Mountain Rd #1304-182
San Diego, CA 92128

Visit the authors' website at: CuringCancerBook.com

First Edition: August 2016

Figure credits are found on page 295
Authors' photograph by Eddie Kwan
Illustrations and cover design by Rene Chee

ISBN: 978-0-9978200-1-0

Printed in the United States of America

To Lloyd Old, M.D. (1933–2011)

You gave us conviction to pursue immunotherapy.

With vision and grace,
you have propelled humanity to the verge of a cure.

You will forever be remembered.

and

To Ravin Agah, M.D., Ph.D.

Because of your unwavering support,
we dared to pursue the impossible.

Contents

A Few Words About This Book

This is a work of nonfiction. It is the culmination of seven years of research and thinking through high-stakes medical decisions. Those decisions directly determined whether one of the authors, Rene, would survive an aggressive cancer.

All details of our story are factual accounts supported by medical records, personal notes, emails and photographs. Much of the dialog has been recreated from recordings, in compliance with state laws, or else from personal notes, emails and memory.

Stories of other patients are either first-hand accounts (supported by emails and recollections of personal conversations) or else derived from academic and news publications. All names of modern day cancer patients and certain identifying features have been altered to protect privacy, unless already published. The true names of Dr. William Coley's patients from a century ago are used.

This book is written for a general audience, with a focus on facilitating a broad understanding of cancer immunotherapy and how it can be used. To achieve this objective, we've simplified scientific explanations of the immune system. For example, we've left out the role of antibodies, B cells and the complement system, choosing instead to focus on T cells. Nor do we explain the different T cell subtypes.

Although written for a general audience, a priority of this book is to help cancer patients. Given the fast-evolving state of cancer immunotherapy, patients wishing to take advantage of it may have to make treatment decisions beyond the standard of care. From personal experience, and from interacting with other patients, we've found that making such decisions requires clear conviction, grounded on a solid understanding of the pros and cons. To build that conviction, we spend a lot of time in this book walking the reader through our own evolution of assessing the benefits and limitations of conventional therapies, discovering immunotherapy, and forming a treatment philosophy. We take time to elucidate thought processes surrounding medical decisions, especially those involving difficult trade-offs.

Knowing first hand that those in the early throes of cancer may be overwhelmed by treatment, we've tried to keep the book simple and focused. To achieve this, we chose the narrative form for most of the book, narrated through the eyes of one of the authors. At strategic locations, we transition into scientific expository to develop a practical understanding of the immune system. To keep the book a readable length, we forgo in-depth scientific discussions, but provide copious references for those interested.

Outlined boxes contain extra reading. Gray boxes highlight lessons learned along our journey. Figure credits, a glossary of terms and a reading group guide are provided at the end of the book.

To reflect the intensely personal nature of this book, we've chosen to use contractions throughout.

The claim of this book—that cancer can be cured—is a bold one that may be hard to believe. From firsthand experience, we know how damaging false hope can be. To that end, we strive to responsibly represent what immunotherapy offers—its strengths and limitations—using scientific explanations, modern-day clinical data and modern and historical case studies. Still, given the competing priorities and limited space, we weren't able to develop certain aspects as much as we would have liked, such as exploring still-evolving science, or scrutinizing additional case studies of long-term remissions. We hope readers will forgive such omissions.

CURING CANCER
with
IMMUNOTHERAPY

Introduction

In December of 2011, a leading surgeon at Memorial Sloan Kettering Cancer Center (MSK) in New York told me I was going to die from my cancer. He pointed to the location of my tumor with a model skull. Listing reason after reason, he convinced me why no surgeon could fully extract the recurrent cancer in my head. He said there were "thousands of microscopic tumors" waiting to grow. The best I could hope for was to buy some time by cutting out the fast-growing tumor—and along with it, my right jaw.

Meanwhile, three lesions in three areas of my lungs were advancing. A leading oncologist at the MD Anderson Cancer Center in Houston (MDA) agreed that my cancer—a rare and aggressive sarcoma—had invaded my lungs. A fourth lung tumor materialized, growing rapidly. The accelerating tumors threatened to riddle my body and take my life.

Despite my dismal prognosis, I believed I could beat my cancer. For over three years, I'd been studying how to harness the immune system against cancer. I was determined to exploit this—not just to live longer, *but to attempt a cure.*

I was first diagnosed in early 2008, a year after I married. My husband, Eddy, and I met as master's students at Stanford University. After seven years working for my Ph.D. at the University of California, San Diego, I was back at Stanford as a postdoctoral scientist, studying the inner workings of bacteria. At the prime of our lives, we were ready to build a future together. Instead, I found myself at the Stanford Cancer Center, my future in peril.

My symptoms began with strange headaches, then pain in my teeth. A doctor diagnosed a disorder of the jaw joint. Hearing loss came next, followed by expanding numbness on my tongue, then chin. A neurologist ordered an MRI and the culprit was revealed—a bulging tumor abutting my jaw, the size of an egg.

By the time I saw the surgeon, the pain was unbearable. I could barely speak or eat. I endured a year of debilitating surgery, radiation and chemo-therapy. Radiation scorched my mouth. I needed painkillers to drink water. Chemotherapy ravaged my immune system, putting me at risk of death by infection.

At the end of that torment, my oncologist congratulated me on clear scans, encouraging me to return to "normal life." But when I asked for my survival odds, she provided no concrete predictions.

Because of my job, I had access to medical and scientific papers. Scrutinizing the data, I discovered I faced a high risk of recurrence, with no effective treatments should my cancer return. One study indicated 100 percent of patients with a disease like mine would die from their cancer.

It was then, in 2009, that I knew I had to do something more to eradicate my cancer. As conventional medicine offered nothing, Eddy and I turned to complementary and alternative medicine. In desperation, we bought books, vitamins and exotic supplements. I followed intensive juice diets and saw alternative doctors. I received infusions of Vitamin C, acupuncture and natural compounds that strengthened the body's innate defenses.

While researching the science behind these alternatives, we identified a recurring theme: strengthening the immune system. We then learned of numerous cases of spontaneous disappearances of cancer—and how some scientists attributed them to the immune system.

And then, we discovered a 100-year-old immunotherapy—a treatment that harnessed the immune system against cancer. Known as Coley's Toxins, it was an injection of two dead strains of bacteria, developed by a Harvard-trained surgeon in New York, in the late 1890s.

Intriguingly, most of Dr. William Coley's patients had advanced sar-comas, similar to mine. Despite their advanced disease, many survived for years—without any chemo or radiation. Some survived *decades,* dying of natural causes. One woman with terminal cervical cancer—a disease still incurable today—lived 30 years cancer-free, dying of pneumonia at 79.[1]

Elated, we brought this information to my oncologist. But she gently dismissed it as belonging to the realm of "alternative" medicine. Even so, we believed it was a mistake to ignore the historical anecdotes, and that science could explain the miraculous healings.

In the midst of our research, my professor at Stanford connected us with Lloyd Old, M.D., a leading cancer scientist at Memorial Sloan Kettering Cancer Center. Considered by many to be the "Father of Modern Tumor Immunology," Dr. Old affirmed our thinking about Coley's Toxins and the power of the immune system to destroy cancer.

Guided by Dr. Old, we embarked on a quest to destroy the invisible cancer in my body. Using a vaccine, he first trained my immune cells to target my cancer. Then, to weaken the cancer's defenses, he wanted me to receive Yervoy, a powerful immunotherapy being tested in clinical trials. I didn't qualify for the trials, but all was not lost—Dr. Old thought Coley's Toxins might achieve the same results.

There was no way to get Coley's Toxins in the U.S. as the FDA prohibited its sale—even though American doctors had used it 100 years earlier. Undaunted, Eddy and I traveled to Mexico to get it.

Despite our efforts, in 2011, my cancer returned in my head and spread to my lungs. My doctors recommended surgery, but we didn't rush into treatment. Instead, we consulted two oncologists and three surgeons. Confirming our fears, they said the chances of a cure with surgery and chemo were low—around 20 percent. One of them—the leading surgeon at MSK (who showed us the model skull)—asserted that the odds were zero.

Resolute, we still believed the evidence showed an immune-based cure was possible. Eschewing conventional treatment, we doubled down on immunotherapy and battled my cancer for another three years.

It would take absolute resolve. Immunotherapy was still highly experimental. We faced opposition from doctors who thought we were pursuing quackery. And we had to go through great lengths to obtain immunotherapy as there was a dearth of clinical trials.

We devised strategies to prevent my cancer from evading the immune system. We had a doctor insert special needles into my tumors to freeze them. The freezing killed the tumors while sensitizing my immune system to proteins in my cancer—like a broad vaccine. We flew to Germany every six weeks, where I received injections of immune cells that could directly kill cancer. We legally brought Coley's Toxins back to the U.S., but no doctor would administer it, so, Eddy had to. For over two years, I received over 200 infusions of the dead bacteria, causing chills and fevers reaching 104°F. We performed these wherever our adventures took us—San Francisco, Detroit, Houston, New York and Germany—in hotels, motels and in my bedroom at home.

My jaw tumor shriveled at first, but then it regrew. I decided to have my jaw amputated. But then, my tumor was discovered to be teeming with T cells—immune cells that destroy cancer! The T cells signified my immune system had begun to attack my cancer.

Galvanized, we forged ahead to eradicate the thousands of micro-tumors in my head. With trembling hands, Eddy stooped over me, surgical mask donned, to inject Coley's Toxins into the crater where my jaw once existed. Sitting by my bed, he held my hand as I endured the transient but intense pain cause by the surge of immune cells.

•。•• •。• •• •。

We had both grown up sheltered and studious. Our lives had followed safe and predictable paths in school and work. On weekends, we preferred having friends over for meals instead of venturing into the wilderness on hikes or camping trips. When it came to medicine, we had always submitted to doctors. How then did we end up defying our doctors, abandoning our careers, traveling the world for treatment and injecting dead bacteria to survive?

The answer? Objectivity, grounded on science.

An objective analysis of medical studies convinced us: should I rely on conventional therapies, I would die.

Objectivity told us I had to act before my cancer returned, because the best time to attack cancer with immunotherapy was when the cancer was still microscopic.

Objectivity told us that if we didn't already have a plan in place (and gleaned some experience with immunotherapy), there'd be no time to learn the ropes once my cancer returned—in which case I'd likely go along with chemo in a panic, and then die anyway.

Objectivity told us Dr. Coley's century-old cures weren't flukes—patients who had terminal cancer were presented before panels of doctors, alive and well decades later.

Guided by Dr. Old, our study of the immune system told us Coley's Toxins wasn't some mystical "alternative" therapy. A wide body of science supported the plausibility of an immune-based cure.

So, facing death in my early 30s, objectivity drove us to step out of our comfort zones, look past man-made constraints of what can or cannot be achieved and pursue a cure.

Our faith, hope and hard work have been rewarded. The expert surgeon said my cancer would kill me. But my scans have stayed silent for the past three years, and I am alive eight years after diagnosis. For a high-grade sarcoma that was twice-recurrent, metastatic and accelerating, that silence speaks volumes. It compels us to believe that immunotherapy has kept me alive against all odds.

On the Verge of a Cure

We believe a cure for cancer will be achieved through immunotherapy. Some of Dr. Coley's patients were cured 100 years ago. And some patients who've participated in modern immunotherapy trials are now alive 16 years later—effectively cured. We believe modern science will soon unlock the secret formula to make these cures reproducible on a widespread scale.

Unlike other drugs, immunotherapy works on the immune system, not on specific types of tumors. If you can activate the immune system against cancer, it should work for any type, not just those it's approved for.

As an example, the modern immunotherapy drugs Keytruda and Opdivo, also known as PD-1 inhibitors, first demonstrated benefit in patients with melanoma, a form of skin cancer known to respond to immunotherapy. About 25 percent of terminal patients responded, leading to rapid FDA approval. Shortly after, researchers were amazed to find that it worked for lung cancer—a cancer they didn't think would respond to immunotherapy. Within two years, the FDA approved PD-1 for lung cancer, kidney cancer, bladder cancer and lymphoma. Approval is likely soon to come for gastric cancer.

It will take time for clinical trials to play out among more cancer types.

But these early signals already confirm what logic tells us: immunotherapy—which works on immune cells—is not specific to one type of cancer.

Since 2009, we have staked my survival on the belief that immunotherapy can cure my sarcoma. But it wasn't until the later half of 2014, after decades of research and testing, that clinical trials for two modern immunotherapies demonstrated revolutionary results, forever dispelling the misconception that the immune system is useless against cancer.[2]

Skeptics turned into believers. Doctors who didn't take our efforts at immunotherapy seriously now do. All across the country, cancer centers are racing to establish immunotherapy programs. Patients formerly facing certain death now enjoy stabilization or even complete remission. The excitement is so palpable that the federal government, under the leadership of Vice President Joe Biden, has launched an ambitious "moonshot" to *cure* cancer. Only a short while ago, uttering the word "cure" would have evoked skepticism and ridicule.

Former President Jimmy Carter's success with immunotherapy justifies this optimism. In the summer of 2015, doctors removed a cancerous spot in his liver. On August 20, 2015, Carter announced the cancer had spread to his brain. Carter's prognosis was dismal, with an average four months survival.[3] "I just thought I had a few weeks left," he said at a news conference.[4]

Hours later, 90-year-old Carter underwent treatment. Carter's doctors, likely apprised of the latest research, cleverly gave him the immunotherapy drug Keytruda (the PD-1 inhibitor) in combination with radiation. Six months later, Carter announced he no longer needed treatment. His cancer was gone.

While it's possible that radiation itself could have eliminated his tumors, it's more likely that PD-1 *in combination* with radiation produced the success. Powerful synergies between the two are being observed by researchers nationwide; tumors resistant to radiation or PD-1 suddenly shrink when the two are combined.[5]

Despite accelerating approvals, it will be years before most patients will benefit from immunotherapy. The majority will first be given chemo, even in cases where immunotherapy has been approved. Many will die, never even hearing about immunotherapy.

In February of 2016, my uncle told me of his childhood friend, Harry. Harry was in his 60s, and his stomach cancer had spread to his lungs. Two oncologists told him there was nothing left to do. They failed to inform Harry about the large PD-1 trial for his cancer. Nor did they tell him about the early stage trial that showed a third of patients with his cancer had responded to PD-1.[6] Harry was still well enough to take part in the trial. Alternatively, his oncologists could have prescribed PD-1 *off-label* (a legal option where they could give a drug that's approved for other cancers). But they didn't. Harry resigned himself to a hopeless prognosis. Three months later, he passed away.

Perhaps Harry's oncologists weren't apprised about immunotherapy or didn't fully appreciate its potential. But just because your doctor isn't apprised, that doesn't mean you can't benefit from immunotherapy.

We know patients who have reversed terminal cancer because they pursued immunotherapy—even though it was "experimental" and not yet approved.

In March of 2014, I met Mary, a young woman in her 30s, battling a highly resistant form of Hodgkin's lymphoma. She'd received radiation and many different chemotherapies. These failed to shrink the large mass in her chest. As a last resort, her oncologist prescribed a risky procedure that could have killed her—a stem cell transplant—even though studies had shown it was unlikely to work. He gave her treacherous doses of chemo, which demolished her immune system. For months, she was confined to the hospital. A simple infection could take her life. Luckily, she recovered. But in November 2014, she learned the procedure had done nothing for her cancer; her oncologist suggested hospice.

Then, a miracle happened. Mary had been asking her doctor about PD-1 ever since we told her about it in March. Even though scientific studies strongly suggested it would work, her oncologist had deemed it too "experimental." But in December, a Phase 1 clinical trial showed encouraging early data. Unlike Harry's oncologists, he didn't wait for FDA approval. Instead, he gave the drug to Mary *off-label*. Like Jimmy Carter's doctors, he *combined* radiation with PD-1. No hospitalization was required.

Three months later, Mary's tumors had vanished. "Experimental" immunotherapy had succeeded where multiple "proven" chemo regimens had failed. The side effects? Some itchy skin.

The Power of Knowledge

Mary is alive today and back at work because of knowledge married with action. She researched, then obtained immunotherapy *17 months* before FDA approval. Had she waited, she'd be dead.

In these pages, we'll share with you how I survived the dismal prognosis of my cancer with immunotherapy. As Patrick Hwu, M.D., Head of Cancer Medicine at the largest cancer center in the U.S. (MDA), once told us, *knowledge is power*. We will share what we learned from working with Dr. Old and other researchers and physicians, from thousands of hours studying scientific papers, and from lessons learned making difficult choices that determined my survival.

We will distill the complex immune system into understandable concepts. We will show you how the current immunotherapy results—as revolutionary as they may be—can be improved upon. And we'll describe the science and strategies on how to mobilize a more complete immune response against cancer for better results.

Part 1 of the book describes how we found immunotherapy. **Chapters 1 and 2** describe my diagnosis and initial treatment with conventional therapies, the limitations of these approaches and how they can hurt the immune system. **Chapter 3** describes the critical decision to examine the data for ourselves, which enabled us to discern my true prognosis and conclude the need to do more. **Chapter 4** catalogs our foray into alternative therapies and relates some stories of miraculous cures that steered us toward immunotherapy. **Chapter 5** describes the amazing world of Coley's Toxins that inspired our efforts.

Part 2 describes our pursuit of immunotherapy. We write of adventures obtaining treatment, mishaps that offer valuable lessons, and stories of patients met whose successes inspire and instruct. Specifically, **Chapters 6 and 7** describe current immunotherapies such as adoptive T cell procedures, cancer vaccines, PD-1 and CTLA-4 inhibitors. **Chapters 8 and 9** recount our adventures in Mexico where I received Coley's Toxins, then describe the dangers of an immune system gone haywire. **Chapter 10** highlights how tumors respond differently to immunotherapy compared to chemo, and why we need to give it time to work. **Chapters 11 and 12** describe how we attempted to mobilize different aspects of the immune system against cancer through combination strategies, including employing surgery in **chapter 13**. **Chapter 14** focuses on the historical precedent and rationale for injecting tumors directly, as William Coley had done a century ago. **Chapter 15** explores the fascinating relationship between what we eat, how it affects inflammation, and how inflammation enables tumors to subvert immune cells for their growth and protection.

Finally, **chapter 16** summarizes our point of view and provides practical tips and ideas on how to take advantage of immunotherapy today.

We are at a critical juncture. It will take time for clinical trials to verify what we believe will be proven: that immunotherapy can work for most cancers, if not all. It will take time for physicians across the country to appreciate the full potential of immunotherapy and incorporate optimal combination strategies.

But patients with advanced cancer cannot afford to wait years for formal approval. An average of 1,600 patients die from cancer in the U.S. *every day*—almost 18 times the number who die from car crashes.[7,8] We feel many of these deaths can be averted—if only the patients or their doctors are more informed about immunotherapy.

For the moment, it is up to patients to educate themselves and drive their own care if they wish to leverage immunotherapy. It will take time, effort and money. But thankfully, immunotherapy has become exponentially more accessible within the past two years.

A century ago, Dr. William Coley cured patients with his rudimentary vaccine. Of over 1000 patients treated, 500 obtained near-complete regression.[9] For decades, he was maligned by other physicians who couldn't reproduce his results. But today, long-term clinical trial data proves an immune-based cure isn't wishful thinking or quackery. An ever-expanding arsenal of clinical trials and off-label immunotherapies offer informed patients the tools to unleash their immune systems against cancer.

We sincerely hope this book will inspire and inform you in your journey to cure cancer with immunotherapy.

PART I
Drawn to Immunotherapy

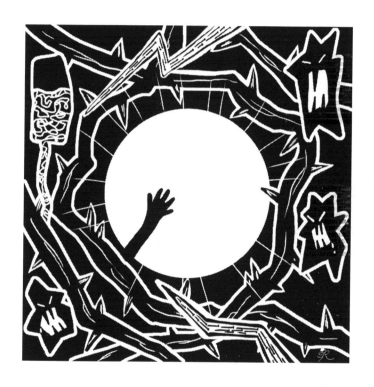

CHAPTER 1

Pain and Numbness

EDDY AND I HAD MUCH TO LOOK FORWARD TO. After seven long years, I had finally earned my Ph.D. in biology. I then accepted a postdoctoral research position to study the inner workings of bacteria at a research lab at Stanford University. Eddy was living out his dream of starting his software consulting business. Life was good. It had always been good for as far as I could remember.

We'd been married for six months when the headaches began. I'd rarely had headaches, so I attributed them to tiredness, probably from juggling work and maintaining our new household. They occurred sporadically, pain jolting along the right side of my face and racing upwards, from cheek to temple. They were bothersome, but a cup of coffee usually banished them—at least until the next morning.

Soon, I began to feel pain in my upper right molars. Eating became a problem. Chewing triggered a terrible shooting pain. Biting on a tender piece of chicken felt like trying to gnaw on the shell of a crab claw. I adapted by chewing only on the left. *It must be a cavity or a crack in my tooth*, I figured. Strangely, my dentist couldn't find anything to explain my agony.

Then, my right jaw began to click and pop whenever I opened my mouth. The noises were loud and disconcerting. When I looked in the mirror and gaped wide, my right jaw would jut out—as if dislocated at the joint. *Aha! It had to be temporomandibular joint disorder (TMJ)*, a dysfunction of the jaw often caused by clenching or grinding of teeth during sleep. A quick internet search affirmed my hunch. Same symptoms, same pain.

But what was causing me to grind my teeth? The wedding? The new job? Moving in with Eddy? Were they all subconsciously stressing me out somehow?

In an attempt to isolate this possibility, I purchased a do-it-yourself moldable mouthguard and began wearing it to bed, hoping the cushion would realign my jaw and stop the pain. But the symptoms didn't improve, and only worsened with time. Eventually, I saw an Ear, Nose and Throat (ENT) specialist who ordered a CT scan of my sinuses. It revealed no abnormalities. Based on my symptoms, the ENT diagnosed me with TMJ, a common malady for those with *bruxism*: the involuntary grinding of teeth during sleep. I patted myself on the back for guessing correctly.

Months passed. My symptoms worsened. I became dependent on ever-increasing amounts of coffee. The brew tamed my headaches and the pain in my teeth. I faithfully wore the mouthguard during sleep, hoping it would eventually allow my jaw to heal.

On Christmas Day, my right ear began to throb. *Yet another symptom? What's going on with me? Was this related to my jaw?* At the time, we were visiting Eddy's family in Singapore. At a walk-in clinic, a doctor peeked into my ear canal and noticed signs of infection—nothing major. He prescribed antibiotic drops. As we left the clinic, I felt relieved, satisfied with the diagnosis.

After some days of antibiotics, the throbbing subsided. Then, all of a sudden, a numbness nested on the right side of my chin. *The right side again,* I observed. The numbness spread to my lower lip. Soon, I could no longer feel the right tip of my tongue.

But the ENT said it was TMJ ... so all this is probably referred pain or numbness from the jaw, I rationalized.

After the long trans-pacific flight home, the pressure in my right ear refused to equalize. Again, I rationalized it away as a case of "airplane ear"—perhaps some trapped mucus was blocking my Eustachian tube. The right side of my head felt perpetually underwater, all sounds muted. Within days, I lost all hearing in my right ear.

Despite the crescendo of perplexing symptoms, I was glad to be back stateside, surrounded by the comforts of home. I knew it would take some days to get over jet lag. But late into the second week, I still felt constantly fatigued—even after a long night's sleep.

It was the day of our first wedding anniversary! I had been eagerly awaiting this excuse for a nice meal out with Eddy. But the pain from my teeth had become so intense that I had no appetite. We ended up going to a nearby food court, where I picked at my food.

My escalating symptoms deeply troubled Eddy. Unable to take it any longer, he refused to accept that it was just TMJ. Right then and there, he insisted we go see a doctor. I didn't think my symptoms warranted an immediate visit. But the discomfort and fatigue compelled me to comply.

So, the rest of our first anniversary was spent at the urgent care clinic—a rather unromantic setting. But it would eventually turn out to be the best anniversary gift I could have received from Eddy.

The Path to Diagnosis

A critical turning point, the urgent care visit finally set me on the path to correct diagnosis.

At first, the doctor suspected some sort of inflammation was causing my symptoms. She started me on Motrin. I quickly maxed out at the highest permitted dose. Anything lower would conjure an immediate resurgence of pain. I frequented the drugstore, where I repeatedly cleaned out their stock of Children's Motrin: I needed a liquid version, as I had difficulty swallowing pills. At the maximum adult dose, a bottle lasted less than a day. I quickly became dependent on the Motrin, faithfully downing medicine-cup shots every few hours, afraid that the pain would rear its ugly head were I to miss a dose.

Meanwhile, the urgent care doctor put in a referral for me to see a neurologist; she wanted someone to follow up on the facial numbness. When I finally got to see the neurologist, he was concerned that my symptoms were limited to one side of my head. He said there were certain nerve conditions that might cause similar symptoms—but that they should also manifest in other areas of the body. As a precaution, he ordered an MRI.

By now, it was obvious that teeth grinding couldn't sufficiently explain my symptoms. Eddy and I had done our own research on the side. We wondered if I had a stubborn bacterial infection. Perhaps it would explain the ear infection, the inflammation and the swelling.

The clinic's MRI machines were fully booked for weeks, so we opted to drive an hour to a branch across the San Francisco Bay. The sooner I got the scan, the sooner I'd be referred to the next expert who could help unravel this mystery.

I had just gotten back to my work lab after the MRI and a quick lunch when my phone rang. It was the neurologist.

"You have a large tumor in your head! I'm having you see a head and neck surgeon immediately!"

A tumor in my head? I thought I'd heard incorrectly. My heart began to pound. With the cell phone glued to my good ear, I dashed out of the lab and hid in the stairwell.

Incredulous, I asked if it could be an infection or an abscess masquerading as a tumor. I hoped the neurologist would acknowledge the possibility, but he asserted that wasn't the case.

I was shocked. *It was a tumor all these months? How could this be?* At the same time, I was strangely relieved to have an answer to my mystery. The symptoms had bewildered us for almost half a year, disrupting dates and outings and had spoiled the simple pleasure of eating. It took a while for reality to sink in, for me to accept that the cause of my misery was a large mass in my head—about the size of an egg.

Terrifying thoughts crept in: *Could this be cancer? Am I going to die? I'm still young, and we've been married for only a year. Our life together is just beginning . . .*

But a tumor isn't necessarily cancer, I consoled myself . . . *There's still a chance they can cut this out . . . I'll be rid of the pain and symptoms, and I'll go right back to life.*

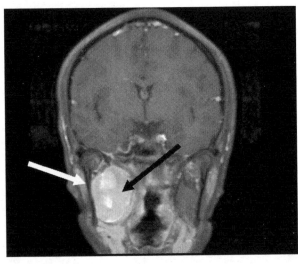

Figure 1: Front view MRI shows 5 cm tumor in my head (black arrow), pressing against my right jawbone (white arrow). (January 2008)

First Time in a Cancer Center

The neurologist had me see a surgeon at the community clinic later that afternoon. The surgeon felt my case was beyond his expertise, so he referred me to Stanford Cancer Center—just a stone's throw away from the lab where I worked on campus. I had walked past it day after day, never giving a thought to what went on inside.

My boss, Professor Lucy Shapiro, did everything she could to have me see the right doctors. Her research lab was part of the Stanford Medical School. She made sure my case wasn't lost amid the administrivia that sometimes plagues large hospitals. She got me an appointment with Dr. Michael Kaplan, chief of head and neck surgery. Without her advocacy, I would probably not be alive today.

I'd hardly been sick throughout my life. The only time I'd seen a doctor was for coughs and colds. It was surreal to be seeing someone for a tumor in my head.

The day of my appointment with Dr. Kaplan arrived. The physician's assistant came in first and took a detailed history. I recounted the progression of my symptoms, careful not to leave out anything. Not long after he left, Dr. Kaplan entered and introduced himself. Cheerful and witty, he cracked a joke to lighten the mood. If I'd been in a better state, I would have joined Eddy in nervous laughter.

My case had been discussed at the weekly multidisciplinary tumor board, a meeting where a number of doctors—experts in different specialties—convene to review and discuss the best treatment for patients. The details of my case had been analyzed by a medical oncologist (one who prescribes chemo and understands the growth behavior of my cancer), a radiation oncologist (who delivers radiation therapy to tumors), a surgeon, a radiologist (who interprets scans), and a pathologist (who analyzes tumor tissue to pinpoint the type of my cancer).

Since I had not undergone any prior biopsy or surgery, there was no pathology information to clarify what was in my head. All they had to go by was my MRI.

●₀ ●● ●₀● ₀● ●₀

Despite the lack of pathology insight, the board believed that my tumor was most likely a *benign schwannoma*, a type of nerve tumor—because it was round, clearly delineated and appeared *well-encapsulated*. Most cancers are not so "neat and round." Their uncontrolled, haphazard growth causes them to form careless, sloppy borders as they drunkenly invade surrounding tissues.

I had never heard of a schwannoma. But the only thing I could think about was that Dr. Kaplan had said schwannomas are **benign**. Eddy and I clung to that word.

When normal cells mutate and no longer play by the rules, they multiply uncontrollably, disregarding the normal balance between growth and death. When enough of these cells amass, they form a tumor. If the tumor is benign, these cells stay in that one spot in the body. But in cancerous tumors, malignant cells break free from their normal confines and are swiftly carried away in the bloodstream or lymphatic system to distant parts of the body where they form new colonies. This diaspora of cells from the mother tumor is known as *metastasis*.

In the majority of cases, it is metastasis that kills cancer patients. The new colonies grow into full-fledged tumors, creating havoc around the body. Death can come when tumors block or annex organs critical to life (such as the lung, liver, brain, intestines), or when tumors damage blood vessels, causing irreparable internal bleeding. But if my tumor was indeed benign, there was no risk of metastasis—and removing the solitary mass could cure me.

When cancer is suspected, doctors often obtain a *biopsy* sample—a small amount of tissue from the patient's tumor. They insert a needle into the tumor, guided by real time CT or ultrasound imaging, then suck out some tissue for pathology analysis. They do this to gain information about the tumor *before* cutting it out.

Depending on the size and location of the tumor, it may be important to first shrink it with radiation or chemotherapy. This is called *neoadjuvant* therapy. Neoadjuvant therapy can loosen a tumor's death-grip on adjacent critical organs or blood vessels, strengthening the odds that subsequent surgery would thoroughly remove the tumor.

In my case, the tumor was causing so many symptoms that the impetus to immediately remove it was irresistible. Immediate surgery would relieve my symptoms. As the tumor board felt my tumor was benign, they didn't think a biopsy was needed, nor did they prescribe neoadjuvant radiation or chemo. We jumped at the board's recommendation. All we could think about was getting that thing out of my head—and extinguishing the pain.

Surgery was promptly scheduled for a week later. I was grateful for Dr. Kaplan's willingness to operate so soon, and grateful that my boss, Professor Shapiro, had gotten me to see him so quickly. For the first time in months, I felt optimistic.

I had stopped taking Motrin a few days earlier. I wanted to know—I wanted to feel—what the tumor was doing in my head. More importantly, the active ingredient in Motrin is Ibuprofen, which thins the blood, and can lead to dangerous bleeding during surgery; it was imperative that I expel it from my system in time for the operation.

During that week before surgery, as the Motrin wore off, the pain unleashed all at once. I knew that Motrin was a pain-reliever, but I didn't realize how much it had masked. I became instantly bedridden, devoid of all energy. I began to vomit frequently and experienced persistent nausea. Whenever I could muster enough strength to speak, it would be in bare whispers.

Such was the effect of this throbbing invader pushing hard against nerve, muscle and bone. It besieged all vital structures: my throat, making it difficult to swallow; the roof of my mouth, causing extreme pain in my teeth when I ate; my jawbone, making it difficult to open my mouth; my *trigeminal* nerve, causing the right-sided facial numbness; my Eustachian tube, making me deaf in one ear; and the base of my skull, causing fatigue and pain.

In that state of unabating pain and suffering, I could see myself closing my eyes, letting go, losing consciousness and leaving it all behind.

But I clung on. If I could endure this misery for just one more week, it could be gone in the blink of an eye. All I needed was for the tumor to be benign.

Surgery

Surgery was supposed to be straightforward: remove the entire tumor with minimal damage to bone, muscle or nerve, then sew me up. The procedure would last only a couple hours. By hour four, Eddy feared something was amiss.

Dr. Kaplan and his chief assistant emerged from the operating room. Pausing at the edge of the waiting area, they beckoned Eddy aside, away from the other families anxiously awaiting news of their own loved ones. Dr. Kaplan said I was stable, but there'd been some complications. In the middle of surgery, I'd begun to bleed uncontrollably. An emergency intravenous line was inserted into my ankle to transfuse in unit-after-unit of blood—more than half the entire blood volume in my body had to be replenished.

In the intensive care unit, I groggily emerged from my anesthesia-induced slumber. The immediate sensation—an intrusive tube stuck down my throat—was horrible. It prevented me from speaking and caused me to continuously retch. I was weak and heavily sedated. Still, I managed to motion for somebody to get the tube out. But it'd been left in place for an important purpose—to protect my airway in case my throat were to close from surgery-related swelling. I continued to retch for a few hours before someone finally extracted the tube. But by then, I'd already vomited a few times—with the tube still down my throat. *Ugh!*

I instantly noticed the absence of pain in my head. *Wow, what a difference from before,* I thought. I'd almost forgotten how it felt to be without pain. A surge of optimism coursed through me. *Dr. Kaplan must have succeeded in getting it all out.*

When I was stable enough, I was relocated to the surgical ward, where I would spend the next few days recovering. I was so happy when Eddy and my family arrived. But I fatigued easily and slept through most of the next two days.

My energy slowly returned. Aside from a little weakness, I felt well. My face looked quite normal, considering the scope of the surgery and the risk of nerve damage. The *trigeminal nerve,* a large and important nerve bundle that exits the brain not far above the jaw joint, had to be carefully protected while removing the tumor. Fanning out from the trigeminal—like distributaries in a river delta—are a complex set of nerve branches that control sensation and movement for that entire side of the face. Thankfully, my right eyelid opened and closed just fine. The corner of my eye didn't droop—something the medical residents kept probing for during morning rounds. The right corner of my mouth, though, refused to cooperate, making my smile lopsided.

The only other visible evidence of my surgery was a four-inch incision—extending from under my chin, up and back toward the angle of my jaw. Dr. Kaplan had thoughtfully made his entry point along a crease line on my neck. And in closing me up, he'd sutured it impeccably. Even the nurses couldn't help but pause and admire his handiwork. I was so happy and relieved to be on the path back to my normal self, blissfully unaware of the emotional truck about to blindside me.

The Final Diagnosis

The assistant surgeon popped in without warning. In a matter-of-fact way, he informed me that my tumor was *not* benign; it was highly malignant. Known as *synovial sarcoma*—it was one of the rarest forms of cancer: only 800 people in the entire United States are diagnosed with it annually.

And then he left.

As I sat on the hospital bed, surrounded by Eddy and my family, the emotion welled up and gushed all at once. I sobbed uncontrollably. The sobs crescendoed into a wail of anguish. I couldn't breathe. My chest ached. My body went limp as Eddy held me tight.

This diagnosis meant that surgery would no longer be the quick fix Eddy and I had hoped for. This diagnosis meant the risk of death had increased dramatically. This diagnosis implied I'd have to run through the gauntlet of high doses of radiation and chemotherapy. This diagnosis marked only the beginning of a long and difficult road ahead.

To my further dismay, I also found out the tumor had broken apart during surgery, spilling its malignant contents all around inside my head and neck—as if loads of toxic, polluting, cancerous cells had been suddenly dumped into the rivers of my bloodstream. Also, the *surgical margins* were found to be positive, meaning microscopic cancer remained at the edges of the surgical cuts. It was a matter of time before these would regrow into numerous *satellite* tumors.

So, I had started off thinking this was TMJ, then a bacterial infection, then I had been diagnosed with a benign tumor, and then told it was cancer, which had then broken apart and spilled inside my head during surgery, and finally, I received the news that it was an exceedingly rare and highly aggressive cancer. Was all this really happening? What more could go wrong?

Messed up Chromosomes

Before surgery, I had asked the assistant surgeon if he would take a picture of my tumor. Some might consider this morbid, but, as a biologist, I wanted to visualize what was causing all of that physical and emotional anguish.

The assistant surgeon had been unable to comply. But I didn't give up. If I couldn't see how it looked to the naked eye, I wanted to know how it appeared microscopically. I contacted the pathologist, who graciously provided me with pictures of the cells. One picture showed the tumor's *chromosome spread.*

The human body is made up of trillions of cells. Within the nucleus of each cell, there is a master program, encoded in DNA. In a normal healthy human cell, this DNA is organized into 23 pairs of chromosomes. Each pair comprises strands that are identical in length and pattern, except the sex chromosomes in males. A chromosome spread involves taking a cell that's about to divide, cracking it open, taking a picture of the chromosomal content, then analyzing the copies and pattern of each chromosome.

When the chromosomes from my tumor were spread, hardly *any* matching pairs were found! Instead of two identical copies of each chromosome, there were anywhere from one to four copies—each exhibiting different lengths and patterns.

They say a picture is worth a thousand words. I knew this well, as I had spent most of the past decade studying cells and bacteria under the microscope. The grotesque anomalies in the genetic material meant these cells would never submit to the myriad mechanisms that regulate normal growth behavior.

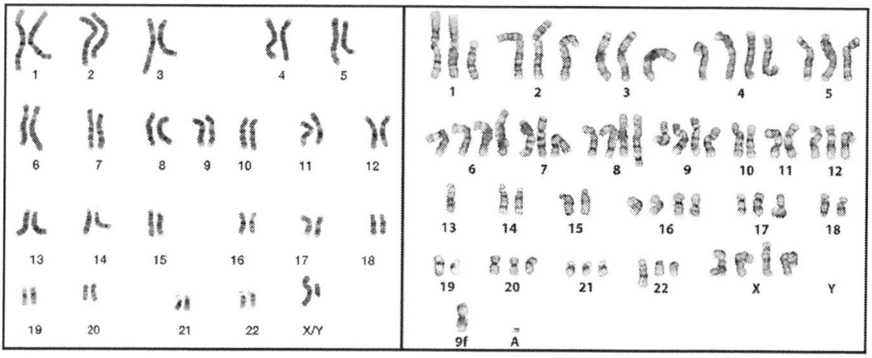

Figure 2: LEFT: Chromosomes of a normal human cell: 22 matching pairs + X/Y sex pair.[A] RIGHT: Chromosomes from a cell of my tumor: gross deviation (1, 3, or 4 strands instead of paired strands).

The pathologist had also analyzed how quickly my tumor was growing by measuring its *mitotic index*—a measure of how fast the tumor cells were cloning themselves. The index registered at 14/10 high power fields (hpf). Wondering what this meant, I looked it up on the internet. The search yielded a study done at the Dana-Farber Cancer Institute in Boston. The study showed less than one in seven synovial sarcoma patients whose tumors had that mitotic index would still be alive in ten years.[1]

The chaos within my tumor instilled in me the gravity of my situation. How could I fight this enemy that would never play by the rules? Alarmed by the one-in-seven survival statistic, I searched for more information about my prognosis, but the rareness of my cancer meant there was little data. Most of the medical websites offered only murky descriptions, disclaiming "it all depends on the individual situation." Yet, at every turn—every website and research paper that I could find—a constant, undeniable refrain reinforced my new reality—the ominous two words: poor prognosis.

The large size and tight location of my tumor, the contaminated margins and tumor spillage, the monstrous disarrangement of DNA, the rapid rate of multiplication, and the droning message of a poor prognosis all conspired to convince me that modern medicine could not protect me. The bright future that Eddy and I had barely envisioned together—the culmination of five years of courtship and decades of education and hard work—transmogrified into darkness, uncertainty and a sense of impending death.

CHAPTER 2

A Damaged Immune System

I WAS FINALLY HOME, RELEASED from the confines of the hospital. The familiarity and comforts instilled a sense of normalcy—an illusion that I had made it through the fire, and could finally relax. But Eddy and I both knew it was a facade.

I lay in bed, memory foam cradling my tired body. I turned toward Eddy, who was exhausted from the intense nights of staying by my side at the hospital. He stroked my hair as we smiled sadly at each other. "Get some rest," he whispered, turning off the lamp.

As I lay staring into the darkness, vivid thoughts of death filled my imagination. I saw myself at my own funeral. Eddy was there, his anguish inconsolable. Mom sobbed quietly. Dad held her hand, expressionless. Matt and Ethan, my younger brothers, flanked Eddy, their arms around his shoulders. They were all there: my grandmother, my aunts, uncles and five younger male cousins.

Tears streamed down my cheeks as I lay contemplating death. But I wasn't crying for myself. I had peace and assurance of where I was going to be. Instead, I was sad for Eddy and for my family, sad I couldn't comfort and assure them they need not mourn for me.

The tears soaked my pillow. I felt the wetness against my ears. I was tempted to dry them, but decided not to stir as I didn't want to rouse Eddy. He deserved his much-needed rest. Quietly, I cried myself to sleep ...

Little did I know that Eddy was still awake, unable to fall asleep despite his exhaustion. He, too, lay in the dark, quiet as a mouse, also not wanting to rouse me. He had his own anguish to deal with, as he would later share:

One year of happiness together? Is that all we get?

It doesn't seem fair ... How can this happen to someone like her? From the first we met, I wanted to spend the rest of my life with her. So gentle and giving. Always thinking about others ...

She's the best thing that's ever happened ... I moved to San Diego ... waited five years for her Ph.D. Now I have to watch her destroyed by chemo and radiation?

And that poor prognosis ... Does it mean I'll watch her die?

Quietly, without tears, Eddy lulled himself to sleep.

In the days after surgery, we drew closer than ever before, holding each other tighter than ever before. The sweet sadness that permeated our time together was broken only by visits from family and friends. Their presence made us forget, for a moment, what lay ahead. In those days, we discovered who our true friends were. Many journeyed from great distances to comfort and encourage us. Some who were near stayed silent and distant.

During those weeks of defining solitude, something began to stir within. We had often read about cancer patients summoning the will to fight for their lives. But we never understood what that meant until now. A seed of determination had begun to germinate: a resolve to survive, no matter how poor the odds or how hopeless the cause.

We were going to fight—I for Eddy, and Eddy for me. If there were difficult decisions, we were going to make them together and bear the consequences together, with no regret. Whatever the treatment prescribed, I was ready to endure it—no matter how difficult, debilitating or dangerous.

The Medical Oncologist

Two weeks after surgery, it was time to see the medical oncologist. Aside from prescribing chemotherapy, she best understood the behavior of my cancer—how fast it was growing, how likely it was to spread, how effective chemo would be against it and whether it made sense to employ focal therapies such as radiation.

"As you know, you have synovial sarcoma," said Dr. Jacobs. "The good news is we don't see any regional lymph nodes lighting up on the recent PET scan. Nor is there any evidence of spread to other parts of your body."

"That's awesome!" I said, breathing a sigh of relief.

Lymph nodes exist throughout the body. They act like filters, trapping foreign particles and cancer cells. None of the nodes in my head or neck had lighted up, which would have signified a spread of cancer. Even better, the rest of my body was clear.

"Yes," replied Dr. Jacobs. "But that doesn't mean there's no cancer in your body. It just means there aren't any *detectable* tumors."

"Now, the tumor in your head *was* quite large—and it broke apart during surgery—so, estimating the size is tricky … but adding all the pieces together, I'm going to say it was a five-and-a-half centimeter tumor."

My heart sank as I began to recall the numerous studies warning that sarcomas larger than five centimeters have a greater propensity to spread—and a much poorer prognosis.

"Also, the margins were positive, meaning there's still microscopic tumor left in your head, surrounding the area where your primary tumor was. We need to go after those remaining cancer cells—get them now before they grow back. So what we're going to do is first have Dr. Quynh Le over at Radiation Oncology treat you. Rest assured, she's very good at what she does.

"After you receive high-dose radiation, you'll come back to me for chemo. Unlike radiation that can only treat one area, the goal of chemo will be to go after cancer cells throughout your body—cells that may have broken off and settled in distant organs."

"What organs does synovial sarcoma usually spread to?" I asked.

"The most common site is the lung. It can sometimes go to the brain or liver, or nearby lymph nodes. But by far, the lung is where we see it most.

"Again, the good thing is your PET scan doesn't show any evidence of tumor anywhere in your body. The chemo will address any metastatic cancer still too small to be seen on the scans."

Dr. Jacobs said nothing about my prognosis. But she instilled within us a sense that things were under control. She was going to go after my cancer while it was still invisible. That sounded like a winning strategy. She was emphatic, reassuring and authoritative, and the consultation left me hopeful. Despite the rarity of my cancer, it felt good to know I was being treated by a sarcoma expert.

I determined to cooperate with Dr. Jacobs and the rest of my team. I would become the perfect patient. I would do anything they asked of me.

Burning Radiation

Six weeks after surgery, it was time for my first dose of radiation.

Like a thick clump of crabgrass ripped from a lawn, only to leave thousands of invisible seeds in the immediate boundary, surgery had failed to eradicate the cancer in the margins. Radiation would burn those invisible cells, as if a gardener were to set a small sterilizing ring of fire in and around the dirt patch that remained. In all, I was to receive 66 grays of radiation—*3.3 million* times that of a normal chest X-ray.[1]

Radiation works by damaging cell DNA. Like a master program, DNA controls how a cell grows, develops and acts. But a cell can repair its own damaged DNA. So, in order to kill it, the rate of damage must overcome the ability for self-repair.

The radiation prescribed for me was to be spread over 30 *fractions*. By splitting into smaller doses, normal cells get a day of rest in between the ten-minute, daily irradiations. The break gives them time to heal and repair. But cancer cells, with their diminished ability to self-repair, accumulate damage day after day and eventually die.

The stakes were high; sarcomas are known to develop resistance to radiation. Dr. Le had one chance to kill the remaining cancer in my head with the thirty doses. She had to irradiate me with the highest possible amount. The 66 grays would be my lifetime limit. Beyond that, morbid side effects—non-healing ulcers, infections and tissue death—could occur. If my cancer were to return, further radiation would be out of the question.

The daily irradiations were, at first, easy, quick and non-invasive. I felt nothing. But as the days passed, side effects took their toll. I began to fatigue, finding it difficult to keep my eyes open after the ten-minute sessions, as if I'd been out all day in the sun. We worked hard to keep up my strength. I ate as much as I could, despite increasing pain in my mouth and throat. My sense of taste disappeared. It was a strange experience. I had always luxuriated in nuanced flavors, but now, I savored nothing.

Then, I began to have difficulty eating altogether. I stopped producing saliva. It hurt to eat with such a dry mouth. I developed excruciating mouth sores and blisters. We had moved in with my parents before radiation began; Eddy tag-teamed with mom to prepare juices and liquefied foods. Even the tiniest particles felt like sandpaper. Meals became painstaking but necessary. I sat in front of the TV for hours with my gray sludge of flavorless calories. Eyes glued to the screen, I watched enticing food shows and imagined delectable flavors supplanting the tasteless nectar I reluctantly sucked through a straw.

It was critical that I finish every drop of the liquid meals. The radiation sent my body into a *hyper-metabolic* state. I needed large amounts of calories just to maintain weight. Dr. Le had ordered me to consume at least 2000 calories per day. We diligently recorded every calorie, adding energy-dense foods like avocados and bananas to meet daily goals. Thankfully, in the weeks following surgery before radiation, I had worked hard to bulk up to a hulking one hundred pounds. Despite my efforts, I was already back down to ninety-three.

My doctors advised me to drink Ensure, a common protein drink full of sugar. But we were leery of the possibility that dietary sugars could feed cancer and make it grow faster. The breakneck growth of tumors requires a constant supply of energy. Unlike other cells, cancer cells don't produce energy by burning glucose with oxygen. Instead, they convert glucose inefficiently, wasting 95 percent of available energy. To make up for the loss, they perform the conversion 100 times faster. This unrelenting binge of profligate consumption can be seen with the PET-CT scan, the gold standard for identifying active tumors, which works by detecting their rapid sugar uptake.

The idea that sugar can accelerate cancer is commonly dismissed as myth or naiveté—the argument being all cells in our body need sugar, and therefore, there's no practical way to reduce intake just to slow down cancer. But what if this was a case where science might validate myth, given enough time? There were valid scientific questions behind the sugar "myth," such as how it increases insulin and other hormones that can feed tumors.[2] In any case, we didn't see the need to risk it. So, instead of Ensure, we blended chunks of meat into soup for protein, adding tablespoonsful of oil to satisfy my calorie needs. In between meals, Eddy fed me eight cups of freshly squeezed vegetable juice.

Toward the end of radiation, the side effects became unbearable. I took painkillers just to sip water. Counting down the days, I doubted I would complete the thirty sessions. By now, my weight had dropped precipitously, breaching the ninety-pound minimum I had set for myself. I was chronically fatigued and slept most of the day, waking only for agonizing nourishment. Just when I thought I couldn't go on, radiation concluded.

Amazingly, within days, my mouth and throat began to heal. I could soon eat and drink without painkillers. Despite warnings of permanent loss, my sense of taste returned! Dr. Le was surprised at how well I healed. Perhaps the eight daily cups of vegetable juice had done some good? As I graduated from liquids to solids, I vowed never to take for granted the ability to eat without pain.

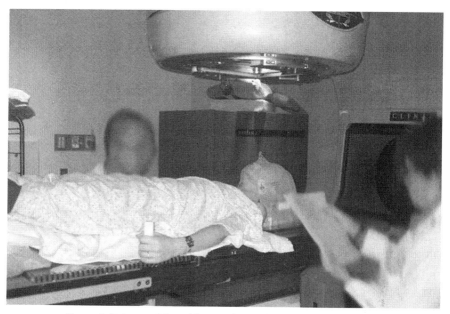

Figure 3: Being positioned for a radiation session. (March 2008)

Caustic Chemo

Two months after radiation, my mouth and throat had healed enough to begin chemo. If the goal of radiation was to burn a ring of sterilizing fire around the crabgrass crater, the goal of chemo would be to poison the entire yard with herbicide—just in case the wind had carried and distributed its seeds to distant areas of the lawn.

For the chemo, Dr. Jacobs prescribed an older generation of deadly *cytotoxics*—drugs that killed fast-dividing cells in the body. I would receive a combination of two: doxorubicin and ifosfamide. Newer targeted therapies block specific mechanisms within certain cells, but these older drugs indiscriminately kill any rapidly dividing cell—not just cancer cells, but also hair follicle, reproductive, skin and bone marrow cells. The wholesale destruction poses a risk of serious—and sometimes deadly—side effects.

Doxorubicin was developed around the 1970s from a natural antibiotic.[3] Known to some as "Red Death" for its color, it carried a long list of side effects, including turning one's urine red, which was benign (albeit disconcerting). "Milder" effects included nausea, vomiting, mouth ulcers, diarrhea, swelling and numbness in the feet and hands. More dangerous were liver damage and a resurrection of radiation symptoms. But the most serious and lethal consequence was irreversible damage to the heart—a progressive side effect that can appear decades later.[4] To reduce the odds of these sequelae, Dr. Jacobs carefully tailored the dosage to my body weight, making sure I wouldn't receive anywhere close to my allowed lifetime limit of doxorubicin.

Ifosfamide, a derivative of mustard gas, was first approved for use in the U.S. in 1988. The latter was used in chemical warfare by German troops during World War I, causing horrific blisters, sores, vomiting and bleeding in the lungs. Poisoned soldiers died slow and painful deaths and were later found to have very low numbers of white blood cells. This led to experimentation with treating lymphomas, a cancer of the blood. In 1967, a German pharmaceutical company eliminated many of the toxicities from mustard gas, introducing the new compound as ifosfamide.[5] Despite the "improved" toxicity, ifosfamide had an even longer list of side effects than doxorubicin. The milder ones included nausea, vomiting, diarrhea, hair loss and mouth sores. More serious were chest pain, confusion, hallucinations, shortness of breath, bloody stools and bladder damage leading to bloody urine. But the scariest consequence was permanent destruction of bone marrow—where the cells of our immune system are produced. Without enough immune cells, my body would fail to fight off infections; microbes normally present in our bodies would become a mortal threat.

It didn't help that we had just read of a young woman in her thirties—treated just months earlier for cancer—also at Stanford. She died suddenly, her heart ravaged by "Red Death."

Many other cancer patients receive chemo at the outpatient clinic and are able to go home the same day. Some are sent home with portable pumps; a father of a friend played golf while the chemo infused into him.

In my case, the high concentrations of toxic drugs were too treacherous. I was to get five rounds of chemo. Each round required a week's stay in the hospital, during which I would receive 24-hour-long infusions. I would be closely monitored for serious side effects. I wouldn't be allowed to walk beyond the ward because accidental spillage posed a major safety risk to others. The nurses who came to administer the chemo would have to wear protective clothing and clear plastic face shields when disposing the used chemo bags. And yet, these poisonous drugs would be infused into my body.

Infusing the toxic drugs directly was too damaging to my veins. So, there was one last thing I needed before I could start chemo: a peripherally inserted central catheter (or PICC line) needed to be placed into my upper arm. A specially trained nurse cut an opening in my skin and threaded the long, flexible catheter from my upper arm all the way into my heart. In essence, the snaking tube was a shielded channel through which caustic drugs could be infused. It would protect the sensitive walls of my veins. Once within the heart, the poisons would be diluted by a larger volume of blood, then swiftly dispersed to the rest of the body. The catheter also served as a portal for other medications and supportive fluids, reducing my need to be stuck with a needle.

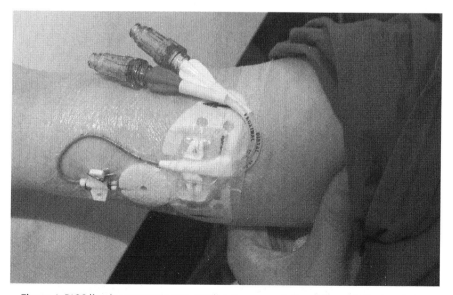

Figure 4: PICC line in my upper arm. Medications were infused through the two hubs and traveled through thin tubing all the way into my heart.

The first day of chemo arrived. I waited hours for a hospital bed to become available, and more hours for the pharmacist to mix the drugs. It was past midnight before the chemo finally started coursing through my veins. I drifted off to sleep, exhausted from the long day and from the anticipation leading up to this moment.

Fifteen minutes in, I was jolted awake. A terrible, heavy sensation pervaded my chest. I felt sick. Eddy was fast asleep, his body limp and awkwardly slumped in an uncomfortable-looking chair next to my bed. I paged for my nurse, and she came rushing in.

She was stunned; almost all of the doxorubicin had infused into me. Instead of safely entering over a 24-hour period, it'd sped into my body within a span of fifteen minutes. By then, Eddy was up, groggily trying to make sense of what had transpired. As the reality of the nurse's panicked words sunk in, our mental grappling was replaced by horror. Was "Red Death" going to kill me, just as it'd killed the other young woman?

What had caused the chemo to infuse so quickly? As is policy when administering toxic drugs, two nurses had cross-checked the drug names, the drug concentrations and the infusion pump settings. So, why the error? As it turned out, the doxorubicin had raced into my body not because of human error. The culprit was a faulty infusion pump.

The next morning my oncologist came in to see me. She told me that doxorubicin is sometimes given as a quick *bolus*, where the full amount is injected within a short period of time. She assured me I would be all right. Yet, I somehow wasn't entirely comforted.

From then on, we began to take ownership over my safety. We started asking questions. We made it a habit to double check all medication, making sure I was being given the right drug at the right dosage. To ensure that the accident didn't recur, we visually tracked the drip rate of my chemo. We would count the number of seconds between each drop, then watch for obvious deviations. No more trusting the machines. If there were any medical mistake or machine malfunction, I would be the one to suffer the real consequences.

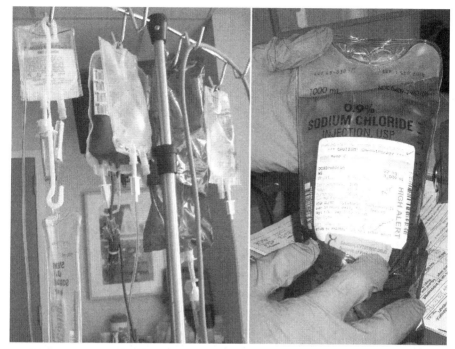

Figure 5: LEFT: Bags of chemo, blood and saline infusing into me. RIGHT: Saline bag containing "Red Death" (doxorubicin), wrapped up in dark plastic to protect it from light.

The Consequences of Chemo

Between rounds of chemo, I was sent home for two weeks of rest. I quickly lost all hair. The mouth sores I suffered during radiation flared up, resurrected by the twin toxic drugs. Fatigue set in, and I spent increasing portions of the day in bed. But the most devastating impact occurred in my bone marrow.

Bone marrow, the spongy, inner core found in the larger bones of our body—such as the hips, thigh bones, arm bones and breast bone—is where blood cells are produced. Within this spongy core, special immature blood cells (stem cells) transform into different types of cells: red blood cells, platelets and white blood cells. These white blood cells make up the immune system. They protect our body against foreign invaders, infectious pathogens and even cancer. There are many kinds of white blood cells, but the ones most important for defending against pathogens are called neutrophils. My chemo weakened these the most.

Neutrophils are the most abundant white blood cells in our body. A normal healthy adult produces a hundred billion every day.[6] They circulate in the bloodstream until they detect inflammation, which marks the presence of an infection. Highly pliable, they escape the bloodstream by squeezing through small gaps in between the walls of tiny blood vessels. Having landed in the infected tissue, they wiggle their way toward the source of infection, where they engulf invading microbes and pump them with deadly substances, finally digesting them using enzymes. While a hundred billion neutrophils may sound like a lot, there are about a hundred *trillion* microbes in the human body to subdue. If left unchecked by a dearth of neutrophils, these normally benign microbes can overwhelm the body, leading to serious infection or even death.

After each round of chemo, my *neutrophil count*—the measure of neutrophils in my blood—would begin to drop. In theory, the count would stabilize in about ten days, then climb (signifying recovery). Before the next round of chemo, my blood had to be tested. If my bone marrow had sufficiently healed, the count would register above a threshold, making it safe to proceed.

In order to help my bone marrow recover faster, I was prescribed Neupogen, a stimulant. The active ingredient in Neupogen is G-CSF—a protein normally produced by immune cells to summon reinforcements against invading pathogens. Injections of G-CSF can prod the bone marrow to produce more white cells. In 1991, doctors began using it to rescue chemo patients from fatal infections.[7]

The Neupogen came in small, single-use syringes, but at a big price—it wasn't covered by insurance and cost thousands of dollars. We were surprised at this first experience of having to pay thousands out-of-pocket for medicine; in the years to come, we would end up paying hundreds of thousands more.

The nurse instructed me to self-inject the Neupogen into my thigh for seven days straight after each round of chemo. I couldn't bear the sight of the needles, so Eddy assumed the responsibility. It was Eddy's first experience injecting medicine; in the years to come, he'd inject me hundreds of times more.

Unfortunately, after the first round of chemo, the Neupogen failed to sufficiently raise my neutrophil count. To allow my neutrophils to recover, my rest period was doubled, and the second round of chemo was delayed. After the second round of chemo, Dr. Jacobs instructed me to increase the number of Neupogen injections. The increased injections allowed me to start my third round of chemo on time. But the damage to my bone marrow was accumulating, and the fourth round of chemo was again delayed. Concerned that the delays were giving the cancer too much time to recuperate, Dr. Jacobs reduced my chemo dosage by a quarter. Finally, in a desperate attempt to coerce my bone marrow to produce more neutrophils, she instructed me to inject Neupogen for two weeks straight—from the day the fourth round ended to the start of the fifth round. The tenuous recovery of my neutrophils was an omen of what was to come.

After the fifth round, my neutrophils refused to rebound. They dropped further despite my having stopped all chemo. The implications were serious—and potentially deadly. A complete failure of the bone marrow meant my body would soon succumb to the trillions of microbes currently peacefully coexisting within me. Had I survived five rounds of noxious chemo only to die from bacteria or fungi rampaging through my body, no longer held in check by neutrophils?

Concerned, we kept in close touch with Dr. Jacobs, hoping she could do something for me beyond the weekly blood tests. Dr. Jacobs referred us to the hematology department. But they merely confirmed the obvious: chemo had damaged my bone marrow; there was nothing to do but wait and hope for the best.

A month passed, then two. My count kept dropping. Every Monday we drove to the cancer center for blood work, praying that the latest test would finally reveal signs of recovery. But none came. My neutrophil count lingered in the range of "mild" danger. When it dropped to "moderate" danger, our concern became anxiety. Then, it suddenly plunged to the boundary between "moderate" and "severe" danger.

I received a call from Dr. Jacobs that morning.

"I'm really sorry," she said. "There's nothing we can do for you."

CHAPTER 3

Deciding to Do More

JUST WHEN MY NEUTROPHIL COUNT HAD PLUNGED to a level of "severe" danger, Eddy came down with the flu. The exhaustion from the traumatic year of treatment had weakened him. He feared that the virus would endanger my defenseless body, so he moved out to live with my brother across the San Francisco Bay, entrusting me to my parents. He hated that he couldn't be with me. He had been by my side almost every day since diagnosis 11 months earlier. And it was two days to the new year, a time when most long to be with loved ones. But most of all, he desired to soothe my fears concerning my faltering bone marrow.

Our second wedding anniversary arrived in the middle of Eddy's flu. He came to see me that day, bearing a bouquet of white and purple daisies with pink carnations. We sat in the backyard with face masks on, a few feet apart, unwilling to get too close. Despite the difficult year and my flailing neutrophils, we were glad to be alive, and happy to have this moment. The masks muffled our voices, but accentuated our eyes and the unspoken sentiments they conveyed. The scene was even more memorable than our first anniversary at the urgent care clinic.

It was wise of Eddy to have moved out. The flu lasted over two weeks with epic fits of coughing and sneezing. Despite his sickness, he began a feverish search to unearth a panacea for my ailing bone marrow.

As science and conventional medicine had nothing to offer, he turned to the world of complementary and alternative medicine. Over the phone, and later in person, he consulted a dietitian, a naturopathic doctor and two alternative M.D.'s, all of whom had experience helping patients survive the ravages of chemoradiation. He gleaned ideas on how to support my body with vitamins, supplements, living foods (like raw vegetable juice), and rich sources of minerals (like bone marrow soup). Without studies to validate these recommendations, we had no assurance they would work. But they seemed harmless, and we were willing to try anything.

I began taking the recommended vitamins and supplements. Eddy made me the vegetable juices when he recovered and ordered marrow bones over the internet from a farm in Missouri, which mom boiled into soup. To our relief, after a month, my neutrophil count stabilized. It approached the safer plane of "moderate" danger by February, and by March, "mild" risk.

Had the vitamins, supplements, juice and soup helped? Perhaps the extra nutrition made the difference? The answer felt inconsequential; the terror had passed. Even so, my neutrophil count would stay anemic, ping-ponging between "mild" danger and low-normal. This oscillation would persist for years. Chemo had forever robbed my bone marrow of its full capacity to produce immune cells.

Clear Scans

Fourteen months had elapsed since the surgeon removed my head tumor. It was time for scans—an MRI to watch for recurrence at the primary site, and a chest CT to inspect for tiny lung nodules that would illuminate any spread of the cancer.

The passage of time can change one's outlook. At the onset of diagnosis, all we could think of was my "poor prognosis," how our future together would be cut short. But as we endured radiation and chemo, the drive to finish treatment quelled the sense of foreboding and replaced it with optimism. Surely the toxic, debilitating treatment had obliterated those puny remnants of cancer? If radiation could excoriate my throat, and if chemo could damage entire organs, why wouldn't they destroy those measly cells? That logic—whether grounded or not—was followed by concerns for my faltering bone marrow. These thoughts had hijacked our attention away from the question of prognosis.

But now, with those twin diversions fading into the past, we could again fixate on my survival. We planned to ask Dr. Jacobs about my prognosis at the next follow-up.

"Congratulations, your scans are clear," said Dr. Jacobs, as she entered the exam room.

Relieved, Eddy and I thanked her for seeing us through the difficult year.

"See, chemo wasn't all that bad, right?" said Dr. Jacobs. "Don't you think radiation was worse?"

"I guess so ..." I said, recalling how it hurt even to drink water.

As she examined me, she asked, "Have you noticed any new growths on your body?"

"Err ... no," I said, somewhat taken aback. It was a logical question, though. Sarcomas are aggressive cancers, known to sprout tumors with little warning. But no one had ever instructed me to inspect my body. *Was I supposed to be checking myself? How often?*

She then asked if I'd felt any numbness or weakness in my limbs. I had not. As I answered, I tried to recall which of the chemo drugs caused these effects.

Inspired by her inquiries, I inventoried every recent symptom, just in case they were early indicators of late-occurring side effects of chemo. I told her about the slight pain and nasal congestion in my right sinus, noting that it seemed to improve with nasal sprays; I described the pain in my upper and lower molars, which I'd assumed were the continuing effects of radiation; I mentioned the slight discomfort just below my ribs on both sides, and of the slight numbness in the lower-to-middle part of my back by my spine. But Dr. Jacobs didn't seem concerned about any of these symptoms.

As the examination drew to a close, it was time for Eddy to broach the question: "Dr. Jacobs, now that Rene has completed radiation and chemo, if you take into consideration all factors such as her tumor size, that it broke apart during surgery and spilled its contents, what do you think her true prognosis is?"

We hoped for a cogent answer, but instead received an encouraging-yet-nebulous admonition not to worry about the future. She emphasized I was in remission and doing well. She assured me that if my cancer were to return, we would deal with it then. She ended the appointment with the exhortation, "Now that you're done with treatment, try to return to a normal life."

For a moment, we were reassured by Dr. Jacobs' declaration of my remission. But her soothing words created the opposite of their intended effect. If chemoradiation were effective, why didn't she give me a clear number? Was I going to live another year? Another five? Ten?

We left the appointment that day, calm but unsettled. My bone marrow had stabilized. I'd survived a year of tribulation—and then some. Though constantly fatigued, and though my neutrophils were impaired, I was otherwise well. But uncertainty persisted. How likely was it that those embers of malignancy remained? And now that the stream of chemoradiation had been shut, when would they burst into flame?

If only there were a way to interrogate my body for vestiges of cancer. Blood tests fail to detect traces of sarcoma, and scans detect tumors only of a certain size. By the time they are caught, tumors are pregnant with malignancy—a CT scan can detect a 2.0 mm tumor, which has roughly one million cells, and a chest X-ray can detect a 1.0 cm tumor, comprising *one billion cells*.[1]

We were thankful that nothing showed up on my scans. But we knew it didn't mean I was "cancer-free"—a common refrain associated with clear scans. To be cured, every last microscopic cancer cell in my body had to die. Otherwise, it was a matter of time before they multiplied and spread.

Uncovering my Prognosis

After we saw Dr. Jacobs, we began to research my prognosis in greater detail, hoping to clarify my survival odds. But, due to the rarity of my cancer, the studies were few and the sample sizes small.

In 2015, 12,000 sarcoma cases were diagnosed in the U.S. But those cases comprised over 70 types of sarcomas, making each subtype exceedingly rare. The table below puts the case count in perspective and compares it to more common cancers, such as breast, lung and colon.

Number of new cases	Cancer type	Number of cases versus all sarcomas combined
231,840	Breast cancer	19 times
221,200	Lung cancer	18 times
132,700	Colon/Rectum cancer	11 times
73,870	Melanoma	6 times
54,270	Leukemia	4.5 times
11,930	All sarcomas (70 types)	
800	Synovial sarcoma	1/15 of all sarcomas

Table 1: Number of diagnosed cancers by type. (2015 U.S. data from seer.cancer.gov)

Of the 800 synovial sarcoma patients, head tumors are rarer still. Most of the studies we found were of sarcomas of the limb, where "definitive" surgery—such as amputation of a hand or leg—could be done. But the location of my head tumor made this impossible. It meant that the results of these studies might overstate my chances at survival.

The concentration of rare cases at high-volume cancer centers provided enough data to perform meaningful analysis. So, we looked for studies from the two largest cancer centers in the country—Memorial Sloan Kettering Cancer Center in New York (MSK) and the MD Anderson Cancer Center in Houston, Texas (MDA). One of the "larger" analyses from MSK examined the factors that influenced survival of 112 patients with sarcomas of the limb over a 14-year period from 1982 to 1996.[2]

The MSK study suggested I had a 40 percent chance of remaining alive five years after treatment. Two "risk factors" placed me in the group with the worst prognosis. The first was a tumor larger than five cm. The second was bone invasion. (My tumor had invaded the adjacent jawbone.) But all the patients in this study had limb tumors and profited from "curative" surgery; their surgeons were able to cut wide swaths around the tumors to achieve better margins. I wasn't so fortunate.

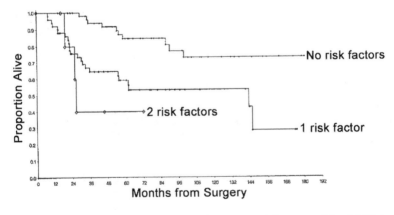

Figure 6: Tumor-related mortality of synovial sarcoma of the extremities. I fell into the "2 risk factors" category. Only 40% of these patients survived five years (60 months).[B]

Revisiting the analogy of crabgrass weed, the sarcoma experts at MSK are akin to experienced gardeners, who have tended to thousands of lawns (patients) over many decades. Through their collective wisdom, they've learned the growth behavior of a specific type of invasive crabgrass (synovial sarcoma). They've come to realize that even after they rip out the aggressive weed, perform a controlled burn around the dirt patch and spray powerful herbicides over the entire lawn, many of the lawns remain infected. Over time, these lawns sprout baby weeds, now resistant to herbicides. Ripping out or burning each baby weed is not an option, as it sacrifices too much lawn. The progeny multiply, spawning further offspring of their own. No matter what the gardeners do, within five years 60 percent of the lawns end up being choked to death by the proliferating weed. Wait longer, and even more lawns succumb.

A high-volume sarcoma center such as MSK has nine medical oncologists on staff, reflecting the number of sarcoma cases they treat. In contrast, Stanford's sarcoma unit had two or three. If the MSK study had accrued a mere 112 synovial sarcoma patients (with localized disease of the limb) over a 14-year period, it stands to reason that Dr. Jacobs may have seen only a small number of similar patients with my disease. I now understood why it was difficult to prognosticate my survival.

Finally, we found a study that focused on patients with head and neck synovial sarcoma treated at MDA between 1968 and 2004.[3] Over that 36-year period, the authors identified only 40 patients. This suggested that the largest cancer center in the U.S. saw an average of 1.1 patients like me every year. The authors aptly state in their abstract: "Synovial Sarcoma of the head and neck is extremely rare [emphasis mine], and our results should be viewed with caution given the relatively small group size and treatment over a 36-year period."

Although the sample size was tiny, the data seemed to match the prognosis from the MSK study of sarcomas of the limb. Within five years, only 40 percent of patients with tumors larger than five cm were alive. By 12 years, no one was left.

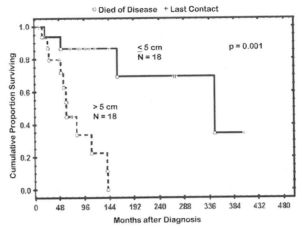

Figure 7: Survival of patients with synovial sarcoma of the head and neck by tumor size. Patients with tumors greater than five cm have significantly worse prognosis (dotted line).[c]

Furthermore, the graphs failed to capture the patients' quality of life, or the ordeal they suffered in the years before they died. The graphs merely showed how many patients were still alive by certain years.

I tried to put myself in these patients' shoes and imagine what life would be like, should I relapse. I pictured myself going back to Dr. Jacobs for a routine scan two years in the future:

I'm complacent after two years of clean scans. I'm expecting her to congratulate me on my second anniversary of being "cancer-free." But as she enters the room, I notice a somberness. She gently breaks the news that my cancer is back. I'm devastated. But there's no time to process these feelings as she catalogs the plan of action.

Dr. Jacobs tells me that radiation is out of the question; I've had my lifetime limit. She sends me back to Dr. Kaplan, the expert head and neck surgeon. In a desperate bid to exterminate the local recurrence, he meticulously gouges out a large chunk of flesh and bone, leaving my face lopsided and disfigured.

And then comes more chemo. The studies are clear: chemo doesn't cure; it only prolongs life. But I'll take it. Like radiation, "Red Death" has a lifetime limit, so further dosing is out of the question. Praying that my bone marrow doesn't collapse from higher doses of ifosfamide, I consent with trepidation, wondering how long my body will withstand it.

I make it through year three, but it takes a toll. As in first-line therapy, *nausea and fatigue set in. As expected, my bone marrow weakens, but some-how I evade total failure. By the middle of year four, my neutrophil count again teeters at the border of "severe" danger. Dr. Jacobs stops the ifosfamide.*

With nothing else proven to work, she offers a drug off-label. It's a drug used for treating pancreatic cancer, but she says some oncologists have tried it for sarcoma. I consent to it, praying it works. My tumors remain, but they seem to be growing a little slower.

In between rounds of chemo, I go for open-chest lung surgeries. The pro-cedures are intensely painful. The surgeon cracks open my chest to get at the tumors. The largest is 10 cm wide, in my lower left lobe. Recovery after each surgery is debilitating and protracted. I'd read of sarcoma patients who en-dured five, even 10 surgeries to weed out unrelenting disease. I wonder how many I can tolerate.

Year five arrives. By now, the effects of chemo and surgery have devastat-ed my body. My spirit flounders. My lung tumors continue to sprout. After seven lung surgeries, there's not enough lung left to cut. The surgeon tells me she's sorry—there's nothing else she can do. At Dr. Jacob's office, we discuss the pros and cons of trying yet another experimental chemo.

In the middle of the discussion, I pause, out of breath. As I listen to her describe the chemo, I stare at the wall. More side effects ... more pain ... more prolonging the inevitable. I decline, opting to spend my last month of life with Eddy and my family.

Both the MSK and MDA studies meant that something like the above scenario would happen. With a 60 percent probability, my death would culminate by year five.

The MDA graph was more incriminating. It dropped to zero. This meant that all synovial sarcoma patients (yes, *all*) with head and neck tumors larger than five cm died by year 12.

The MDA survival curve foretold my future. My disease was going to return. At that point, life becomes a downward spiral of suffering. And then I'll die.

The Limitations of Conventional Therapy

That the curve went all the way to zero meant radiation and chemo were not as effective as we'd hoped. The authors of the MSK study noted that radiation helped prevent local recurrence, but patients were still killed by the spread of their disease. The authors also warned that while chemo could shrink tumors, there was "no evidence of a survival benefit." This suggested that, when the tumors came back, they grew even faster, negating *any* overall benefit. It was disturbing to think that the months of chemo—the hair loss, the nausea, the numbness in my fingers, the chronic fatigue and the permanent impairment of my immune system—might not make any difference in how long I got to live.

So, why are radiation and chemo limited against sarcoma and many other cancers? What stifles their benefits? A major reason is that cancer cells constantly mutate. Early rounds of chemoradiation kill off susceptible cells, but the hardy survivors flourish and sprout new tumors.

If caught early before it's spread, localized cancer has a good chance of being cured—in many cases, with surgery alone. But patients with an advanced disease often cannot be cured. In these cases, oncologists settle to keep the patient alive for as long as possible using radiation, chemo or newer drugs. But as the cancer mutates, these therapies flounder, and side effects accumulate.

For decades, sarcoma oncologists have been constrained by the limitations of surgery, radiation and chemotherapy. In contrast to other more common cancers, targeted drugs with fewer side effects did not exist for sarcoma. (The first targeted drug would only be approved four years later in 2012.[4]) The smaller "customer base" for a rare cancer meant there was less financial incentive for innovation. In an escalating war against the disease, sarcoma oncologists pursued more radical surgery, stronger doses of radiation and higher concentrations of chemo. Their attempt to overcome a tenacious foe with brute force was limited by serious side effects, and even death.

I had a close call with bone marrow failure, which fortunately stabilized; but a former colleague of Eddy's, Frank, was not so lucky. An engineer in his mid-forties, Frank was diagnosed with osteosarcoma two years after I'd received my diagnosis. Osteosarcoma, a type of cancer of the bone, is known to affect teenagers, but adults are not exempt. Curiously, it began in Frank's hip—right at the spot where he wore his cell phone for many years. Frank endured an eight-hour surgery to remove the cancerous tumor, followed by a bone transplant. But his cancer had spread to the opposite hip. So, after he'd healed from surgery, Frank's doctors started him on chemo. They gave him two of the same drugs I'd received, doxorubicin and ifosfamide, as well as a third, cisplatin. Frank tolerated the earlier rounds well enough. But a month before he was to complete chemo, he experienced sudden heavy bleeding in both lungs. The bleeding was a side effect of chemo. (Frank had no tumors in his lungs that could have caused the bleeding.) A week later, Frank died in the hospital—from the side effects of chemo.

Survival for cancer is represented as a five-year statistic. Spend a few minutes at the National Cancer Institute's SEER website (*seer.cancer.gov*). Pick any cancer. Then look at the survival statistics for patients whose cancer has spread, labeled as "distant" cancer. Five-year survival tends to be around 10 to 20 percent, with a few cancer types in the 30s. This means that once the cancer has spread, only one, two or three out of 10 patients will still be alive in five years.

As an example, I include below the five-year survival for colorectal cancer. For patients with metastatic cancer, survival is 13.5 percent. That means only 1.35 out of 10 patients remain alive by the five-year mark.

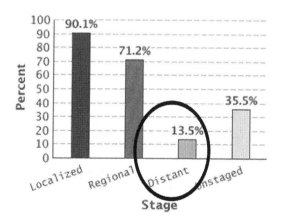

Figure 8: SEER five-year survival data for colorectal cancer. The five-year survival for metastatic (distant) colorectal cancer is 13.5%.[D]

What happens *after* the five years? What do the 10, 15 and 20-year survival numbers look like? The SEER website doesn't supply that data. Nor is it readily found elsewhere. The lack of such data hints that not many patients with metastatic disease make it to 10 years or beyond, reflecting the limitations of chemotherapy.

> **The Difference in Survival Between Localized and Metastatic Disease**
>
> The survival for localized disease (cancer that hasn't spread beyond the primary site) tends to be much higher, reflecting the potential of "getting it all" with surgery, while highlighting the limitations of chemo. For example, the five-year survival for patients with localized colorectal cancer is 90.1 percent, in contrast to 13.5 percent for metastatic cancer. (Note that the five-year survival for my localized sarcoma was only 40 percent, meaning that most patients with localized sarcoma likely already have undetected metastatic disease, or that their localized cancer is more likely to return and kill them.)

Realizing the Need to Do More

Taken as a whole, the medical papers, the statistics, my aggressive head tumor and the limitations of chemoradiation gave us a realistic expectation of our future. The "normal life" Eddy and I hoped to return to—pursuing a career, starting a family, watching children grow—would never happen, unless we veered from the scope of regular medicine.

We couldn't accept Dr. Jacobs' offer to return to a normal life. We had to do more.

We brought our research to my doctors, but it proved futile. Some suggested that the numbers "didn't matter." They argued that statistics only capture the outcome for a pool of patients. They said the only thing that mattered was *my* specific lot. What if I was one of the lucky ones? What if chemo and radiation had eradicated every last cell? Later on, we'd meet other doctors and patients who'd repeat this dictum and downplay the importance of statistics.

We understood. What patient wants to hear, "There's a 60 percent chance you'll be dead in five years" right after completing a hellish year of treatment? What good is it for doctors to convey dismal numbers if they have no weapon left in their arsenal? I'd received the standard of care. No other treatment would increase my survival. Therefore, there was no reason to burden me with statistics. So, why not encourage me to re-engage in normal life?

We intensified our research. All the information we needed was accessible over the internet. For hours a day, we sat glued to our laptops. We studied the standard and experimental treatment protocols for patients with recurrent disease, seeking to understand the risks and benefits. We pored over the details, translating cryptic medical-speak into tangible terms of how much longer I'd live and what side effects I'd have to endure. We learned that if my cancer were to return, the only drug that could reliably shrink it was a *much* higher dose of ifosfamide. Fear struck: if regular-dose ifosfamide had led to a brush with bone marrow failure, high-dose ifosfamide—*five times* more toxic—would demolish my immune system, leaving me forever defenseless against infection. In harsher terms, it'd kill me.

My inevitable demise seemed more certain. The studies indicated my cancer was likely to spread to my lungs by two years after chemo. Waiting for it to return was a losing strategy. Why not find new ways to attack it right now? We reasoned that a microscopic tumor—with fewer cells to destroy, and not yet fortified by an established blood supply—would be easier to kill. Finding that extra preemptive weapon became our compulsion.

Exploring Other Ways to Kill my Cancer

To kill my cancer, we sought to understand its genetic makeup—what was driving its aggressive behavior. We shipped a sample of my tumor to a company that could identify the misbehaving genes.

The gene profile yielded promising information. It listed genes found in my tumor that were known to be involved in many cancers. Along with the misbehaving genes, the profile recommended various drugs believed to be effective against them. These drugs were available; the FDA had approved them for other cancers. In theory, I could receive them off-label. Although not specifically approved for my cancer, my doctor could still prescribe them. They might not be covered by insurance, but at least I could get them.

We brought the report to Dr. Jacobs, but she wouldn't prescribe off-label drugs as I exhibited no evidence of disease. If I had active disease—and had failed high-dose ifosfamide—then she might consider them. But for now, from a safety, legal and ethical standpoint, prescribing drugs not-yet-approved for sarcoma was too risky.

Main specimen, excision: Sarcoma most consistent with monophasic synovial sarcoma.

POSSIBLE AGENTS THAT MIGHT INTERACT WITH CANDIDATE GENE TARGETS:

Assay	Candidate Target	Significant Result	Possible Agent(s)
IHC	SPARC	(increased +2, 90%)	paclitaxel albumin-bound
Microarray	SPARC	(increased 5.58)**	paclitaxel albumin-bound
Microarray	SSTR2	(increased 11.20)**	octreotide
Microarray	HIF1A	(increased 3.35)**	sorafenib, sunitinib, bevacizumab
Microarray	SRC	(increased 2.34)**	dasatinib
Microarray	GART	(increased 2.12)**	pemetrexed
Microarray	DNMT3A	(increased 1.93)**	azacitidine, decitabine
Microarray	SSTR3	(increased 1.82)**	octreotide
Microarray	NFKB2	(increased 1.48)**	bortezomib
Microarray	RRM1	(decreased 0.58)**	gemcitabine, hydroxyurea
Microarray	MLH1	(decreased 0.57)**	gemcitabine, oxaliplatin
Microarray	RRM2B	(decreased 0.52)**	gemcitabine, hydroxyurea
Microarray	MGMT	(decreased 0.39)**	temozolomide
Microarray	RRM2	(decreased 0.30)**	gemcitabine, hydroxyurea

* IHC = Immunohistochemistry
** Increased or decreased are relative to normal controls.

Figure 9: Results of my tumor analysis, showing abnormal gene expression and potential drugs to target them.

With off-label drugs no longer an option, we then turned our attention to experimental drugs being tested in clinical trials. We found out about these trials from other sarcoma patients over the internet, and also by searching the National Institutes of Health's (NIH) clinical trials website (*clinicaltrials.gov*). We studied the side effects and converged on those with better safety profiles. But the trials required patients to have at least one measurable tumor. My scans were clear. With no tumors to follow, how would the investigators know if the drug was working?

These dead ends demoralized us. With each passing month, the sense of urgency grew stronger. My fatigue dragged me down, forcing me to take long naps throughout the day. But I couldn't give up.

Eddy was my pillar of strength. He went with me to every medical appointment. He nursed me back to health. He sat by my side for hours on end, scouring medical websites with me, sometimes reading aloud medical papers while I laid in bed, often continuing his searches late into the night after I'd fallen asleep. He'd abandoned his career to fight alongside me. With his strength, I became a little more fearless.

Despite the setbacks, we weren't about to give up. Just because conventional medicine didn't have answers, it didn't mean there weren't any. Having exhausted all avenues, we found ourselves again turning to the world of complementary and alternative medicine.

CHAPTER 4

Exploring Alternative Cures

MOST OF THE DAY, I sat in the kitchen. I liked it there. It was bright, warm and large. A long Scandinavian dining table dominated the space. It stood by the glass sliding door that opened into the expansive backyard. An olive-green, faux leather couch leaned against the wall. Strewn across the large center island were two households' pots, pans and cooking devices—ours and my parents'.

I didn't mind the mess. My parents' presence made it worthwhile. Mom was always preparing a pot of soup full of rich meats and vegetables—nutrients to aid my still-recovering body. We couldn't have gotten through the year of treatment without my parents' support. And now, with an uncertain future ahead of us, we were grateful to be living under the same roof with them.

I was still fatigued—a side effect of chemo. Six months had gone by since the final infusion. My neutrophil count had stabilized but still dipped below normal, with transient drops into the range of "moderate" danger. During these plunges, my fatigue would worsen, and I'd take long naps on the green couch, often dreaming of food and occasionally awakening to the smell of freshly baked cakes.

Eddy would often join me in the kitchen. I'd foreseen my demise with conventional medicine; we were intent on exploring other ways to escape my prognosis. Side-by-side, we scoured the internet for stories of alternative cancer cures on our laptops. Whenever we found an interesting story, we'd debate the authenticity and plausibility of the science. Estimating we had a year and a half before my cancer returned, we were driven to thoroughly survey the prodigious list of panaceas that the internet offered.

We were drawn to testimonials of patients who proclaimed their cancer had vanished with alternative treatments. They offered an attractive premise: that I could influence my outcome, without harming my body with toxic drugs or radiation.

But how would we know if the anecdotes were valid? Some of these testimonials were written with persuasive and compelling detail, albeit tricky to interpret. A patient may attribute disappearance of her cancer to an alternative treatment but fail to mention other herbs or vitamins used. As the benefits of chemoradiation can sometimes come late, she may mistakenly ascribe tumor shrinkage to the alternative therapy instead of chemoradiation.

We kept an open mind as we scrutinized the anecdotes. How else would we find an answer outside the box? At the same time, we kept probing for a clear correlation between the alternative treatment and the disappearance of cancer.

A Frenetic Search

We studied the curious candidates: the Gerson Protocol, a vegetable juice diet and detoxification regimen that requires the cleansing of bowels with coffee enemas; the Budwig Diet, which uses flaxseed oil fine-blended into cottage cheese; infusions of vitamin C or ozone straight into the blood; traditional Chinese medicine and acupuncture; the drinking of alkaline water; low doses of naltrexone, a medicine used by drug addicts to stay clean; laetrile, a chemical from the pit of apricot seeds that converts into cyanide; the Rife machine, a device that beams electromagnetic and radio waves into the body; curcumin, an anti-inflammatory compound found in curry; the oil of the cannabis plant; and various protocols used in Mexican cancer clinics that offered everything from calf-liver injections to specialized vaccines—just to name a few.

Two different people referred us to an acupuncturist based in Cupertino near Apple's headquarters. Even though we hadn't studied acupuncture much, we knew it was a key part of Chinese medicine, practiced for thousands of years. It's also used in integrative medicine. Cancer centers sanction it for the side effects of chemoradiation, such as nausea or fatigue. There's no evidence it would cure cancer, but friends and internet sources suggested it might "balance" my immune system. We didn't understand what this meant, but perhaps it could restore my neutrophils? Seeing that the clinic was close by, and thinking it could do no harm, we thought *why not give it a try?* The experience turned out to be unforgettable.

The first session was predictable. The acupuncturist swiftly placed thin needles in my scalp, forehead, stomach, legs and feet. I looked like a pin cushion, tense at the thought of the protruding needles, but I didn't feel them at all. Afterwards, I didn't notice a difference in my health, but we kept an open mind.

At our second session, as we waited in the treatment room, the acupuncturist's assistant dragged in two large potted cactus plants. We assumed she was rearranging the office plants. Upon closer look, we realized they weren't decorative—there were acupuncture needles stuck in them. *This is getting strange*, I thought, exchanging a furtive glance with Eddy.

The acupuncturist had me lie down on the treatment table. He inserted needles into me—all fine and expected. But then he did something unexpected: he used wires to connect the needles on the cacti to those on my body. Summoning his assistant for help, he rotated the table on which I was lying, explaining he needed to align my body with the sun. Finally, the assistant—in all seriousness—implored us to give thanks to the cactus plants for the healing they were about to bring upon me. We decided this acupuncturist was not for us.

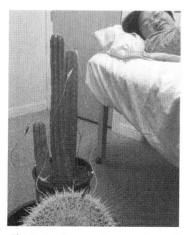

Figure 10: *Acupuncture session with the cactus plants.*

Our frenetic search for alternative treatments seemed to be a common experience for other cancer patients we'd gotten to know. By now, Eddy had befriended three sarcoma patients over the internet: Martha, Charlie and Joe. These valiant warriors were battling sarcomas that had spread around their bodies. Having failed different combinations of chemo, their tumors were advancing. All they wanted was a chance to live a while longer. As conventional medicine had little to offer, each turned to alternative medicine.

Martha was receiving intravenous vitamin C three times a week, along with infusions of alpha-lipoic acid, a common vitamin. She also received infusions of ozone and silver into her blood. In addition, her doctor prescribed low doses of naltrexone, the aforementioned anti-narcotic. She was flying from California to Arizona for treatment, which cost her $11,700 for a three-week course.

Joe was using vegetable juices, traditional Chinese medicine and bloodroot, a paste made from a medicinal plant. He claimed that he'd successfully eliminated a tumor from his stomach with bloodroot and drinking two liters of organic juice daily. A large scab formed over the area where he had applied the bloodroot paste. After 38 days the tumor detached and fell off. He went back to his doctors, who performed a biopsy. When it came back negative, his doctors claimed he had been misdiagnosed.

Charlie, desperate to suppress the dangerous tumors growing in his abdomen, went all out. His strategy? Attack the cancer from different angles. Like me, he had a sample of his tumor analyzed to identify mutations. He then searched for vitamins, over-the-counter medicines and even prescription medicines to attack every mutation listed in the report. He took 30 different vitamins and drugs daily. To keep them in his blood at all times, he spaced them out throughout the day, forcing himself to wake up every two hours at night.

There were no operating manuals, no guides. Like ours, their searches were frenzied. But Martha, Joe and Charlie had formulated strategies to survive.

We had to find our own approach. For a while, we continued without focus, feverishly sampling every claim of tumor shrinkage. But the expanding list of alternative therapies threatened to overwhelm us. It was impossible to try them all. We needed to narrow our search. But how would we identify the best candidates?

We looked for stronger anecdotes, giving priority to case studies written by physicians. We noticed the tendency for patients to try many things all at once, which made it difficult to know what worked. So, we looked for cases where patients took only a small number of clearly listed therapies.

To further streamline our search, we focused on compounds that were studied by scientists.

Alternative compounds are often investigated for their medicinal properties and long histories of use by man. Some of these compounds are later refined into drugs.[1] For example, the origin of aspirin can be traced to a folk remedy, the bark of willow trees, used to reduce pain and fever as far back as the time of Hippocrates (400 BC). The active ingredient, salicylic acid, was isolated in 1763 and led to the birth of aspirin in 1897.[2,3]

Spontaneous Regression

Amid our research, we encountered a commonly used medical term: *spontaneous regression*. Physicians use it to describe the unexpected disappearance of cancer, often in cases of poor prognoses. The word "spontaneous" connotes an unknown cause: doctors don't know what to attribute the regressions to. But we believed there was a scientific explanation behind these phenomena—even if modern medicine had yet to decipher it.

We found evidence of spontaneous regressions from centuries ago. As early as 1742, French physician H. F. Le Dran reported on a 15-year-old girl with extensive cancer of her left breast. The inoperable tumor ulcerated. Gangrene developed. Within two days, the entire tumor sloughed off with profuse bleeding and pus formation. After five weeks, the wound healed, leaving no trace of cancer. Unfortunately, the cancer recurred and the young lady died eight months later.[4]

We discovered that spontaneous regression may be more common than otherwise thought. Just months earlier, as I was recovering from my final round of chemo, Dartmouth Medical School researcher, H. Gilbert Welch, M.D., M.P.H., published a thought-provoking paper in collaboration with two Norwegian researchers. They studied two nearly identical groups of over 100,000 Norwegian women over a period of six years. One group was scanned with a single mammogram at the end of the six years. The other was scanned more frequently, every two years. The researchers found that the incidence of invasive breast cancer was 22 percent *higher* in the actively screened group over the six-year period.

Given the conventional thinking that invasive breast cancer always progresses, the total number of cancers in each group at the end of six years should've been similar, considering the huge sample sizes. The discrepancy led the researchers to conclude that some of the cancers, left untreated in the single mammogram group, had spontaneously regressed and were no longer detectable by the end of six years.[5]

In a *New York Times* article on Nov 24, 2008, Dr. Welch was quoted as saying, "There are some women who had cancer at one point and who later don't have that cancer."[6] In this study, about 350 patients of 100,000 may have experienced spontaneous regression. It hinted that spontaneous regressions may be more common than thought.

In a review of cases between 1900 to 1987, the authors state that spontaneous regression is viewed as a "relatively rare occurrence," with *approximately 20 cases* reported in the world literature each year.[7] Over 246,000 cases of breast cancer were diagnosed in the U.S. in 2016. When extrapolated, the Norwegian study suggests about 860 annual spontaneous regressions of breast cancer in the U.S. That's not counting other countries and other cancer types. It's likely that the number of true spontaneous regressions is far greater than the "20 cases reported" each year.

The existence of spontaneous regression gave us hope. It suggested that something beyond the bounds of conventional medicine could repel an otherwise invincible cancer. Regressions resulting from alternative medicines now seemed more plausible.

A Case of Spontaneous Regression with a Medical Mushroom

Queen Elizabeth Hospital in Kowloon is the largest acute care hospital in Hong Kong. With around 1,800 hospital beds and 4,800 medical staff, it serves an effective population of 900,000 and cares for about one-third of all cancer patients in Hong Kong.

In January 2003, a 47-year-old man named Mr. Wong walked into Queen Elizabeth Hospital. He'd been experiencing gastric pain in his upper abdomen just below the ribs. On January 30, a surgeon examined the insides of his stomach and duodenum (beginning of the small intestine) using a thin, flexible endoscope. Finding a large ulcer in the area where the stomach connected to the duodenum, he took a small biopsy specimen.

In addition to the biopsy, the surgeon gave Mr. Wong a urea breath test. The test checked for *H. pylori*—a bacterium found in over two-thirds of the world's population[8]—and a common cause of ulcers and pain.

The Nobel Prize Winning Doctor Who Experimented On Himself

As recently as the 1980s, scientists believed that ulcers were caused by spicy food or stress. But Australian physician, Barry Marshall, had suspected otherwise. He believed that stomach ulcers and stomach cancer were caused by bacteria. An associate of his, pathologist Robin Warren, noticed that many gastric ulcer patients had a mysterious bacteria clinging to the tissues of their biopsy specimens. Their theory was greeted with skepticism and ridicule by the scientific community. It'd been a long-held maxim that no bacteria could survive the strongly acidic environment of the stomach.

Prohibited from experimenting with people, a frustrated Dr. Marshall cultured *H. pylori* from a patient with stomach inflammation. Then, in a bold move to prove his theory, he drank the broth. Within days, he became seriously ill and developed massive inflammation in his stomach—a precursor to ulcers. In 2005, Drs. Marshall and Warren were awarded the Nobel Prize in Physiology or Medicine for proving that *H. pylori* causes inflammation and ulcers in the stomach. Their discovery paved the way for millions around the world to be treated for *H. pylori*. It also demolished the once-held dogma that bacteria cannot survive in the stomach and illustrates the importance of keeping an open mind.

Mr. Wong's breath test came back positive, so the surgeon prescribed a course of antibiotics to eradicate the bacteria. But more serious was the biopsy—it revealed diffuse large B-cell lymphoma, an aggressive cancer. The presence of *H. pylori* had led to chronic inflammation in Mr. Wong's stomach, which in turn likely gave rise to his cancer.

There was no time to lose, as the cancer was a fast-growing form of non-Hodgkin's lymphoma. On February 10th—11 days after the biopsy—surgeons removed the cancerous segment of Mr. Wong's stomach. But, to their amazement, when examined under microscope, the stomach tissue showed no evidence of cancer!

Perplexed, the surgeons asked him if he'd done anything else in the 10 days before surgery. They discovered that Mr. Wong—driven by the sudden diagnosis of advanced cancer—had ingested mega-doses of a medicinal mushroom known as Reishi. Reishi, also known as Lingzhi or *Ganoderma Lucidum*, has been used in traditional Chinese medicine for over 2,000 years. The spores are thought to be more potent than the mushroom itself. Almost immediately after the initial biopsy, Mr. Wong began consuming a powdered product which contained the spores of Reishi mushrooms. He did this for five straight days. Besides the spores, Mr. Wong had taken no other medicines except for the antibiotics for his *H. pylori*.

The surgeons were intrigued by the spontaneous regression of Mr. Wong's cancer. They analyzed the surgical samples of his stomach. In the immediate layers of tissue surrounding the ulcer, they found incredibly dense concentrations of T cells—a type of immune cell. They concluded that Mr. Wong's immune system had attacked the cancer and eradicated it. In 2007, they published a paper documenting the case.[9] At the time of writing, Mr. Wong had been cancer free for two-and-a-half years.

Mr. Wong's remarkable remission after just five days of Reishi spores is one of many anecdotes we found of cancer regression triggered by medicinal mushrooms (such as Reishi, Maitake or Turkey Tail). But Mr. Wong's case was well documented and clear-cut: the short duration between diagnosis and surgery didn't give him time to try other herbs or medicines. It supported the view that the Reishi spores caused the regression.

A Case of Complete Regression with the Gerson Therapy

Max Gerson was a German-born American physician who designed a complex diet and detoxification regimen for cancer. Originally developed to treat tuberculosis, his protocol involved hourly consumption of organic vegetable juice, the use of dietary supplements and the elimination of toxins using coffee enemas.

Among alternative cures, the Gerson protocol provokes fierce controversy. Supporters of the therapy point to the large number of anecdotes and testimonials. Many have traveled to Mexican clinics to get it, and some claim to have been cured of cancer for many years. But patients who obtained Gerson therapy in Mexico likely received other therapies such as vaccines and intravenous vitamin C. The addition of other therapies made it tricky to objectively assess the anecdotes.

Eddy first became interested in the Gerson therapy when my bone marrow began to fail after chemo. In search of an antidote, he read testimonials of amazing healing after the drinking of vegetable or carrot juice. Seeing no harm in it, he spent two hours daily washing and juicing vegetables, including red and green leaf lettuces, romaine, endives, escarole, beet tops, watercress, red cabbage, green bell peppers, Swiss chard and tart green apples. Every day, I faithfully drank the slightly bitter, bile-colored elixir. My bone marrow did eventually stabilize and partially recover. But there was no way to know if the juices had contributed to the restoration, as I had taken other supplements.

Now that we were looking for something to kill my cancer, Eddy remembered he'd bought Dr. Max Gerson's book, which chronicled the healing of 50 terminal patients.[10] Browsing through the cases, he found them almost convincing. But Eddy could see why a National Cancer Institute review had concluded there wasn't enough evidence to validate the therapy: The patient accounts weren't as clear-cut as Mr. Wong's success with Reishi. Nevertheless, Eddy felt it was worth a closer look.

One of the more convincing cases that stood out was that of eight-month-old baby, R.S. In 1950, R. S. was found to have a lump on his left shoulder. His concerned parents brought him to see a surgeon at St. Joseph Hospital in Elgin, Illinois, who excised the lump, unaware it was an aggressive cancer. The pathologist diagnosed it as a sarcoma. After the surgery, R.S.'s shoulder swelled again and began secreting pus. As sarcomas are known to aggressively spread along muscles, the surgeon concluded the tumor had regrown. He recommended drastic measures—amputate the arm and shoulder.

Distraught at the thought of amputation, his parents sought a second opinion at the Children's Memorial Hospital in Chicago. Given the infiltrative nature of sarcoma, the second surgeon felt that even an amputation would fail to extract all of the cancer. Radiation therapy was too dangerous and ineffective. Instead, he recommended a more conservative approach—cut a wider area of tissue around the original site to remove as much tumor as possible and hopefully buy some time.

But swollen glands appeared in baby R.S.'s left armpit and neck. The lumps implied that his cancer had spread from the shoulder to the armpit and upwards into the neck, and had invaded his lymphatic system. At this point, a radical amputation was again recommended, but his parents again refused.

Dr. Max Gerson started treating R.S. in late July 1950. At first, he refused to drink the colorful vegetable juices, as he was probably used to the white of milk. His mother cleverly disguised the bottles with white paper. At the initial consult, Dr. Gerson had noted the deep operation wound, two-and-a-half inches long, covered with pus. A month later, the wound had closed. Remarkably, all the swollen glands in his armpit and neck resolved. Baby R.S. went on to recover fully. He was last seen by Dr. Gerson in July 1957—seven years later. He'd grown to be a healthy, strong child with no sign of cancer.

R.S.'s complete remission struck Eddy; he understood the implications of regionally spreading sarcoma. An entrenched sarcoma does not stop invading and spreading its sinister tentacles of malignancy unless drastic measures are taken. R.S. hadn't been treated with radiation nor chemotherapy; his parents had refused amputation. The Gerson therapy was the only treatment he received.

Dr. Gerson had taken blood samples from R.S. every three weeks from July 1950 to March 1951, observing that his lymphocyte count was significantly higher than normal, with spikes in August and December. (Lymphocytes are a type of immune cell known to attack cancer. The T cells mentioned in Mr. Wong's case are a type of lymphocyte.) The presence of lymphocytes hinted at an immune mechanism behind R.S.'s regression. Perhaps Dr. Gerson's therapy had stimulated his immune system against his sarcoma?

The sarcoma in R.S.'s shoulder was confirmed. But the swollen lumps in his armpit and neck hadn't been biopsied, so we can't be sure they were cancerous. There were two plausible explanations for the lumps. First: his cancer had invaded the lymph nodes in those regions, causing them to bulge with disease. This is what his doctors believed had happened. Second: he had a bacterial or viral infection that occurred in the area of the cancer. In response, his lymph nodes swelled up, pregnant with immune cells. In either case, the lymphocyte count hinted that R.S.'s immune system had been activated—either by the cancer or by an infection. The activated immune system correlated with his remission.

We understood the tenacity of sarcomas. They didn't vanish without reason. There had to be a scientific explanation for his remission, and the clues hinted at an immune mechanism.

A Common Theme?

With every day that passed, I slid a little further down the survival curve, and my expiry date drew a little closer. Mr. Wong's success convinced us to purchase expensive bottles of Reishi spores. And Eddy continued making me the Gerson juices, which I faithfully endured.

We discovered that some scientists were actively studying intravenous vitamin C (IVC).[11] Clinical trials combined IVC with chemotherapy for pancreatic cancer.[12] Testimonials and local news reports told of patients who testified that IVC had put them into remission. We decided to give it a serious try. For many weeks, three times a week, Eddy drove me from San Jose to Santa Rosa, California to obtain the infusions. The drive was two hours each way, over the Golden Gate Bridge. By the end of the day, he'd be completely spent. Aside from some transient fatigue, I didn't feel any different on IVC. There was no way to know if it was destroying my cancer. It was an exercise of faith.

It was a full-time job studying alternatives, trying different therapies like intravenous vitamin C and vegetable juices, all the while going in for weekly blood draws and dealing with administrivia—calling doctors, paying bills, dealing with insurance. But amid this turbulence, we managed to eke out time to study and ponder the role of the immune system in controlling cancer.

We couldn't stop thinking about the dense presence of T cells in Mr. Wong's stomach and R.S.'s high lymphocyte count. We continued our study of spontaneous regressions and learned that some scientists believed that the elimination of cancer by the immune system might explain the mysterious regressions observed throughout history.[13,14]

I needed to learn more. Although I was a biologist, I wasn't versed in immunology. My main area of study had been the inner workings of single cells. In contrast, the immune system is a byzantine network of cells.

The Immune System

The human immune system protects our bodies from things that don't belong in it. These include foreign invaders such as bacteria or fungi, as well as cells gone bad—such as cancer cells or virus-infected cells.

Hundreds of billions of immune cells exist in our body—many times more than the number of people in the world. Some cells engulf foreign invaders directly, digesting and killing them. Other immune cells secrete proteins that perform key functions. Some of these proteins stick to foreign invaders to puncture holes in them, weakening and killing them. Other proteins attract additional immune cells to join the fight. Still others cause foreign invaders to clump together, making them more easily recognized and devoured by immune cells. It's amazing how complex the immune system is, and how the different cells and proteins work together to repel invaders.

The immune system consists of two branches—the innate immune system and the adaptive immune system.

The Innate Immune System

The innate immune system consists of cells and proteins that stand always ready to attack invading pathogens, such as bacteria, viruses or fungi. A single bacterium that enters through a cut on our finger can reproduce into tens of millions of progeny within a few hours. In the first critical hours and days of infection, we rely on the innate immune system to defend us.

Macrophages (or "big eaters") are large immune cells that sense and eat invading microbes. They loiter in strategic places where they are likely to encounter microbes, such as the gut, lung or under the skin. To detect these microbes, they feel for identification markers on the surface of microbes. Once identified, they engulf the microbes, pump them with poisons and kill them.

The macrophages then sound the alarm, secreting proteins that call for other immune cells. This creates a state known as *inflammation*.

The inflammatory proteins stop other patrolling immune cells in their tracks, beckoning them to join the fray. Within the bloodstream, these proteins help immune cells break free from rushing rivers of blood by helping them stick to the walls of blood vessels. Once stuck, the immune cells then push and squeeze through gaps in the walls, entering tissues and advancing toward the site of danger.

The first responders rushing to defend the borders are the *neutrophils*— the most abundant immune cell in our body. They are our key line of defense against the trillions of bacteria that would overcome us otherwise. Like their larger cousins, the macrophages, these "small eaters" are able to recognize, engulf and kill microbes. Billions of neutrophils overwhelm the site of infection, turning the tide against the microbes.

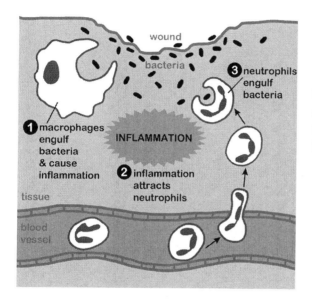

Figure 11: Innate immune cells responding to invading bacteria, attracted by inflammation.

But how does the innate immune system deal with viral infections like the flu? When a flu virus invades the body, it infiltrates cells and hides deep within. How is the innate immune system able to detect these viruses if they cannot be touched? Here's where *natural killer* (or NK) cells become important.

Normal cells have a certain protein on their surface known as *MHC Class 1*. But some virus-infected cells (and some cancer cells) don't. This difference allows NK cells to differentiate between normal cells and virus-infected cells. NK cells identify virus-infected cells by touch, looking for the absence of the MHC Class 1 protein. When the absence is detected, they punch holes in the surface of the infected cell. They then release enzymes that enter through those holes. Once inside, the enzymes cause the cell to self-destruct, taking down the virus along with it.

In the early days of infection, bacterial, fungal and viral invaders are held at bay by the innate immune system as described above. There are other mechanisms involved, but we will not describe them here.

The Adaptive Immune System

The innate immune response can still be outsmarted or overwhelmed by bacteria, viruses or cancer cells. Thankfully, we have a second layer of defense called the adaptive immune system.

The adaptive immune system seeks to mark an enemy for death, then creates a large army of immune cells to demolish that specific enemy. But it takes a few days for the army to be born, during which the body relies on the innate immune system to hold the fort, keeping invading pathogens at bay.

While the frontline cells of the innate immune system are busy suppressing the invading horde, the *dendritic cell* is hard at work. Dendritic cells bridge the innate and adaptive systems. Like macrophages, they guard tissues that contact the external environment, such as our skin, lungs and intestines. They constantly feel around for dangerous adversaries. When a dendritic cell contacts an enemy, such as a bacterium or cancer cell, it engulfs, then digests the hapless victim.

Now pregnant with fragments of the enemy, the dendritic cell has one more important job to do: find its way to a training ground, where it will cultivate an army of soldiers to further destroy this foe. The destination is the lymph node—a bean or oval shaped structure that can be thought of as a crossroad town, through which billions of immune cells flow and mingle. In our bodies, there is a sprawling interconnected network of lymph nodes from head to toe. Migrating to a nearby lymph node, the dendritic cell holds out fragments of digested pathogen on arm-like structures known as *dendrites*. And then it waits, patiently, to meet with *just* the right *T cell*.

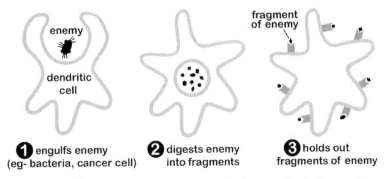

Figure 12: Dendritic cell capturing pathogen and presenting its fragments.

The T cell is the foot soldier of the adaptive immune system. Billions of these exist in the body. Each T cell can only recognize one fragment of an enemy. But collectively, the T cells in our body can recognize all possible fragments of any foe they'll ever encounter—a remarkable fact of nature.

In the lymph node, throngs of T cells come in contact with dendritic cells. But it's only that rare T cell that can recognize a *specific* pathogen fragment advertised on the arm of a dendritic cell. When the match is made, this T cell stops and bonds to the dendritic cell. Now activated, the T cell goes on to multiply, making thousands of copies of itself within three to five days. The process is repeated to create a massive roaming army of T cells targeting that specific pathogen. It can take a few days to generate the army and bring an infection, such as the flu, under control.

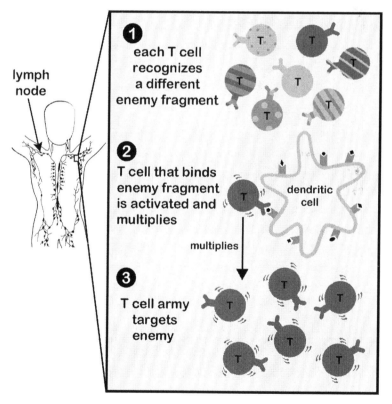

Figure 13: In lymph nodes, dendritic cells activate a T cell army to target the enemy. Only the T cells that bind to enemy fragments on dendritic cells are activated. Once activated, the T cells are cloned into large numbers to repel the current threat.

After the threat has been eradicated, the marauding T cells die off, their life purpose achieved. But a small number of *memory T cells remain.*[15] These and their progeny have one purpose—stand ready to repel the pathogen, should it dare reappear.

In this way, the adaptive immune system constantly "adapts" to the threat at hand, creating transient armies of T cells and long lasting memory T cells to wipe out invading bacteria, virus-infected cells and even cancer cells.

An Ancient Clue

We were fascinated to learn about the immune system—a complex microscopic army that exists within each of us. As Eddy and I delved deeper into the inner workings of the immune system, we were awestruck by an intriguing alternative cancer immunotherapy known as Coley's Toxins.

Coley's Toxins was named after its inventor, Dr. William Coley, a Harvard-trained surgeon who practiced at Memorial Hospital in New York at the turn of the 20th Century. The hospital would go on to become the world-renowned Memorial Sloan Kettering Cancer Center. Dr. Coley was said to have treated around 1000 patients with this century-old immunotherapy.[16] We were excited to discover that most of his patients had some form of advanced sarcoma—similar to my disease. But more astounding was that up to half of these patients survived for many years—*some still alive many decades later, with no tumors left in their bodies.*

The long-term survival of these patients suggested that a possible cure for sarcoma may have existed for over 100 years. If not for the indisputable evidence of spontaneous regressions throughout history, we would've thought this to be a hoax. But the premise of an immune-based cure made sense: if the immune system is capable of rejecting entire organs that are transplanted into patients, why couldn't it eradicate tumors?

Sitting in the kitchen one night—the aroma of mom's fresh-baked green tea chiffon cake filling the room—Eddy and I shivered with excitement and anticipation.

This was it. We knew we'd found our preemptive weapon.

Putting aside all other alternative therapies, we resolved to pursue Coley's Toxins with undivided focus.

CHAPTER 5

Coley's Toxins:
A 100-Year-Old Immunotherapy

In the summer of 1890, a young lady from New Jersey by the name of Elizabeth "Bessie" Dashiell, was riding a passenger train. Seventeen, bold and adventurous, her railroad trip would take her across the continent and up to Alaska. She was a close friend of the young John D. Rockefeller, Jr., the only son of Standard Oil founder, John D. Rockefeller, who would become the richest man in U.S. history. "They took carriage rides together, rode horses along the Hudson Palisades, and exchanged long, thoughtful letters."[1] He thought of her as his "adopted sister."[2] He had three sisters, one of whom was also named Bessie.

In a bizarre accident, Bessie's right hand got trapped between the seats of the train. It left a common bruise on the back of her hand. Some pain and swelling occurred, after which the injury seemed to improve. But after a week, the symptoms resurged. To alleviate the discomfort, Bessie placed her hand and wrist in a splint. By September, the pain had become constant. Occasional sharp flashes interrupted her sleep. Her family decided to take her to New York City to see a specialist, and Bessie was referred to a young surgeon by the name of William Coley.

Twenty-eight-year-old William Coley, a graduate of Yale and Harvard, had just completed surgical training at New York Hospital. Dr. Coley was in his first year of practice when Bessie was referred. On October 1, Dr. Coley examined his young patient. He noticed a small mass, "about the size of half an olive,"[3] above the knuckle joint of her small finger. When he pressed down hard to see if it could move, she expressed pain. Suspecting an infection, he felt for swollen lymph nodes under her armpit, but found none.

Days later, thinking the culprit was inflammation of tissues around the bone, Dr. Coley made an incision to drain the swelling. A few drops of pus emerged—nothing suggestive of an infection. Perplexed, Dr. Coley noted that the tissue "seemed abnormally hard and more of a grayish color than normal."[4] He closed and sterilized the wound, then placed her hand back in the splint.

In late October, Bessie returned, her pain unbearable, her symptoms expanding. With no clear idea of the cause, Dr. Coley made a larger incision, scraped off the "grayish granulations"[5] and again closed the wound. After a couple of days of temporary relief, the pain came roaring back. Bessie began to lose sensation in several fingers.

Finally, the fledgling surgeon realized this could be cancer. A biopsy revealed it to be "round cell sarcoma."[6] On November 8, 1890, after further consultation with his mentor, Dr. William Bull, Dr. Coley amputated Bessie's arm below the elbow.

It was too late. Her sarcoma had spread.

Tumors began to sprout all over her body. On December 11, a lump the size of "a small almond"[7] appeared on her right breast; the very next day, two smaller lumps materialized on her left breast. One week later, the cancer had spread to the lymph nodes under one armpit, and even more breast tumors sprouted. She became anorexic. By Christmas, she could no longer go out to walk. Her pain so severe, she needed constant morphine. "She began to lose sensation in her lower lip and chin, then in some lower teeth."[8] Her liver started to fail, causing jaundice. Two weeks after Christmas, a huge tumor about the size of "a child's head"[9] occupied the abdomen above her stomach.

In these last stages of suffering, the breast tumors grew to the size of avocados, the abdominal tumor continued expanding, and her entire body—"from head to toe"—became riddled with small tumors that Dr. Coley described as "buckshot or split peas."[10]

On January 23, 1891—four months after she had first seen Dr. Coley, Bessie Dashiell died in her home, at the age of 18. Dr. Coley, by her side, signed her death certificate.

Mr. Stein

Traumatized by his first encounter with a vicious sarcoma, the young Dr.

Coley began to contemplate devoting his career to the study of cancer. A friendship grew between him and Rockefeller, Jr., as Bessie's death deeply impacted both men and spurred them to devote themselves to the cause of cancer research.

Rockefeller Jr. and his family went on to become a major source of support for the first hospital in the U.S. dedicated to treating cancer. The New York Cancer Hospital, where Dr. Coley would eventually move to, is now known as Memorial Sloan Kettering Cancer Center and is consistently ranked as one of the top two cancer centers in the country.

Dr. Coley's life-long devotion to cancer research began with the files of Dr. William Bull. In scrutinizing his mentor's records, he was taken by the remarkable case of a German immigrant named Fred K. Stein.

In the fall of 1880, Mr. Stein had developed a small red lesion on the side of his face, in front of his left ear. It grew steadily to "the size of a hen's egg."[11] In June 1881, it was surgically removed. After only three months, Mr. Stein needed a second surgery to cut away a fast-growing recurrence "the size of a pigeon's egg"[12] (about two-thirds that of a chicken's). Two years later, it returned yet again, just below the left ear. By the time he saw Dr. Bull, it measured four-and-a-half inches wide, and looked like "a bunch of grapes."[13]

On June 5, 1884, Dr. Bull removed the large tumor. As the wound was large, skin grafts were needed to cover it. Several attempts were made but failed, leaving the wound exposed to infection.

Three months later, Dr. Bull attempted a final surgery on the relentless tumor, which had become infected and ulcerated. During the procedure, he found that the tumor had attached itself to Mr. Stein's carotid, a crucial artery that supplies blood to the brain. It was impossible to remove all of the cancer. Mr. Stein was left with a five-inch-long by four-inch-wide wound: a veritable hole in the side of his neck barely held together by sutures. Pathology revealed it to be round cell sarcoma. Dr. Bull declared the case "absolutely hopeless."[14]

Another skin graft was attempted to cover his wound, but again failed. One week later, on October 12, Mr. Stein developed a high fever. A bright red rash bounded across his face. Diagnosed as *erysipelas*, it was caused by the bacteria *Streptococcus pyogenes*, commonly known as "Strep"—the same bacteria that causes strep throat.

This was 1884. It would be another 44 years before Sir Alexander Fleming would discover penicillin and spark the era of antibiotics. Erysipelas was a deadly scourge that killed scores of patients in 19th-century hospitals. Hospitals in England contaminated by erysipelas and other bacteria were occasionally demolished and rebuilt to bypass unsuccessful attempts at decontamination.[15]

Mr. Stein, facing dual threats of death from erysipelas and sarcoma, now had to be isolated so as not to infect other patients. But then, something extraordinary happened—after each attack of erysipelas, his tumor shrunk and the ulcerating wound rapidly healed. To the amazement of Dr. Bull, the cancer eventually vanished and the wound healed, leaving a "healthy scar."[16] By late February 1885, Mr. Stein was discharged.

As the young Dr. Coley studied the miraculous account of regression, a surge of enthusiasm must have possessed him. Scouring the immigrant housing tenements of New York's Lower East Side, Dr. Coley finally located Mr. Stein. With his own eyes, he verified that Mr. Stein was cancer free and in good health—seven years after Mr. Stein's fatal sarcoma had magically melted away.

At the time, radiation and chemotherapy didn't exist. Surgery was the only weapon against cancer. If tumors couldn't be safely cut out, the patient faced certain death. With visions of Bessie Dashiell's tumor-riddled body fresh in Dr. Coley's mind, Mr. Stein's miraculous triumph over death ignited a fire within the young doctor. It marked the beginning of a lifelong quest to unlock the secrets of an apparent cure for cancer.

Coley's Toxins

After the encounter with Mr. Stein, Dr. Coley began injecting patients—at first, with live bacteria.

His first patient, Mr. Zola, an Italian immigrant, "had only a few weeks to live."[17] His inoperable neck

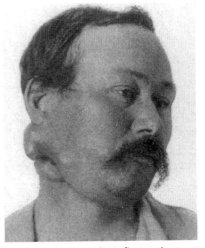

Figure 14: Dr. Coley's first patient, Mr. Zola (1891).[E]

sarcoma had spread to a tonsil, obstructing his throat; he was emaciated from malnutrition. In May 1891, with Zola's consent, Dr. Coley infected him with live erysipelas—often lethal in this pre-antibiotic era. Erysipelas was highly contagious, so Dr. Coley went to the lower Manhattan tenements where Zola lived to infect him. Mr. Zola's reactions were mild; the infections weren't taking. Still, one month into treatment, the tonsil tumor had "appreciably diminished in size."[18]

By October, Zola's tumors had rebounded. A friend of Dr. Coley visited Europe and brought back a virulent strain of erysipelas, which Dr. Coley injected into Zola's neck tumor. Zola's body "shook violently with severe chills."[19] Nausea, vomiting and pain followed. He developed a fever of 105°F. A red rash spread across his neck, face and head. By the second day, the neck tumor began to disintegrate, spewing dead tissue. By two weeks, it had vanished, and the tonsil tumor had shrunk further. Over time, Zola grew stronger. His neck wound healed. The tonsil tumor didn't disappear, but stayed small.

Four years later, Dr. Coley saw Zola, noting he was "in excellent condition,"[20] his tonsil tumor kept in check. Zola later returned to Italy and reportedly died there, eight-and-a-half years after first treatment, purportedly from a local recurrence. He had outlived his prognosis of a few weeks by almost a decade.

Encouraged by early successes such as Mr. Zola's, Dr. Coley grew bolder and more convicted. Between 1891 and 1893, he treated 12 patients. But two died from erysipelas. To make the toxins safer, he killed the bacteria, inactivating them with heat. Seeking to refine and strengthen his toxins, he collaborated with pathologists and bacteriologists to produce the most virulent strains possible. His final concoction consisted of two strains of heat-killed bacteria: *Streptococcus pyogenes* and *Serratia marcescens*.

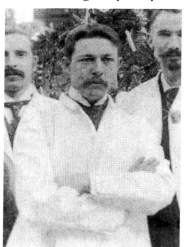

Figure 15: Dr. William Coley (1862-1936) in 1892.[F]

Hired by Dr. Bull, Dr. Coley moved to the newly opened New York Cancer Hospital. He now had the resources of a hospital to support his research. There, Dr. Coley held the position of attending surgeon until he retired in January 1933.

Over the course of 40 years, Dr. Coley treated over 1000 patients with his toxins. About 500 of these patients experienced near-complete regression.[21] Decades later, some were documented alive and disease-free. His toxins became known worldwide; physicians in the United States, England, Belgium, and even China began to use them.[22]

As the science of immunology was still in its infancy, these early pioneers of immunotherapy practically worked in the dark. Even today, modern immunotherapy yields variable results. It's no surprise then, that these physicians—some of whom concocted their own versions of Coley's Toxins—saw wildly different results. Some reported complete regression; others reported no benefit whatsoever.

The Monographs

Having studied the remarkable history of Dr. William Coley's toxins, Eddy and I wanted to read, first-hand, the stories of his patients. We fixated on those who survived twenty, thirty or forty years after treatment. Long-term survival was the ultimate test. The shrinking of tumors wasn't good enough—even chemo and radiation could achieve that. A patient alive and well decades later—that was the mark of an effective cure.

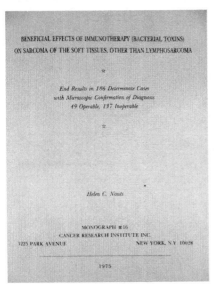

Figure 16: Copy of monograph 16 by Mrs. Helen Coley Nauts, the late daughter of William Coley.

Scouring the Stanford Medical Library catalog, we hunted down copies of monographs that described Dr. William Coley's patients in detail. These monographs were compiled by Mrs. Helen Coley Nauts, the late daughter of Dr. Coley. A housewife and mother with no formal medical training, Mrs. Coley Nauts taught herself record keeping, oncology and immunology, with the singular focus of preserving her father's work for mankind.

The monographs contained case after case of patients her father had treated. They were old, yellow and faded. Many of them hadn't been checked out since acquired in the 1970s! For four decades, these treasures had stayed hidden in the basement of the Stanford Medical Library. Quivering with excitement, impatient to uncover the secrets of a possible cure for cancer, we turned the aging pages.

The monographs chronicled Dr. Coley's heroic attempts to save the lives of his patients. Late into the night, we pored over the cases, scrutinizing the nuances of each account. What we found astounded us. Either Dr. Coley had fabricated the patient records—or the treatment was truly capable of creating miracles.

Mrs. Gruver

The majority of Dr. Coley's patients had sarcomas. This was not surprising as he'd begun his research with sarcomas and eventually became the head of the bone sarcoma unit. But Dr. Coley and other physicians treated other cancers as well. One such case—a patient with carcinoma of the cervix—demonstrates how Coley's Toxins can bring about long-lasting cures.

In 1891, Mrs. R. Gruver, a 41-year-old woman in the small town of Stroudsburg, Pennsylvania, began to experience pain in her lower abdomen. Over the next two years, her symptoms—vomiting, headaches and so forth—gradually worsened, and by May 1893, she checked into New York Hospital.

The left side of her abdomen hurt when pressed. Her cervix was "very hard,"[23] and the external orifice of her uterus was "surrounded by a ring of hard nodules."[24] She was diagnosed with cancer and surgery was scheduled. Dr. William Bull operated on her, removing a mass the size of a small avocado, along with her cervix. Surprisingly, pathology showed the growth to be "normal cervical tissue,"[25] and she was discharged.

All was well for three years. But then her symptoms recurred with occasional bloody discharge. For another three years, she endured worsening symptoms: nausea, retching and even vomiting feces.

This time, Mrs. Gruver was seen at a hospital in Scranton, Pennsylvania, a little closer to her hometown. Taking note of her history, Dr. Charles Thompson decided to operate to see what was causing her symptoms.

Making a large incision in her abdomen, he discovered suspicious looking masses. The mass in the lower right abdomen was deemed inoperable. He sent a tissue sample to James Ewing, an up-and-coming pathologist at the Medical College of Cornell University. The pathology revealed that she had cancer, a carcinoma.

In July 1899, Mrs. Gruver again checked into New York Hospital. A doctor examined her and found two masses attached to her intestines on "each side of her abdomen."[26] These twin tumors had been rapidly growing for six months. "The region of the cervix was hard and eroded, her uterus enlarged and firmly fixed."[27] Mrs. Gruver's cervical carcinoma had metastasized to her intestines. With surgery out of the question, chemotherapy not yet invented and radiation therapy barely in its infancy, Mrs. Gruver was sent home and told she had less than 18 months to live.

At that point, she was informed about Dr. Coley's work. Seeing that she had nothing to lose, Mrs. Gruver consulted Dr. Coley, who confirmed the diagnosis and dismal prognosis. Despite the hopeless situation, Dr. Coley was willing to let her try his toxins.

One of Mrs. Gruver's three children was a doctor himself, recently out of medical school. With instructions from Dr. Coley, the young Dr. Charles Gruver, along with another physician, began injecting Mrs. Gruver with the toxins.

The injections began in August 1899. Dr. Gruver injected the toxins through his mother's abdomen, using a long needle to reach deep into the tumors. For six months, twice-weekly, he perhaps held her hand, as she endured the acute swelling at the injection sites. Perhaps he comforted her as her fever rose and covered her with blankets when her body shook violently with the chills.

As a physician, Dr. Gruver would've wished to alleviate his patient's discomfort. But as a loving son who wanted to see his mother survive, he had to help her look past the transient discomforts of the high fevers and fix her gaze on the prize of a cure. Intent on living, both mother and son persevered—the mother enduring the painful injections, the son watching her fight for life. Their determination would soon be rewarded.

Before the young Charles began injecting his mother in August, her tumors had been growing rapidly. The injections halted their expansion, and the tumors gradually shrunk. By December, he could barely feel them when he pressed on her abdomen.

Along with the tumor shrinkage, Mrs. Gruver's general condition began to improve. The injections necessitated that she stay in bed for many hours. But in between, she resumed her normal activities and was able to perform all of her own housework.

Dr. Gruver continued injecting his mother twice weekly until January 1900. Thereafter, to ensure thorough extermination of the cancer, he injected her once a week for another full year, rested, then resumed injections, making the total duration of treatment about three years. Their persistence was rewarded.

Mrs. Gruver went on to live for another three *decades*, enjoying "unusually good health,"[28] never to experience further recurrence of cancer. In January 1929, while visiting her son in Asheville, North Carolina, she caught the flu, came down with pneumonia and died. Had she lived a little while longer to witness the infamous stock market crash in October of that year, she would've been 80 years old. The Coley's Toxins injections had effectively cured her of terminal metastatic cervical carcinoma—a feat still unattainable with modern conventional therapy.

Was There a Scientific Basis?

Dr. William Coley stumbled upon his toxins by studying the end effects of erysipelas on Mr. Stein's sarcoma. He had no science to rely on when he injected his first patient. It'd be another 17 years before German Nobel laureate, Paul Ehrlich, proposed that the immune system could protect against cancer. The only guides Dr. Coley possessed were observation and trial and error.

Through years of experimentation, Dr. Coley derived some "best practices" that achieved superior results. These included direct injection into tumors, injecting enough toxins to elicit high fevers (above 103°F), frequent injections (every one or two days), prolonged injections (six months minimum), and injecting before and after surgery.

But how did Coley's Toxins work? What was the science behind it? Scientists have postulated different theories. One theory says it activates enzymes that dissolve the protective layers around tumors.[29] Another theory is it prevents the formation of blood vessels in tumors.[30] But most scientists believe it works by activating immune cells to attack tumors.[31,32,33,34] Scientists have yet to decipher the inner workings. Meanwhile, Dr. Coley's empirical observations may offer some clues.

Direct injection into tumors intrigued us the most. After much research, Eddy and I believed that the sudden introduction of dangerous-looking bacterial fragments raises an alarm, causing innate immune cells to invade the injected tumor.[35] In a frenzy, neutrophils, macrophages and natural killer cells inflict death on some tumor cells. The violent cell death provokes dendritic cells to create T cell armies against the cancer.[36] An adaptive immune response mounts, where T cells target and destroy remaining tumors. Memory T cells then protect against recurrence, leading to long-term cures in some patients.

In one sense, the lack of scientific insight allowed Dr. Coley to chase the "impossible." Mr. Stein was a living testament that a cure was attainable. In contrast, modern medicine can sometimes develop myopia. Decades of failed drug development had conditioned a demoralized medical community to settle for meager improvements.

For example, Votrient, a drug that inhibits key enzymes that affect cancer growth, was approved for advanced soft tissue sarcomas in 2012. It was hailed as the first drug approved for sarcoma in decades. How much more life did this revolutionary drug buy? Using the gold standard of overall survival (time between initial treatment and death), patients on Votrient lived an average of two months longer than those given placebo.[37] In contrast, some of Dr. Coley's patients lived for decades, seemingly cured of advanced sarcoma.[38]

Consider Avastin, a drug that slows the growth of new blood vessels. It was approved in 2014 for recurrent or metastatic cervical cancer—the same disease that Mrs. Gruver had. Approval was based on a modest increase of four months of life.[39] In contrast, Coley's Toxins had given Mrs. Gruver 30 years of cancer-free life.

While single case reports can't be compared against large-scale randomized trials, these data highlight the dramatic contrast between drugs that buy a little time versus a therapy that can cure.

Why Had Coley's Toxins Disappeared into Obscurity?

If Coley's Toxins could shrink tumors, why did it disappear from the landscape of American medicine? Having studied the historical context, we believe there was an answer—albeit, a complex one.

Despite the successes of Dr. Coley and his colleagues, other physicians failed to reproduce his results. One major problem was production consistency. The Parke-Davis company, a subsidiary of Pfizer, attempted to manufacture the toxins. But they made it too weak, and it showed equivocal benefit.[40] Other physicians tried to culture their own toxins, but, failing to get results, concluded the toxins were useless. Without a standardized production process, it was impossible to achieve consistent results.

Coley's Toxins often took months—sometimes over a year—of injections to achieve success. What doctor could afford to spend that much time on a patient?

Coley's Toxins was a therapy ahead of its time. In the late 1800s, scientific understanding of the human immune system was in its infancy; the germ theory of disease was still nascent. Many doctors didn't accept the controversial view that microbes were the true agents of infectious diseases. Instead, they believed infectious diseases were somehow transmitted through the air, caused by "bad smells that emanated from filth, decay or rotting plants and animals," or through direct contact with a sick person.[41] Some European doctors had already accepted germ theory, but it was challenged by American physicians until 1876, when German microbiologist Robert Koch finally proved that anthrax was caused by a bacterium. Such was the medical atmosphere in which Dr. Coley struggled to explain his cancer-shrinking toxins.

In the early decades of the 1900s, radiation therapy became ascendant. Newer machines delivered stronger doses deep into the body, making treatment of deep-seated tumors possible. Then came chemotherapy in the 1950s. The impressive, tumor-shrinking capabilities of chemoradiation overshadowed the difficult-to-reproduce benefits of Coley's Toxins. Both these therapies were also quicker and easier to administer. Results came sooner. Efforts were made to standardize them; doctors nationwide could achieve reproducible results.

Who could've predicted that chemoradiation would mainly delay the inevitable? Not until the 1960s would the medical community realize that the initial dramatic shrinkage from chemoradiation wouldn't, as a whole, translate to long-term survival benefit, especially in advanced cases of solid tumors.[42]

What about the long-term benefits of Coley's Toxins? Shouldn't the cures have silenced the skeptics? Unfortunately, without well-controlled clinical trials, it was impossible to compare long-term outcomes against chemoradiation. The debate degenerated into a war of philosophies: On the one side stood a handful of faithful adherents—Dr. Coley and a few colleagues, convinced by incredible decades-long disappearances of cancer, obtained through painstaking months of injections. On the other side, stood the juggernaut of chemoradiation, with growing legions of doctors galvanized by the quick and reproducible results, unaware of the long-term inadequacies of these powerful, new modalities.

This philosophical war could be seen in the strained relationship between Dr. William Coley and his new boss, James Ewing, the pathologist who had diagnosed Mrs. Gruver's cervical cancer. In 1913, Dr. Ewing became Medical Director of New York Hospital. (Then renamed to Memorial Hospital.) But he also became a zealous supporter of radiation and rejected competing therapies.[43] He and Dr. Coley often exchanged heated letters and engaged in public attacks. Dr. Ewing criticized Dr. Coley's diagnostic skills, saying the cures he'd obtained through the toxins had not been for sarcomas, but for other cancers. He constantly deprecated the toxins in public. Dr. Coley openly accused Dr. Ewing of assigning cases to be treated with radiation, despite the lack of data to support long term efficacy.[44]

As if these factors weren't enough, in 1962 the FDA was given expanded authority under the Kefauver-Harris congressional amendments.[45] Known as the "Drug Efficacy Amendment," it forced manufacturers to provide proof of efficacy and safety before approval. Other traditional medicines in prior existence—such as aspirin and Tylenol—were "grandfathered," their continued use allowed. But Coley's Toxins was not. This nail in the coffin made it unlawful to manufacture the 70-year-old medicine for sale, until proven in clinical trials.

To make things worse, in 1965, the American Cancer Society (ACS)— seeking to protect citizens from all manner of quackery—added Coley's

Toxins to its list of "Unproven Methods of Cancer Therapy."[46] The black-listing dissuaded mainstream researchers from studying Coley's Toxins, for fear of being associated with charlatanism. Most modern doctors wouldn't even have heard about Coley's; the tarnish of quackery would ensure they would never.

Approaching the 21st century, the cost of clinical trials skyrocketed; it cost $800 million to approve a product in clinical trials.[47] Even if brave academics could obtain funding for early-stage trials, only for-profit companies had the wherewithal to see a therapy through FDA approval. The toxins comprised two unpatentable strains of natural bacteria—a fatal handicap in the world of commercialized medicine. What company would risk hundreds of millions without exclusivity rights to protect their investment?

While all of the above was happening, Dr. Coley and the other adherents had either passed away or retired. It would be up to Dr. Coley's daughter to keep the flame burning: Mrs. Helen Coley Nauts, who fought to preserve her father's gift to humanity.

A second figure carried the legacy—a prominent scientist by the name of Dr. Lloyd Old, who had fought to remove Coley's Toxins from the ACS' blacklist. Dr. Old had pioneered the use of Bacillus Calmette-Guérin (BCG)—a live bacterial vaccine, similar to Coley's Toxins—in cancer, establishing it as a standard-of-care therapy for superficial bladder cancer.[48] Dr. Old's staunch support suggested the possibility of scientific validity. Why else would a distinguished scientist jeopardize his reputation to defend a "quack" therapy?

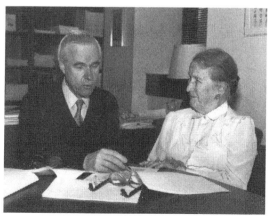

Figure 17: Lloyd J. Old, M.D., seated with Cancer Research Institute founder Helen Coley Nauts, c. 1990.[G]

Was There Supporting Data?

The large number of physician-documented case reports, not just by Dr. Coley, but also by his peers, were almost enough to convince us to get treatment. But one question remained: was there supporting clinical trial data to affirm these reports?

We discovered a handful of trials had been run between 1962-2002.

In 1988, researchers at Temple University in Philadelphia published results of a trial where 13 patients with various far-advanced cancers were given Coley's Toxins. Despite receiving small doses of the toxins, one patient with lung cancer experienced partial tumor shrinkage, and "many had stabilization of disease."[49]

In 1990, researchers from Shanghai Medical University, China, published a paper in collaboration with Temple University researcher, H. Francis Havas, and Mrs. Helen Coley Nauts. Eighty-six patients with advanced liver cancer were followed. Half were randomly given Coley's Toxins in addition to standard therapy. Adding Coley's Toxins doubled long-term survival in some patients; shrunk some tumors, making them operable; and augmented the response of conventional treatment.[50]

In 1991, a German trial of 15 patients with metastatic melanoma showed three (20 percent) complete regressions. At the time of writing, these patients had been "cancer-free" for 32, 21 and 15 months, respectively. A fourth patient also had disease stabilization for five months.[51]

These trials (and others not described here) were small and therefore underpowered to show conclusive benefit. Some trials used weak doses of toxins. Even so, they clearly suggested that Coley's Toxins could shrink tumors and slow down cancer, lending support to Dr. Coley's case reports.

How Could I Get Coley's Toxins?

Having contemplated the history and nuances of Coley's Toxins, Eddy and I concluded it was legitimate. Multiple sources confirmed it could eliminate some tumors; perhaps my microscopic disease would be even easier to eradicate?

We found two clinics in Tijuana that offered the toxins. But how would we know if the concoctions were potent and safe? The physicians in Dr. Coley's day struggled to create consistent formulations. Had the Mexican clinics solved these issues?

Eddy toyed with an idea. "Why can't you make it yourself? You're a biologist—it's just two strains of commonly found bacteria, heated and killed ... Dr. Coley made his own, using 19th-century equipment. If your cancer returns, and there's nothing the doctors can do, what's there to lose?" I brushed off the brazen suggestion.

Eddy found a recipe. If the websites were to be believed, for decades, a chemical engineer by the name of Wayne Martin had worked with an alternative M.D. to help patients get the toxins.[52] Visions of poor Bessie Dashiell—covered from head to toe with buckshot metastases—made Eddy's idea seem less radical.

Upon further research, we learned of a fortuitous development. A Canadian company, MBVax, was trying to revive Coley's Toxins. They claimed to have solved the production inconsistencies. We contacted the company, but learned we couldn't get it in Canada or the U.S., as both countries required validation in large-scale clinical trials. MBVax was trying to get the trial process going, but it could take years. However, clinics in Mexico, Paraguay and the Bahamas were legally treating patients with it. MBVax had compiled data from these clinics that demonstrated safety and tumor regressions, and Canadian drug manufacturing standards offered us a layer of protection. Taken as a whole, we felt we had found a safe and reliable version of Coley's Toxins, worth the risk.

Still, we wondered ... how could it be that this potential cure for cancer had eluded doctors for decades? Were we conjuring justifications to rationalize its obscurity? Were we falling into the classic trap of a desperate cancer patient wanting to believe in a miracle cure?

At the next routine follow up, I asked my sarcoma oncologist, Dr. Jacobs, about Coley's Toxins. She gently suggested it belonged to the realm of "alternative" medicine and that there was no proof it worked for sarcoma.

We were impressed she'd even heard about it, given that the toxins had vanished from conventional medicine. Few doctors would have, unless they were researching immunotherapy. Still, Dr. William Coley wasn't an "alternative" doctor. He was the head of the Bone Tumor Service at the first cancer hospital in the country. In addition, most of Dr. Coley's successes had been with sarcomas.

We turned to that second figure—the prominent scientist who had fought to remove Coley's Toxins from the ACS' "quack list." Examining Dr. Old's credentials, we learned he'd uncovered the existence of markers on the surface of immune cells (known as CD antigens). This critical discovery enabled scientists to identify different kinds of immune cells. He'd also discovered key entities in cancer biology, such as p53, a gene mutated in half of all cancers— and TNF, a major group of immune proteins that play a role in killing tumors. These were seminal scientific discoveries.

Dr. Old had been Vice President and Associate Director for Scientific Development at Memorial Sloan Kettering Cancer Center. From 1990 onwards, he was Director of the Ludwig Institute for Cancer Research (LICR), an international non-profit powerhouse with an endowment of $1.2 billion. This organization had the scientific and financial means to conduct its own basic research and clinical trials in cancer immunology, on par with universities and pharmaceutical companies.

Dr. Old's credentials were unassailable. If we could trust anyone to audit our belief in the toxins, it would be him.

Dr. Lloyd Old

It was June 2009, eight months after chemo, 17 months after surgery. I continued to struggle with bouts of fatigue and vacillating neutrophils. I slept 12 hours daily. Aside from occasional trips to the stores, weekly blood tests and daily walks, I spent my energy studying Coley's Toxins and the immune system with Eddy. One positive thing happened: my *lymphocyte* count started to recover. The normal adult range is between 1000 and 4800 lymphocytes per microliter of blood. Chemoradiation had decimated mine to 300. Now, it was up to 700. *Good.* I needed them to keep rising. For Coley's Toxins to work, I was going to need all the immune cells my body could make.

With our growing conviction about the toxins, it was time to update my boss, Professor Lucy Shapiro, on our next step. She'd been a bulwark of encouragement from the day I was diagnosed. I emailed her about our serious intent to go to Tijuana for Coley's Toxins. I also wrote that we'd learned about Dr. Lloyd Old. She immediately replied, saying she knew him personally, promising to inform him of my situation. The very next day, we received a call from Dr. Old.

We were awed by this serendipitous introduction. Dr. Old agreed *now* was the best time to attack the microscopic disease in my body with immunotherapy. Once tumors are detectable, they can contain billions of cells, and are likely to have developed defenses. In that state, they are thought to be more difficult for the immune system to eradicate. Dr. Old's thinking contrasted that of my conventional oncology team, who understandably felt I shouldn't pursue unproven therapy, especially since my scans were clear. Dr. Old's affirmation galvanized the much-needed conviction to stay on the long and lonely road. After all our research, all our efforts, all our questioning and worrying, we felt vindicated.

Dr. Old's interest in Coley's Toxins was deep-rooted and decades-long. Coley's Toxins had inspired him to think about BCG as a possible treatment for cancer, and he began running experiments as far back as 1959.[53] Like Coley's Toxins, BCG is an injection of bacteria. Although alive, the bacteria are weakened and unable to cause disease. In 1991, the FDA finally approved BCG for the treatment of superficial bladder cancer.

Over the decades, Dr. Old persisted in exploring the benefits of Coley's Toxins. His research organization (LICR) began their own clinical trial of the toxins in 2007, shortly before my diagnosis.[54] In a later phone conversation, he'd express his view that Coley's Toxins hadn't been properly evaluated in modern trials—contrary to the other opinions. While fascinated that LICR was running a trial in Germany, I couldn't participate, as I had no evidence of disease.

Eddy and I could scarcely believe what was transpiring. Our journey had begun with gloom and despair. Survival curves declared I was going to die. In desperation, we searched for a miracle cure. It was a long shot, to be sure, but a plausible one. And now, we had direct access to someone who'd personally known Dr. William Coley's late daughter. Someone who had studied the records himself. Someone eminently qualified to speak about the science. And that someone was now advising us and guiding our efforts to beat my cancer.

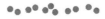

"He-lloooo, Eddy and Rene!" said the voice over the speaker phone. The warmth and kindness it exuded were unmistakable. Huddled over Eddy's cell phone at the kitchen table, we grabbed our pen and paper, absorbing every nugget of wisdom.

Dr. Old agreed that Coley's Toxins was a rational thing to try. But he believed there was a way to increase its chances of working. He said that over the course of history, doctors had difficulties predicting who'd respond to Coley's Toxins. He suspected that patients who had "pre-existing immunity" to their cancer would respond better—in other words, patients whose immune systems had generated the first steps of resistance toward their cancer in the form of T cells and antibodies.

To create this resistance in me, Dr. Old wanted to train my T cells to recognize a protein. That protein would be found only in my cancer, not in normal cells. That protein was called NY-ESO-1.

PART II

Pursuing Immunotherapy

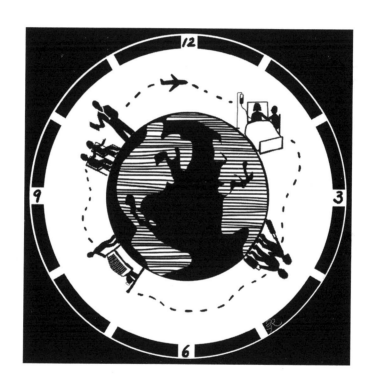

CHAPTER 6

Targeting Cancer with T Cells

AROUND THE TIME WE DISCOVERED Coley's Toxins in 2009, we learned of another synovial sarcoma patient, Heather, who'd achieved stunning success with an experimental immunotherapy. Her husband had shared her story in an online forum for sarcoma patients and caregivers, which Eddy frequented.

Heather was diagnosed two years before I was. Her primary tumor also occurred near her jaw. But what caught my attention was the fact that, like me, she was a scientist at Stanford. Her office was blocks away from my lab. She was treated at Stanford—by the same oncologist who treated me. Of the 320 million inhabitants of the U.S., only 800 people in the entire country are diagnosed with our disease every year. And yet, here were the two of us, diagnosed so close in space and time.

Like me, Heather had surgery, followed by radiation, then chemo. But one year later, the disease invaded her lungs. That same concoction my oncologist had hoped would eradicate the last vestiges of my cancer had failed to prevent Heather's from returning.

This could be me one year from now, I thought to myself. Heather's original tumor was in an easier-to-treat location. Mine was deep and difficult. Moreover, mine had broken apart during surgery and spewed billions of malignant cells.

Heather's travails made a deep impact on me. There were too many uncanny similarities: our workplace, the exceedingly rare disease, the identical treatment. These parallels made the impending return of my cancer more real than any statistic or graph. After one year of debilitating treatment and permanent damage to my bone marrow, would I share her fate?

We were gripped by this palpable foretelling. We read of Heather and her husband's bravery, and how she had endured repeat surgery and chemo. But her sarcoma was relentless, with large tumors rebounding within weeks. Heather's cancer hastened toward the final stages.

Having exhausted conventional therapy, Heather and her husband fought on. Others might have folded. But not them. They abandoned the doomed strategy of more surgery and chemo, instead seeking advice from an experienced sarcoma oncologist at a high volume sarcoma center—the MD Anderson Cancer Center (MDA) in Houston, Texas. The decision proved to be a pivotal one.

Instead of recommending more chemo, the medical oncologist at MDA suggested Heather enroll in an experimental clinical trial. Running the trial was a pioneering immunologist by the name of Steven Rosenberg, M.D., Ph.D., at the National Cancer Institute (NCI) in Bethesda, Maryland. Heather was to receive a form of immunotherapy known as *adoptive T cell therapy*. (I'll refer to it as "adoptive therapy" from here on.)

Adoptive therapy seeks to artificially manufacture what the body naturally creates to repel infections. You'll remember from chapter 4 that, during an infection, the innate immune system is first to deploy. But by day five, dendritic cells activate T cells—those foot soldiers of the adaptive immune system that recognize and attack the invading pathogen. Each activated T cell clones itself into thousands of progeny. Collectively, billions of T cells are made against that single pathogen, reaching as high as 70 percent of all T cells in the body.[1] In this way, the immune system "adapts" to the immediate threat, allocating resources to create a transient but overwhelming force to tame the threat. But tumors fly under the radar, shrouded from the immune system, thwarting the creation of T cells. Adoptive therapy seeks to bypass this problem by manufacturing T cells in the laboratory.

At the NCI, Heather's T cells were extracted from her blood. The cells were genetically modified in the laboratory, enabling them to target her cancer. Once modified, they were cultivated into an army of about 50 billion cells, then re-infused into her body.[2] The T cells instantly went to work and began devouring Heather's tumors.

To our amazement, the modified T cells were able to shrink the diaspora of tumors in Heather's lungs, including large ones that measured seven to eight centimeters wide. A month after the single infusion, most of her 17 tumors had shrunk in half. Two months into treatment, 10 of them had vanished; the largest was now a mere two centimeters. Seven months into treatment, only three tumors remained. The T cells had halted the unrelenting advance of her cancer. Unlike chemo, they continued to suppress

How Heather's T Cells Were Modified to Target Her Cancer

All cells contain DNA. DNA can be thought of as a cell's master program, which controls how the cell grows and acts. It also controls what proteins grow on the surface of the cell. DNA was added to Heather's T cells, causing them to grow unique proteins known as T cell receptors (TCRs) on their surfaces. These TCRs enabled Heather's T cells to lock onto matching proteins found on the surface of her cancer.

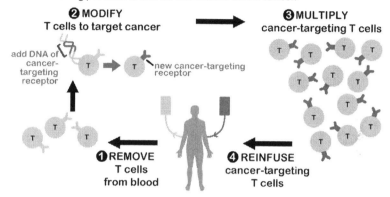

Figure 18: How adoptive therapy manufactures T cells outside the body.

and shrink her tumors months after the single infusion of a living drug. And unlike chemo, she had no side effects beyond the first few days of fever and body aches.

Along with the rest of the online forum, we offered congratulatory posts to Heather and her husband. A short while ago, Heather stood at death's door. Now, almost all of her tumors were gone. Their story beaconed hope for a group that had become accustomed to suffering (caused by the debilitating effects of amputations and chemoradiation) and the overhanging specter of death (advanced sarcoma is incurable).

Decades of failed immunotherapy clinical trials had conditioned oncologists to believe that immunotherapy couldn't shrink large tumors, except in limited cases.[3,4] In contrast, the spectacular tumor shrinkage Heather experienced is vivid proof that the immune system can indeed shrink large and widely disseminated tumors—even those resistant to chemoradiation. Modern medicine was rediscovering what William Coley had shown in the 1890s.

We called Dr. Rosenberg's nurse to see if I'd qualify for the trial but discovered I didn't possess the right "molecular fingerprint." It was frustrating and discouraging not to have access to this powerful therapy. At the same time, Heather's pioneering success solidified our conviction that immunotherapy could liberate me from my dismal fate.

A Precise Target

How had Heather's treatment achieved what conventional chemoradiation couldn't? The answer is in the *exquisite specificity* of T cells. T cells engage in precision, cell-to-cell warfare, attacking *only* cancer cells that express a certain target, known as the *antigen*. Other cells that lack that antigen stay invisible, safe from attack.

The precise targeting allows immunotherapy to destroy cancer cells without harming the rest of the body. In contrast, radiation destroys all cells in the treatment area, and chemotherapy devastates the entire body. The damage done by chemoradiation can cause debilitating side effects and sometimes, it can prove fatal.

For adoptive therapy to work, T cells need a suitable target antigen to home in on. That target must be specific to the cancer, meaning it shouldn't be found on normal cells. If the target is not unique to the cancer (or if too much is found on normal cells) we face the same problem caused by chemo—collateral damage to healthy tissue. In fact, the inflicted harm can be worse. With chemo, the tumor destruction stops when the infusions cease. But with immunotherapy, the long-term memory of T cells can lead to a perpetual attack of healthy organs by T cells, known as *autoimmunity*.

Aside from being unique to cancer, the target antigen must also evoke a robust immune response—meaning that it should lead to the successful attack of tumors by T cells. The immune system is highly complex, and the mere presence of a unique antigen doesn't guarantee the creation of T cells, or that these T cells will attack tumors.

Heather's T cells were modified to target an important antigen known as NY-ESO-1. Discovered by Dr. Old and his colleague in 1997, the

---

Dr. Old's Pursuit of Tumor Antigens

For much of his career, Dr. Old relentlessly pursued the discovery of better tumor antigens for targeting cancer. Among his many distinguished accomplishments, he identified an important group of targets known as *cancer/testis antigens* (or CT antigens). In 1997, the CT antigen NY-ESO-1 was discovered by Dr. Old and his protégé, Yao-Tseng Chen, M.D. at Cornell University.[5] Many current immunotherapy clinical trials target the NY-ESO-1 protein and other CT antigens.

antigen is important because it's found in many cancer types. It is also very specific to tumor cells. It elicits a strong immune response, leading to the spontaneous creation of T cells in many cancer patients. Since NY-ESO-1 proved to be a good target for Heather's synovial sarcoma, perhaps it would work for me? Indeed, Dr. Old would soon use it to go after my cancer.

Dramatic Results and Dangerous Side Effects of Adoptive Therapy

In December 2014, scientists from Memorial Sloan Kettering Cancer Center and Juno Therapeutics, a biotech company based in Seattle, presented data at a conference for oncologists in San Francisco. The data described results of an experimental immunotherapy, given to patients with advanced acute lymphoblastic leukemia (ALL), a type of blood cancer. These patients had failed all treatment, including different combinations of chemo. Most of these patients had been given terminal prognoses of a few months.

The outcome of the trial was astonishing. Of the 27 patients, 24 were put into complete remission.[6] The triumph reverberated across the medical world. The data cracked open the hard shell of fatalism that had long constrained the notion of what can be accomplished against cancer. The oncology community had gotten used to incremental improvements: the prolonging of life by a few months; temporary shrinkage of tumors, only to be followed by rebounding disease; and a paucity of complete regressions. In contrast, the dramatic results of this treatment stood head and shoulders above the historically achievable, putting 9 out of 10 terminal patients into complete remission.

The therapy that achieved this radical result is known as *chimeric antigen receptor (CAR) T-cell therapy*. CAR T-cell therapy is a form of adoptive therapy, similar to what Heather had received. Just as in Heather's case, patients' T cells were extracted, modified to target an antigen found in leukemia, then re-infused. The T cells were able to eradicate large tumors without harming the patients' bodies.

•₀ •° •°₀ •° •°₀

In the case of adoptive therapy for leukemia (ALL), the target antigen was CD19, a protein found on the surface of leukemia cells. But this same protein also abounds on the surface of healthy B cells. B cells are a type of immune cell that produce antibodies—proteins that help our immune system repel infection. So, while CD19-based adoptive therapy can eradicate leukemia, it can also destroy B cells, making patients vulnerable to infection. Fortunately, the collateral damage in this particular scenario can be limited by giving replacement antibodies to patients. But this is not always the case, as can be seen in the following report.

In 2010, a 39-year-old woman named Jane walked into the Surgery Branch of the NCI. Three years earlier, she'd had surgery for colon cancer. The cancerous section of her colon had been removed, but her disease spread to her lungs and liver. Multiple types of chemotherapy failed to stave off the cancer. Death loomed. But Jane came to the NCI for a chance to survive. She was to receive CAR T-cell therapy—a state-of-the-art immunotherapy that few had heard of.

Dr. Steven Rosenberg's team weighed the risks against the benefits. The antigen they planned to use to target Jane's colon cancer was ERBB2, a protein found in many cancers. But there was a slight risk that the antigen could also be present in healthy organs in small amounts. Seeing that her disease was terminal, Jane and her doctors decided that the potential rewards were worth the risks.

Like Heather's, Jane's T cells were extracted, then engineered to target ERBB2. Jane was then infused with 10 billion of her own modified T cells.

Fifteen minutes later, Jane experienced difficulty breathing. Her blood oxygen level plummeted. Forty minutes after infusion, a chest X-ray revealed swelling around her lungs. Doctors rushed her to the ICU and inserted a breathing tube down her throat, ready to connect her to a ventilator should she stop breathing.

In the ICU, Jane's condition worsened. Repeat X-rays showed more swelling in her lungs. Then, her blood pressure began to plummet. The doctors administered drugs to raise it; they pumped her with powerful steroids every six hours, hoping to stem the drop in blood pressure and reduce inflammation. They hooked her up to the ventilator. Despite their efforts, Jane continued to deteriorate. Over the next twelve hours, her heart stopped twice, but her doctors managed to resuscitate her.

Despite the large amounts of drugs, Jane's blood pressure stubbornly faltered. Her heart slowed abnormally. She began to bleed internally, within her digestive track.

After five days in the ICU, Jane's heart stopped pumping.

What had gone wrong? Despite her tumors, Jane had been stable until she received her own innocuous-looking T cells.

An autopsy showed widespread damage to the tiny sacs in her lungs known as alveoli, severely reducing intake of oxygen into her bloodstream. More seriously, her small blood vessels had become leaky, leading to massive internal bleeding. Without proper blood circulation to deliver adequate oxygen and nutrients, muscles all over her body were damaged and her organs failed.

But what was the root cause of the carnage? The answer—as Dr. Rosenberg's team postulated in a case report—was that Jane's CAR T cells had recognized low levels of ERBB2 antigen in the lining of her lungs.[7] Although present in small amounts, it was enough to attract the infused T cells to her lungs. Having found their programmed target, the T cells entered a state of high alert. They began to secrete signals, known as cytokines, to create a state of inflammation, summoning other immune cells as reinforcements. The recruited cells in turn secreted even more cytokines. In an uncontrolled spiral of frenzied signaling, an avalanche of cytokines was born. This *cytokine storm*—as doctors ominously call it—is a tempest of inflammatory signals that can lead to massive internal bleeding and organ failure.

Jane's outcome demonstrates the violence of an untamed immune response—and what can happen if the antigen is not specific enough. Despite the dangers of adoptive therapy, researchers are currently testing ways to make it safer, such as adjusting the dosage of T cells or designing "safety switches" to turn off T cells on demand.

Creating T Cells in the Body with Vaccines

Since the 1960s, cancer immunologists have pursued two major approaches to create T cells against cancer: naturally, within the body using vaccines, and artificially, in the laboratory—i.e. adoptive therapy.[8]

Adoptive therapy is an attractive idea, but there are drawbacks. It's laborious and expensive. T cells are highly sensitive and need to be processed in specialized laboratories (limited to large academic hospitals). How would the treatment be made available to community hospitals around the U.S. and the rest of the world?

Also, unlike the CD19 antigen in blood cancers like leukemia and lymphoma, finding a suitable antigen for solid tumors has proven to be a challenge. If the antigen isn't specific enough, healthy organs are attacked, causing unacceptable side effects. As we've seen in Jane's case, this can lead to major safety risks.

When Dr. Old suggested that we train my T cells against my cancer, we asked what he thought of adoptive therapy. He knew Dr. Rosenberg and strongly supported the idea. He asked us to keep checking with Dr. Rosenberg's team in case a suitable adoptive therapy trial were to become available.

At the same time, Dr. Old believed that the simpler vaccination approach could also generate very large numbers of T cells in my body. In 2001, Dr. Old spearheaded a worldwide collaboration among leading immunologists, establishing the Cancer Vaccine Collaborative (CVC). Hoping to bring a cure to the masses, the CVC has conducted nearly 50 early-phase clinical trials to advance the development of cancer vaccines.[9]

Cancer vaccines are delivered in a manner similar to vaccines for infectious diseases (such as the flu vaccine). Usually, a small amount of tumor antigen is injected into an area of the body—typically into the layer of fat just beneath the skin of the upper arm. Sometimes, the injection is made deeper into muscle. The antigen is usually mixed with an *adjuvant*—a substance that enhances how immune cells react to the antigen. In theory, if done correctly, large numbers of T cells can be generated with this simple injection.

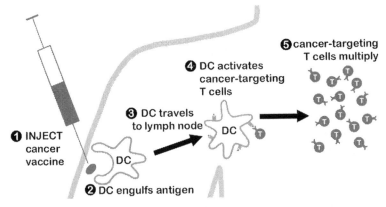

Figure 19: How vaccines create T cells against cancer.

> **How Adjuvants Enhance Immune Responses**
>
> Some adjuvants trap antigen under the skin, slowly releasing it to sustain the "training" of the immune system. Others attract immune cells to the site of the vaccine, increasing the chance of kick-starting the training process. Some adjuvants make dendritic cells (DCs) better able to engulf antigen, migrate to lymph nodes and present the antigen to T cells.

A Clinical Trial for One

Dr. Old wasted no time. First, he wanted to confirm my tumor contained NY-ESO-1. Although found in many synovial sarcoma tumors, not all express it. We sent a sample of my original tumor—that had been removed in 2008—to the New York office of the Ludwig Institute for Cancer Research (LICR). A pathologist tested it and found that almost all of the cells contained high levels of NY-ESO-1.

Having confirmed the presence of NY-ESO-1 antigen in my original tumor, Dr. Old proposed we move forward with an experimental vaccine. At the time, LICR was running an NY-ESO-1 vaccine trial for ovarian cancer. But I didn't qualify for it, and there were no other suitable trials. The only way I could obtain the vaccine was through something called a *single patient protocol*. In essence, we had to set up a clinical trial for one patient—me.

All clinical trials, including single patient protocols, entail a prodigious amount of paperwork. First, we had to find a physician willing to administer the vaccine as part of a research project. Then, safety requirements had to be met at the local (hospital) level, requiring approval from an Institutional Review Board (IRB). Next, the FDA had to be convinced that the treatment was safe—a process that could take months, even years.

Dr. Old suggested we contact an immunologist at Stanford, to see if he'd sponsor my protocol. We followed up on his suggestion, but this burdensome undertaking proved too much to ask. Undaunted, we spoke with a medical oncologist at our local clinic. Although he wasn't as familiar with immunotherapy, he understood what we were trying to achieve. He thought it was reasonable and was willing to go through the process with us. Dr. Old's staff at LICR stood ready to support him with the colossal amount of paperwork needed to get the protocol approved by the FDA.

As my single patient protocol was identical to LICR's ovarian trial, much of the paperwork could be reused, shaving months off the process. The established safety of the ovarian trial would, in theory, lead to swift FDA approval. Given this advantage, we hoped things would move quickly. We were wrong.

The wait for my vaccine dragged on for over half a year. It was early February 2010. Fifteen months had passed since chemo had ended. I was feeling relatively well, except for continuing fatigue. My last scans had been clear. But the survival graphs reminded me that my expiration date drew closer by the day. Eager for news of approval, we watched for every incoming email and listened to every voice message.

Then, one afternoon, Lisa, the nurse with whom we'd been working, called to say that the FDA had approved my protocol. We breathed a sigh of relief. Until now, everything we'd done existed only in our minds or on paper. None of that would stop a rebounding cancer. Now, we could finally get a tangible substance into my body—to wipe out those insurgents of malignancy before they had a chance to regroup.

We had started this process when no tumors were present. Imagine how unnerving the wait would have been if I had actively growing lesions. Later, we met another sarcoma patient who succumbed to her cancer while awaiting approval for her own single-patient protocol. This object lesson taught us the importance of starting things early—especially when putting together experimental therapy.

Lesson learned: When embarking on experimental therapy, expect paperwork and logistical delays of many months, or more.

Receiving the Vaccine

In high spirits, we checked in at the oncology clinic. An assistant ushered us into a treatment room normally used for administering chemo. A few minutes later, nurse Lisa showed up, paper cup in hand. It was half-filled with ice. Sticking out of it were two small syringes, each containing a thick, paste-like substance.

This vaccination was the first of five, to be given three weeks apart. The vaccine consisted of four NY-ESO-1 peptides, which are fragments of the full protein. The peptides were mixed with two powerful adjuvants—PolyIC and Montanide. PolyIC provokes a strong immune response by tricking the body into thinking that a virus has invaded it. Montanide is a thick, water-in-oil adjuvant.

Oil-based adjuvants have long been used in animal vaccines to protect them from infectious diseases. Once injected under the skin, they stay there for years, even decades. The persistency helps keep antigen under the skin—as a slow-release "food source" for dendritic cells. But there is a downside: painful ulcers can develop at the injection site (which is why they are rarely used in humans). Even so, I saw these ulcers as trifling compared to the return of my cancer, and was prepared to endure them should they occur.

Nurse Lisa pushed hard on the syringe to force the thick mixture in. I felt pain as the vaccine squeezed its way under my skin. Within minutes, the underside of my upper arms became red and inflamed. But not much else happened after that. An hour later, I was sent home. That same evening, something exciting happened—I ran a 103-degree fever.

Fevers were classic indicators of immune activation, so I made sure not to suppress it with medicines like Tylenol.

Our excitement that night was just beginning.

It was three in the morning. Everyone in the house was asleep. Suddenly, a commotion stirred us. Bleary eyed, Eddy peeked out the bedroom door. My parents and my brother, Matt, who was also living with us, hustled about in the dark.

"What's going on?" asked Eddy.

"It's an accident … just in front of the house. Mom and I were awakened by the crash," said Matt. "And … there's a car wedged under Rene's SUV."

We dashed out the front door and turned on the driveway lights. It was raining heavily. My trusty SUV, the one I'd had for over a decade, the one with which I'd picked up Eddy from San Diego International Airport the time he flew in for our first date, the one I'd left parallel parked on our street was now straddling the curb, right wheels pushed up into the grass. The rear window was shattered, the frame of the trunk deformed. A red sports sedan was wedged under the rear, its engine pulverized. The impact had hoisted my SUV up onto the sidewalk, ramming it against a utility pole, creating a cleft-palate-like deformation that cut deep into the front of the SUV.

Matt ran to see if the driver, who was standing outside his car, was all right. He looked young, maybe a teenager. Matt called the police. The kid called his mom.

Minutes later, a fire engine, ambulance and two cruisers approached, and the kid took off running. The cops went after him, but weren't able to catch him. Moments later, his mom arrived, exchanged words with the police and left.

After an hour, the rain abated, and we went back to bed.

Eddy and Matt spent the next morning sweeping and picking up thousands of pieces of glass and plastic from the sidewalk. The street had already been cleaned, the red sports sedan towed away. The police had repositioned my poor SUV back onto the road. But it wasn't going anywhere; it was totaled.

The juxtaposition of the dramatic accident with the mild side effects of the vaccine helped imprint the day into memory. Unlike previous chemoradiation, this immunotherapy had virtually no side effects.

●●●●●●●●●●

Later that day, we called Dr. Old, recounting our experience with the vaccine and the fever.

"Oh my, what a vigorous immune system you have!" he said. He was thrilled. To quantify my immune response, he later suggested we send samples of my blood to his team at LICR in Manhattan.

The blood analysis revealed I'd generated large numbers of T cells and antibodies against NY-ESO-1. We now had concrete proof that I possessed T cells capable of targeting my cancer. In theory, as long as the remnant cancer still expressed NY-ESO-1, my T cells would hunt it down.

I completed my fourth vaccination. A few hard lumps had formed on the underside of my upper arms, where Lisa had injected me, but other than that, I had no side effects. The vaccine depots became rock hard over time. Day after day, immune cells swarmed the sites, drawn by the persistent lure of Montanide.

One afternoon, the skin over one of the lumps broke. The accumulation of immune cells had ballooned the site. Yellow pus and blood oozed out. The mobile remnants of the vaccine found its way out, leaving a small crater partially covered by skin. It didn't hurt. It was more of a curiosity. Even so, Dr. Old's team felt I should skip the fifth vaccination—just in case of worsening side effects.

A few years back, as a graduate student, I'd needed antibodies to run experiments. The antibodies came from rabbits. I watched as the poor creatures were injected with antigen, mixed into a similar thick adjuvant paste. In response, they too developed large welts where they were injected, and their immune systems generated the desired antibodies. Now, it was my turn to be the antibody (and T cell) generating machine.

One Advantage of My Vaccine over Adoptive Therapy

Dr. Old had explained the reason for the four peptide fragments in my vaccine: Each person has a set of molecular fingerprints (known as the person's *HLA type*). For some adoptive therapies, the patient's molecular fingerprints limit what her T cells can bind to. Dr. Rosenberg's procedure wouldn't work in me because his modified T cells required a specific fingerprint (which I didn't possess). In contrast, the peptide fragments in Dr. Old's vaccine would generate a spectrum of T cells compatible with all fingerprints. In this way, the vaccine would work for any patient.

I sat in the passenger seat as Eddy drove southbound along the 280 freeway. The smell of our new car was mildly intoxicating. We'd gone to the clinic earlier that morning for a checkup. We'd just passed the Cupertino exit, which led to Apple's headquarters—and the cactus-wielding acupuncturist's office.

Looking out the window, I smiled. It was a perfect California spring day. We were on the way to the same food court where, over two years ago, I'd picked at my food on the day of our first wedding anniversary, unaware of the bulging tumor in my head. But this time, I was going to enjoy my meal.

Things were looking up: My last scans had been clear. It was now almost a year and a half after chemo. I'd received a state-of-the-art vaccine from a leading mind in cancer immunology. Throughout my body, hunter-killer T cells were roving and searching, sensing and interrogating for seeds of malignancy that had overstayed their welcome. Their time was up. The tide was turning. My T cells were going to get them ... or so I hoped.

Advanced Reading: Different Types of Adoptive T Cell Therapies

Adoptive therapies have garnered major publicity due to the dramatic ability to send patients with widespread disease into complete remission. The differences among the three major types can be challenging to understand. But by understanding these differences, patients interested in clinical trials will better comprehend why they may qualify for certain adoptive therapy trials, but not others.

There are different types of T cells, such as helper, killer, memory and suppressor T cells. Killer T cells are the soldier cells that directly attack tumors. Upon contact, a killer T cell punches holes in the membrane of a cancer cell, then pumps it full of poisons.

Adoptive therapy seeks to match up billions of these killer T cells against billions of tumor cells. Once infused, the army of killer T cells roams the body, touching and interrogating neighboring cells. When the lock (receptor) on the surface of a killer T cell matches up with a key (antigen) on a cancer cell, the killer T cell springs into action and delivers death.

There are three main types of adoptive T cell therapies. They have peculiar names: CAR (chimeric antigen receptor), TCR (T cell receptor) and TIL (tumor-infiltrating lymphocytes). We'll just refer to them as CAR, TCR and TIL. Let's consider CARs and TCRs first.

In the case of CARs and TCRs, T cells are extracted from the patient's blood. In the lab, the DNA of the T cells is altered. The altered DNA causes the T cells to generate a certain protein on their surface. This protein is called a *receptor*. Like a lock and key, a receptor (the lock) fits only with a certain antigen (the key) on a neighboring cell. The pairing allows T cells to latch onto their targets.

But how do CARs and TCRs differ? The answer lies in the way their receptors couple with antigens.

For chimeric antigen receptors (CARs) to work, the cancer cells must express a common protein on their surface that the CAR can latch onto.

In contrast, T cell receptors (TCRs) bind to antigen "sitting on" a structure known as the *MHC* (major histocompatibility complex). The MHC is a special molecule that exposes what's within a cell. Proteins found inside the cell are routinely chopped up into smaller fragments by the cell's internal machinery. These fragments are then displayed on the MHC, which advertises them on the surface of the cell. In this way, patrolling T cells are able to discover the proteins within a cancer cell, by using their TCRs to sense the fragments on the MHCs.

Heather's cancer cells were full of NY-ESO-1. But NY-ESO-1 is only found *within* the cell. That is why CARs cannot be used to target internal proteins like NY-ESO-1. Instead, TCRs that match NY-ESO-1 fragments (nested on MHCs) are needed.

In summary, CARs and TCRs are basically different ways a T cell can be modified to match up with a cancer cell, depending on whether the target antigen sits on the surface or lies within.

Tumor-infiltrating lymphocytes (TILs), on the other hand, are T cells found naturally embedded in tumors. Sometimes, the immune system spontaneously creates T cells against a patient's tumors. Although able to target the tumors, these T cells fail to destroy them. Instead, they become prisoners of war, trapped in and around the tumors.

Dr. Steven Rosenberg described the TIL procedure as early as 1986.[10] The procedure involves obtaining a sample of the patient's tumor, most commonly done through surgery. The tumor is then harvested for TILs in the laboratory.

With the TIL approach, there's no need to identify a specific antigen. In fact, a tumor will contain TILs against many different target antigens found within it.

These TILs—regardless of target—are cloned to large numbers, then re-infused into the patient. Once inside the body, they go on to destroy other tumors that express the same targets.

CHAPTER 7

How Tumors Evade the Immune System

IT WAS APRIL 2010, TIME AGAIN for routine scans at Stanford. We were at the clinic to see my oncologist for the results. Dr. Jacobs had retired, and a younger oncologist, Dr. Ganjoo, had taken over her sarcoma patients.

The physician assistant entered first, handing us a copy of the scan reports. In between answering the assistant's standard questions, I glanced at the reports. This time, there were more words than usual.

After examining me, he got up to leave the room, saying Dr. Ganjoo would come in shortly. With Eddy by my side, restive and breathing heavily, we strained to read the words of the lung CT report.

We'd been riding high. The last lung CT scan, taken six months earlier had shown no disease. I'd completed four vaccinations. Dr. Old had verified the presence of tumor-fighting T cells in my blood; we'd been visualizing them destroying micro-tumors before they had a chance to mature. But now, the first line in the CT report read in capital letters, "SUSPICIOUS FOR ... RECURRENCE."

I felt a heaviness on my chest. My heart raced.

The radiologist had found three small masses in my lungs. The lesions were still tiny, each two to three mm. But the growth spurt of one—from barely perceptible six months ago to three mm at present—looked suspicious for cancer. The radiologist urged another scan in three months, as opposed to my usual six.

In addition to the lung lesions, two lymph nodes lit up—one near each axilla (armpit), each about 1.5 cm wide. The radiologist noted these were also suspicious for cancer.

As we pondered the implications of these new masses, Dr. Ganjoo entered. She examined me. She mentioned the lymph nodes, wanting to refer me to Stanford Interventional Radiology for them to be biopsied. But she had little to say about the lung lesions. We wondered why she didn't seem concerned about the lung lesion that was growing—despite the radiologist's warning. (In a post-visit written report, she would merely restate the radiologist's observations.)

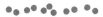

Home from the clinic, we sat in the backyard, attempting to calm our nerves. We sipped blueberry-banana smoothies under the shade of an aluminum gazebo. Eddy had set it up so I could hang out in the open air with visitors who might be sick, as my ability to fight off infections was still compromised.

Seeking guidance, we emailed Dr. Old's team. Their response wasn't what we'd hoped for. None of the ovarian cancer patients who received the same vaccine had responded in the same way. Dr. Old's team took an ethical stance: entertain the possibility that my cancer had returned. They encouraged me to consult my sarcoma oncologist.

We recalled how Heather had received treatment at Stanford when her cancer returned, but how her tumors rebounded within weeks after surgery and chemo. We recalled how she sought a second opinion at MD Anderson, where many more sarcomas are treated. We also recalled how the MD Anderson oncologist referred Heather to the adoptive T cell trial—and how that finally shrunk her tumors. With these in mind, we decided not to have the lymph nodes biopsied at Stanford. Instead, we scrambled to secure a new patient appointment at MD Anderson.

Out-of-state travel would be expensive and tiring. The four-hour flight, car rental and hotel for a week would cost two-to-three thousand dollars. Establishing myself as a patient would take a month or more. We would have to arrange for pathology samples and medical records to be sent over. It would've been far easier to stay at Stanford—a thirty-minute drive from our doorstep. The familiar grounds of our alma mater comforted us. Perhaps there was no need for a second opinion? Even so, we couldn't allow these factors to influence our decision.

A Second Opinion

Houston was a sticky 87 degrees with 80 percent humidity. MD Anderson

Cancer Center occupied several blocks and comprised sprawling buildings 10 to 24 stories high, connected by more than a quarter mile of enclosed overhead walkways that spanned a busy, six-lane Holcombe Avenue. Stopping in at the main cafeteria for lunch, we noticed throngs of cancer patients, some tethered to their IV poles, chemo dripping into their bodies. Every year, over a million outpatient visits, procedures and treatments take place in this virtual city, where malignancy is meticulously managed. But the reason we were here is best summarized by a statement on the center's website: "Our doctors treat more rare cancers in a single day than most physicians see in a lifetime."[1]

At MD Anderson, we saw an experienced sarcoma oncologist, Dr. Robert Benjamin. The first thing he did was to send me for a lymph node biopsy.

I lay on the biopsy table, the interventional radiologist hovering over me. He pressed the ultrasound probe against the clear cool gel slathered over my armpit. I winced as he inserted the needle deep into my armpit. The pain intensified as he repositioned the needle, angling for the right spot. He was having trouble locating the shifty lymph node.

The pain was severe as he sucked out the tissue sample. I breathed again once he retracted the needle. He sent the specimens for analysis. Meanwhile, I had to stay put, just in case he needed to redo the biopsy.

The analysis returned: no cancer was found, nor was there any lymphatic tissue—only muscle and fat. He repeated the procedure on the other side.

Again, no cancer was found. And again, no lymphatic tissue.

Hours had passed. It was a Friday afternoon. We agreed to call it a day. Having failed to extract lymph tissue, the interventional radiologist would later classify the biopsies as "inconclusive."

The following Monday we saw Dr. Benjamin at the clinic. He suspected the lymph nodes were probably a harmless reaction to the NY-ESO-1 vaccine. That they were closely related to the vaccine sites in time and space made this tenable. Also, axillary lymph nodes are not a common site of spread for my disease. Moreover, the interventional radiologist noted that the lymph nodes had shrunk over the few weeks since they were first detected. For these reasons, Dr. Benjamin was willing to bet 10-to-1 they weren't cancer.

In our presence, Dr. Benjamin scrutinized my lung CT images on his workstation. While he agreed the lung lesions *could* be tumors, they were still small, so no immediate treatment was needed. He advised close monitoring, saying a high-resolution CT scan, not an X-ray, should be done every three months. He said I needed to keep doing this for at least *three years* after the last treatment of chemo received, explaining the tendency for sarcomas to suddenly "take off" and sprout tumors, sometimes years later.

Dr. Benjamin's aggressive three-month stance suggested that catching tumors early, while still small, could make a difference in outcomes. Back at Stanford, I'd been getting a CT scan every six months, and there was already talk of decreasing them to once yearly.

Remembering how Bessie Dashiell's sarcoma had consumed her body within three months of amputation, we felt comfortable with Dr. Benjamin's stance. His decades of experience tracking sarcomas carried weight. We felt we'd made the right decision to seek his opinion.

Lesson learned: A second opinion matters, because in medicine, recommendations can differ. Doctors have different philosophies and different levels of experience.

At home in the shade of the backyard gazebo, despite the muted noise of traffic from the busy street out front, we quieted our thoughts.

We were glad that the lymph nodes were unlikely malignant. But the three lung nodules troubled us. It was unlikely that they were a benign reaction to the vaccine. Their random locations suggested a more sinister possibility—the spread of cancer to the lungs. Aside from the spread of cancer, another plausible explanation was "tumor flare," where T cells attack a tumor and cause it to enlarge, and in this case, make a previously indiscernible tumor become visible. But tumor flare would still suggest the presence of cancer in my lungs, and having metastatic cancer would elevate my struggle to a whole new level.

We called Dr. Old to update him on the inconclusive findings.

"We're thinking about you very, very much Rene," he said.

Dr. Old explained that the mere presence of T cells generated by the NY-ESO-1 vaccine may not be enough to destroy cancer, as tumors have ways to defend themselves against the immune system. That cancer could protect itself against immune cells was a relatively new scientific discovery.

It could explain why prior attempts to create T cells against tumors hadn't been more successful. To strip away these defenses, we had two choices. The first was Coley's Toxins, perhaps through the clinical trial in Frankfurt being run by the Ludwig Institute for Cancer Research (LICR). The other was a clinical trial for an immunotherapy known as a *CTLA-4 checkpoint inhibitor*.

Releasing the Brakes of the Immune System

In December of 2014, the *Wall Street Journal Online* published an article titled "Cancer's Super-Survivors: How the Promise of Immunotherapy Is Transforming Oncology." It profiled patients with terminal cancer, alive against all odds. They'd all received a new form of immunotherapy known as a *checkpoint inhibitor*.

One patient, Tom Telford, a New York City high-school teacher, had metastatic melanoma that had spread to his liver and kidneys. Surgery and chemo had failed to stop his cancer. He had less than a year to live. In June 2006, his doctor, Jedd Wolchok, M.D., Ph.D.— one of Dr. Old's protégés—recommended Mr. Telford enroll in a clinical trial at Memorial Sloan Kettering. Mr. Telford was given Yervoy, the checkpoint inhibitor Dr. Old wanted me to have. Made by Bristol-Myers Squibb, it was the first checkpoint inhibitor to be tested in humans.

The protocol called for four infusions of Yervoy, one every three weeks. The doctors hoped to see signs of tumor shrinkage by 12 weeks, but this didn't happen. After Mr. Telford's last infusion, scans showed that the tumors in his liver had enlarged significantly. Dr. Wolchok prepared to deliver the message patients dread: the drug wasn't working; there were no other options.

Despite the tumor growth, Mr. Telford felt well. His night sweats had stopped. His energy had increased. Perplexed, Dr. Wolchok wisely decided to wait another two months to re-scan.

The next scan showed his tumors had shrunk. By May 2007—almost a year after starting Yervoy—all of his tumors had vanished. When the article was published, Mr. Telford had been free of cancer for over seven years and was "still teaching and coaching baseball."[2]

Why did Mr. Telford's tumors gradually disappear after receiving Yervoy? What had the drug done to reverse terminal cancer?

The answer centers around a curiously named protein called CTLA-4.

Found on the surface of T cells, it acts as a "brake." When activated, it causes T cells to shut down, preventing them from multiplying into a tumor-killing army.

The presence of this braking mechanism is not an aberration of nature. It exists for a specific reason: to prevent autoimmunity (when T cells attack antigens found in healthy organs). Up to 23.5 million Americans are affected by autoimmune diseases such as arthritis, type 1 diabetes, multiple sclerosis, inflammatory bowel disease, lupus and psoriasis.[3] The CTLA-4 braking mechanism serves as a failsafe or "checkpoint" that protects against these autoimmune diseases.

You might recall from chapter 4 that dendritic cells (DCs) drive the expansion of T cells, which then attack target antigens. A useful analogy: T cells are cars, and DCs are the drivers. To get T cells to activate and multiply, DCs "step on the accelerator pedal" of T cells. But working against this is the aforementioned CTLA-4 "brake." What good is it to step on the accelerator pedal if the brake is still applied? Yervoy, an infusion of proteins that blocks CTLA-4, effectively "releases the brakes." As a result, Mr. Telford's T cells could "accelerate," that is, they could activate and multiply into a tumor-killing army and attack his tumors.

As the T cells attacked, Mr. Telford's tumors grew, as revealed in a 12-week scan. But these were the early days of checkpoint inhibitor clinical trials: doctors were unaware of the transient "tumor flare" that can occur when immune cells infiltrate tumors, causing them to first swell before shrinking and then vanishing.

Although already documented by Dr. William Coley a century ago, the pattern of initial enlargement, followed by dramatic shrinkage, was an unfamiliar concept to oncologists and researchers accustomed to chemoradiation. With chemoradiation, tumor shrinkage comes quickly. Then, as tumors become resistant, they begin to regrow. Hence, tumor enlargement had been assumed to be a negative sign, associated with advancement of disease. But with immunotherapy, initial enlargement doesn't always imply failure, as modern-day physicians were rediscovering.

Mr. Telford's success foretold the approval of Yervoy in March 2011 for patients with metastatic melanoma. Its approval was an understated-but-critical turning point in the history of immunotherapy. On the surface, only

11 percent of patients experienced tumor shrinkage—a modest figure when compared to chemo.[4] Also, autoimmune side effects were bad enough that 10 percent of patients discontinued Yervoy. Despite the modest response rate and major side effects, Yervoy's true significance lies with the *durability* of tumor shrinkage. The duration of shrinkage achieved by chemo is often measured in mere weeks or months. Yet, a study at the Dana-Farber Cancer Institute in Boston since year 2000 reveals the long-lasting results that immunotherapy can bring about. Of more than 2,000 patients treated with Yervoy, a "vast majority"[5] of patients whose tumors responded were still alive *fifteen years later*.[6]

The ability to confer long-term survival benefit to patients (who'd otherwise die within months) convinced doctors, researchers and drug companies that Yervoy offered an invaluable benefit to some patients. It also convinced them that further efforts to develop immunotherapy were warranted.

Removing Tumor Defenses

Besides CTLA-4, Dr. Old also taught us about PD-1, another immune checkpoint being actively investigated by scientists.

Like CTLA-4, the PD-1 protein is also found on the surface of T cells. PD-1 acts as an "off switch." Tumors can activate this off switch, instructing T cells to shut down.[7] What good is it to create T cells against cancer when tumors can easily neutralize them? This may be one reason why cancer vaccines and older immunotherapies have failed to show greater benefit.

PD-1 inhibitors block the PD-1 protein, thus preventing tumors from sending shutdown signals to T cells. Based on the science, Dr. Old suspected that PD-1 inhibitors would have fewer side effects than CTLA-4 inhibitors. However, clinical trials had just begun in 2010, and it would take years to prove long-term safety. Even so, he said to keep a close eye on PD-1 inhibitors.

In the aforementioned *Wall Street Journal Online* article, some of the patients had received Opdivo, a PD-1 inhibitor. One such patient was David Gobin, a retired policeman from Manchester, Maryland. Lung cancer at 58 was not kind to him. Most of his right lung had to be removed, and he lost 70 pounds amid debilitating radiation and chemo.[8] Two years later, his cancer returned, invading his chest wall. He endured more surgery, chemo and radiation, then a clinical trial of an experimental drug that hinders cells from growing. None of these treatments worked. Doctors told him he had three months to live.[9]

With nothing to lose, Mr. Gobin enrolled in a clinical trial at Johns Hopkins, where he received an infusion of Opdivo every two weeks. Four months into the infusions, Mr. Gobin's tumors began to shrink. He continued to receive Opdivo for two years. Over that period, his tumors kept shrinking and his scans kept improving.

Mr. Gobin then stopped taking Opdivo. Two years later, he was still doing well. His liver tumor had vanished, along with several cancerous lymph nodes. Two lymph nodes still lit up on the scans, but his immune system was preventing them from growing.[10]

"I still have a little cancer. It's still sitting there," said Mr. Gobin, as reported by the *Wall Street Journal*. "It's not doing anything."

Mr. Gobin's success is emblematic of the possibilities of immunotherapy. Unlike chemo, which kills tumors during infusion, immunotherapy seeks to manipulate the patient's own immune system to repel cancer. Even though Mr. Gobin had stopped taking Opdivo, his immune system had become capable of keeping his cancer in check. Not all of the cancer was gone, but he could go on with life, unaffected by his tumors. In short, Mr. Gobin was coexisting with cancer that would've killed him over three years earlier.

In the next four years, clinical trials would show that more patients respond positively to PD-1 inhibitors than CTLA-4 inhibitors. Early trials of very sick patients with melanoma and lung cancer who'd failed chemoradiation showed that 20 to 40 percent experienced tumor shrinkage—a remarkable number for patients who'd otherwise have died.[11,12] In blood cancers like lymphoma, this number would reach an astounding 80 to 90 percent.[13] Patients on PD-1 inhibitors lived longer than if they were given chemotherapy. Most importantly, some like Mr. Telford and Mr. Gobin, remained alive for *many years*—their cancers kept in check by their living immune systems.

Aside from the dramatic efficacy, PD-1 inhibitors cause far fewer side effects than chemo—and fewer than CTLA-4 inhibitors (as Dr. Old had suspected). Eddy and I have known patients who were shocked at the lack of side effects. One patient felt only slight itchiness on her skin, even as all of her chemo-resistant tumors melted away.

In short, PD-1 inhibitors demonstrate superior risk-benefit compared to the existing drugs in use, with the possible bonus of a long-term cure. This has led to swift FDA approvals for melanoma, lung cancer, kidney cancer, bladder cancer and Hodgkin's lymphoma. Meanwhile, a proliferation of PD-1 inhibitor trials for many other cancers is underway.

Are Some Patients Missing Out?

For many decades, it was generally accepted that the immune system couldn't attack tumors.[14] A prevailing train of thought was that cancer cells looked too similar to normal human cells. This inability to distinguish friend from foe was thought to render T cells unable to single out cancer.

Then, as the science advanced, scientists believed that only a few cancers such as melanoma, kidney cancer and bladder cancer were *immunogenic*—meaning they looked "provoking enough" to spark the creation of T cells that can attack tumors.[15] In contrast, lung cancer was thought be one that stayed hidden to the immune system.

In September of 2014, the first PD-1 inhibitor was approved for melanoma.[16] The approval wasn't unexpected, given the acceptance of melanoma as an immunogenic cancer. But just six months later, the FDA approved a PD-1 inhibitor for the treatment of advanced lung cancer (squamous NSCLC), previously thought to be *non*-immunogenic.[17] Seven months later, the FDA expanded approval to include another form of lung cancer (non-squamous NSCLC).[18,19] Doctors and researchers were surprised to learn that immunotherapy could work better than chemo in a cancer once thought unresponsive to the immune system.[20,21]

Lung cancer is the second most common cancer in the U.S., with over 220,000 new cases diagnosed annually. Every year, close to 160,000 patients die from the disease.[22] The PD-1 inhibitor approvals represented a breakthrough for this large community of sufferers, offering longer life and far fewer side effects compared to chemo, with some patients living for years and potentially cured. But in our minds, these approvals represented a more important milestone: they dispelled the once-held misconception that certain cancers (such as lung cancer) couldn't respond to immunotherapy.

The success of PD-1 inhibitors even in "non-immunogenic" cancers begs the crucial question: are patients with other cancers suffering unnecessarily or dying without being given the chance to try PD-1 inhibitors or other immunotherapies? Just because PD-1 inhibitors haven't been approved for their cancers doesn't mean there aren't ways to receive this potentially life-saving drug. Their oncologists can prescribe it off-label, or they can also refer patients to clinical trials. Yet, patients aren't being told about PD-1 inhibitors and continue to believe that chemo is their only option—even when chemo may be less effective and more dangerous.

Mary, the young woman in her thirties (described in the introduction) suffered as a result of this bias. Mary had a highly resistant form of Hodgkin's lymphoma. We met her in 2014, four years after Dr. Old had told us about PD-1. By then, she'd already failed multiple combinations of chemo and radiation—her tumors hadn't responded at all to conventional therapies.

In March 2014, we provided Mary with scientific studies, showing that six years earlier, Japanese researchers had discovered that Hodgkin's lymphoma tumors can neutralize immune cells through the PD-1 off switch.[23] The finding established a solid scientific basis that suggested PD-1 inhibitors would work for Mary's cancer.

We showed her results of a clinical trial of a PD-1 inhibitor in advanced melanoma, proving it could shrink tumors in 40 percent of patients (not just mice).[24] We relayed how the drug was expected to be approved within months due to the dramatic results. Even though there wasn't clinical trial data for Hodgkin's lymphoma, the results from melanoma were likely translatable to her cancer. Unlike chemotherapy, which kills cancer directly, PD-1 inhibitors work on immune cells, in ways not necessarily dependent on the type of cancer.[25]

Finally, we showed Mary the mild side effects of PD-1 inhibitors, compared to chemo. By then, Keytruda (a PD-1 inhibitor) had been approved for melanoma. Mary could receive it off-label.

Mary brought the information to her oncologist, but he didn't offer her off-label PD-1. Instead, he recommended astronomic doses of chemo, which would debilitate her body and obliterate her immune system. To salvage her immune system, she'd be given stem cells from a donor, with the hope that these would repopulate her bone marrow.

We helped Mary research medical studies that showed a stem cell transplant was likely to fail for her highly resistant form of lymphoma.[26,27]

The risk of death from the transplant procedure itself was as high as six percent.[28]

Mary decided to go along with the stem cell transplant—an understandable decision given it was oncologist-recommended. After months of debilitating side effects and solitary confinement (due to an obliterated immune system), Mary got the news. As we'd feared, the stem cell transplant had done nothing for her tumors.

Her oncologist still wouldn't prescribe PD-1. Instead, he offered more chemo—even though all previous combinations of cytotoxics had failed.

Finally, he suggested hospice.

Having exhausted all conventional options, Mary began actively considering immunotherapy clinical trials, all of which were out of state. But the stem cell transplant she'd received excluded her from most of the immunotherapy trials. Also, the large tumor in her chest had become symptomatic. Immunotherapy can take months to work, and delays can occur when enrolling in trials. We feared it was too late for her.

Fortunately for Mary, in December 2014, early data from a phase 1 trial of a PD-1 inhibitor was released at a research conference. The data revealed an *astonishing 87 percent* of Hodgkin's lymphoma patients with similarly chemo-resistant disease experienced tumor shrinkage.[29] The data confirmed the prediction we'd made almost nine months earlier.

Mary's oncologist finally prescribed Opdivo (a PD-1 inhibitor) off-label, in combination with radiation to the large tumor in her chest. Mary experienced no side effects except for some itchy skin. Having gotten used to the debilitating side effects of chemo, Mary feared the treatment wasn't working. But it was.

One moment, Mary was a candidate for hospice. A few weeks after receiving Opdivo, most of her tumors were shrinking. By three months, almost all of her cancer was gone. One year later, Mary went back to work.

Mary was lucky. She'd known about PD-1 and had asked her oncologist about it. The timely release of phase 1 data ultimately convinced her oncologist to prescribe it off-label. Still, why did Mary have to suffer the side effects and risk of death from the stem-cell transplant that required months of hospitalization, when the data had shown it was unlikely to work? Why hadn't her oncologist given her off-label treatment or enrolled her in a clinical trial of the much safer PD-1 inhibitor—a simple outpatient infusion—*before* this drastic measure? He had access to the same supporting studies, which—almost nine months earlier—we'd used to predict the high probability that it would work for Mary with low side effects.

The question is a semi-rhetorical one. It's common practice for oncologists to first exhaust all "proven" therapies such as the stem cell transplant—even though the data shows they may not offer the best balance of efficacy and side effects.

We know many other patients who've passed away, never having been told about PD-1, despite compelling evidence that it can work for their cancer. An example is Harry, my uncle's childhood friend (also mentioned in the introduction). Harry had gastric cancer that had spread to his lungs. Two oncologists told him there was nothing left but to "try some chemo," even though it was unlikely to help. They never mentioned the large, 750-patient PD-1 clinical trial for his cancer.[30] Three months later, Harry died—a travesty, because *two years earlier* a Phase 1 trial had already shown that PD-1 can shrink tumors in 30 percent of patients like Harry.[31]

Missed opportunities like these continue across the country, where untold numbers of cancer patients suffer the debilitating side effects of ineffective traditional therapies, and are then told "there's nothing else."

In 2008, my sarcoma oncologist at Stanford had told me that sarcomas don't respond to immunotherapy. Similarly, other patients who may have heard about immunotherapy are likely still being told today there's no evidence that it works for their cancers. What their oncologists may really mean is that data is still being accrued. But a closer look at early data may actually reveal that immunotherapy holds the best promise of survival.

Why aren't oncologists referring more patients to immunotherapy clinical trials or prescribing PD-1 inhibitors off-label? Some may not know enough about immunotherapy and may not realize the superior risk-benefit it can offer over "proven" chemoradiation. Others may be afraid of lawsuits when they stray from the standard of care. Still others may be waiting for final FDA approval for absolute proof. But patients with advanced cancer don't have the luxury to wait, when the current data may be compelling and the risks low.

Sometimes, other factors such as profit motives may predispose oncologists to stick with prescribing chemo instead of actively exploring immunotherapy alternatives (which might require referring these patients to external doctors or hospitals).

A dear family friend, Mark, in his 70s, was recently diagnosed with stage IV glioblastoma, a fatal brain cancer that took the life of Vice President Joe Biden's son. Even with chemoradiation, Mark's prognosis was dismal.

Before seeing his medical oncologist, I carefully studied the treatment recommendations from *UpToDate.com*—a reputable medical website written by experienced oncologists for other doctors.[32] (Eddy's childhood friend, a gastroenterologist at a large acute care hospital, had suggested the website). Due to Mark's age and weakened condition, the website recommended *against* taking chemo.

Two days later, I went with Mark and his wife, Laura, to see the oncologist. The consultation would be the only one before chemo. The oncologist entered, pulled up the same website on his computer, glanced over the document. "You need chemo and radiation," he said, clearly overlooking the *UpToDate.com* recommendation *against* chemo. He then abruptly rushed off to the men's room. When he returned, he wanted to end the consultation—without telling us when and how to take the chemo pills.

Mark and Laura happened to know a leading neuro-oncologist at MD Anderson who recommended exactly what *UpToDate.com* had suggested— skip chemo, as the benefits weren't worth the side effects. Laura called the oncologist's office to cancel chemo. The next day, the oncologist called back.

"Your husband is going to die if he doesn't take chemo," said the oncologist. Bellicose, he tried to pressure gentle Laura into changing her mind. I'd pre-warned her not to be intimidated. I'd explained that medical oncologists are the only doctors in the U.S. allowed to profit from selling chemo drugs directly to patients—and that this profit often forms the majority of practice revenues, which can lead to a conflict of interest, resulting in the over-prescription of chemo.[33]

A study done by researchers at Dartmouth Medical School reveals the influence of profits on the decision of whether or not to prescribe chemo. At private oncology practices, profits from chemo are directly linked to the prescribing physician's income. But at larger clinics or hospitals (such as Stanford or MD Anderson), the prescribing physician may be paid a fixed salary. In 2005, the Medicare Modernization Act reduced chemotherapy-related reimbursements to oncologists. As a result, oncologists at private practices were 20 percent less likely to prescribe chemo to patients in their last 14 days of life. Oncologists at hospitals didn't reduce their prescriptions. In other words, before the 2005 changes were enacted, some private oncologists may have been over-prescribing chemo to juice profits. Chemo wouldn't help these already dying patients. Rather, it would hurt their quality of life. When there was less profit to be made, the oncologists withheld chemo, focusing on the patients' quality of life.[34]

At age 97, my own grandmother was prescribed chemo and radiation for her localized rectal cancer that was causing her pain and discomfort. The oncologist who saw her had a captive audience of very old patients from a senior day care center. When I asked him how these elderly patients fared after taking the chemo pills, he said "I think they do fine, because I never see them again."

As she had dementia, my grandmother couldn't weigh the risks and benefits. The family decided to reject chemoradiation, especially since they were non-curative, and the side effects could devastate her quality of life. (We'd met a patient with the same cancer who'd had radiation to his rectum. He couldn't sit down because of the radiation-induced pain.) Instead of chemoradiation, we convinced a surgeon to operate. It gave my grandmother two more years of pain-free life. She died at the age of 99 with no evidence of cancer in her body.

My grandmother's case was reminiscent of the Dartmouth study, where monetary factors may creep into play and lead to the "automatic" dispensing of chemoradiation even though it may not be in the best interest of the patient.

Lesson learned: Even if PD-1 inhibitors haven't been approved for a given cancer, their use may already be justified by compelling early data and minimal side effects. Not all oncologists may be aware of these advantages over conventional therapy. Some may continue prescribing ineffective drugs (a decision which may be influenced by profit motives). Until the FDA approves PD-1 for that cancer, the onus is on the patient to do their own research, seek off-label therapy or to enroll in clinical trials.

•ₒ •° •°ₒ •° •°

It was the summer of 2010. Having learned about CTLA-4 and PD-1 from Dr. Old, Eddy and I began to pay greater attention to the ways tumors evade the immune system. We pored over scientific papers, and began to think not only about creating T cells to target my cancer, but also of practical ways to remove tumor defenses.

We also wondered how Coley's Toxins fit into the picture. Dr. Coley didn't have access to these powerful new checkpoint inhibitors. Yet, he was able to cure some patients. Did Coley's Toxins somehow create tumor-killing T cells, and at the same time remove tumor defenses?

As we pondered these thoughts, we felt a growing urgency to take action against my cancer's defenses. Two months earlier—just after my last vaccine shot—suspicious lymph nodes had appeared in my axilla, along with the three lung lesions. What if these lung lesions signified metastatic cancer? What if my vaccine alone wasn't enough?

It was time for another CT scan.

Three days later, I received the results. The first line of the report stated that one of the lymph nodes had decreased in size. *Great! Dr. Benjamin was right: the armpit lymph nodes were probably just a reaction to the vaccine.*

But the second line stated something curious—two of the lung lesions had now become hollow.

The radiologist noted that the hollowing-out could mean progression of my cancer. When tumors advance, they usually just enlarge. But in rare cases, tumors may hollow out.

We called Dr. Old to update him. He wondered if the hollowing-out meant that my T cells were attacking cancer in my lungs. It seemed logical. But there wasn't a practical way to verify the theory.

The conversation veered toward the pressing task: what could I do to strip away the defenses around my cancer and help my vaccine-generated T cells work better?

Dr. Old was eager for me to receive Yervoy in the near future. During the conversation, he was interrupted by another caller. When he returned, he said the caller was Dr. Jedd Wolchok, his protégé, who led the Yervoy clinical trial that Mr. Telford was part of. As Yervoy was not yet approved, the only way I could get it was through a clinical trial. But without measurable tumors, I wouldn't qualify.

There were hints of impending approval, perhaps within a year, after which I could get Yervoy off-label. But without confirmed cancer, few doctors would be willing to administer it for fear that the potential autoimmune side effects would outweigh the unmeasurable benefit. Furthermore, insurance wouldn't cover it, and many hospitals charge a 400 percent markup. Later, we learned that each infusion of Yervoy costs $30,000 wholesale—$150,000 after markup. A starter course requires four infusions, which costs a prohibitive $600,000.

PD-1 was even further behind CTLA-4 in clinical trials. Approval wouldn't come until 2014—four years later. There was no way we were going to sit around and wait. If these things in my lungs were tumors, I probably would've succumbed to my cancer by the time it was approved.

Coley's Toxins and the Fearsome Bodyguards of Tumors

Dr. Old had taught us that immune checkpoints like CTLA-4 and PD-1 are ways by which tumors can evade the immune system. But he also described other mechanisms, one of which is how tumors recruit and surround themselves with a certain ally. This ally is a fearsome agent of the immune system, known as the *regulatory T cell*, or *Treg* (pronounced as tee-reg).

Tregs are a special type of T cell. Unlike their cousins—the *helper T cells* and *killer T cells* that destroy tumors—Tregs play a crucial role in preventing autoimmune diseases. In organs such as the lung or intestines, constant exposure to particles from the air or from food may sensitize the immune system against foreign antigens. The resulting attack by T cells may lead to allergies and chronic inflammation, causing damage to the lung and gut. Tregs suppress immune responses against these antigens, thus minimizing damage to these organs.

Scientists have long known that tumors can surround themselves with Tregs, and that the presence of Tregs is associated with poor prognosis. Tumors secrete proteins that attract Tregs, recruiting them into their fold.[35] The Tregs implant themselves within a tumor and become its bodyguards—killing other T cells that attempt to approach the tumor. Tregs also maim dendritic cells, ripping key proteins off their surface to render them incapable of activating T cell armies.[36] These are some ways that tumors subvert Tregs to their advantage.

For many years, scientists have tried to find ways to eliminate or reduce Tregs. One method is to use low doses of cyclophosphamide, an inexpensive chemo drug. Some immunotherapy clinical trials incorporate it to disarm Tregs.[37] Also, CTLA-4 inhibitors like Yervoy are thought to abolish the suppressive effects of Tregs.[38] But most intriguing was Dr. Old's hypothesis that Coley's Toxins may work by reducing Tregs.

By now, we'd scoped out options for getting Coley's Toxins in Tijuana, Mexico. The Canadian company, MBVax, had been shipping their version of Coley's Toxins to Tijuana clinics. Dr. Old himself had tested their formulation and said it was one of the most potent he'd ever seen.

To us, the choice was clear. Despite the impending approval of Yervoy, not a single therapy in history could claim what Coley's Toxins had achieved—complete remissions in terminal sarcoma patients that lasted for decades.

"Did you get a hold of Elke Jäger?" asked Dr. Old. He'd earlier referred us to one of his colleagues in Germany, Elke Jäger, M.D., Ph.D., who was running LICR's clinical trial of Coley's Toxins in Frankfurt.

"Yes, we have," replied Eddy. We had hoped to glean tips from Dr. Jäger on what to expect were I to receive the toxins in Mexico. Dr. Jäger mentioned the importance of fevers—how they correlated with tumor shrinkage in a patient. Unfortunately, the German FDA prohibited her from increasing the dosage once patients achieved their first fever. The restriction severely limited the effectiveness of the therapy, as patients quickly become tolerant to capped doses. We realized then that the Frankfurt trial wasn't the best option for me.

Dr. Old had a theory: When Coley's Toxins is injected into a tumor, the transient inflammation alters the environment within that tumor, changing it from one that protects tumors into one that allows tumors to be attacked by immune cells. He further explained that Coley's Toxins contains important compounds being tested in clinical trials. These compounds activate the body's innate ability to repel bacteria, tricking it into thinking that an active infection is present. Dr. Old theorized that this trickery may lead to the reduction of Tregs—those fearsome bodyguards of tumors.

"When the body thinks it has an infection, it doesn't need Tregs," said Dr. Old. "It needs one thing—to get rid of that infection. I think that's how Coley's may work: by decreasing the immunosuppressive part of immunity."

⁂

We'd studied Coley's for over a year, talking with researchers from New

York, Canada and Germany. We'd even spoken with a patient who'd received it 14 years ago and was still alive, cured of metastatic melanoma. We'd done our research on how to manage the side effects. It was time to take action and get the toxins into my body.

Before we headed across the border, Dr. Old called again, asking how I felt about getting Coley's.

"I'm so excited I'm *finally* going to get it!" I replied. How could I not be? I was about to undergo a century-old therapy documented to *cure* some patients. Even if it didn't cure me, I hoped it would strengthen the effects of my NY-ESO-1 vaccine.

Dr. Old was glad at my enthusiasm and offered me tender words of encouragement. "You've done all your research, Rene … What's the sense of doing one's research, if one doesn't live to one's conclusions?"

How CTLA-4 Inhibitors Work

How does Yervoy, a CTLA-4 inhibitor, "release the immune system's brakes"? Recall that during the T cell training process, dendritic cells (DCs) extend bits of tumor antigen on their arms, waiting to match with T cells that recognize the antigen and to multiply them into a tumor-killing army.

However, if these matched T cells have CTLA-4 on their surface, the DC will "apply the brakes," shutting down the T cell, instead of activating it.

Yervoy is an infusion of antibodies (proteins that stick to a specific target). When infused into Mr. Telford, the antibodies blocked the CTLA-4 proteins on his T cells. Once blocked, the T cells' brakes couldn't be applied. The antibodies had effectively "released the brakes," allowing the T cells to activate and multiply. The following diagram illustrates the process:

❶ CTLA-4 "brake"

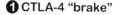

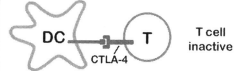

❷ CTLA-4 antibody blocks CTLA-4 "brake"

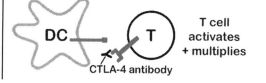

Figure 20:
Abbreviations:
DC=Dendritic cell, T=T cell

(1) During antigen-presentation, the CTLA-4 "brake" prevents activation of T cell.

(2) CTLA-4 antibody blocks CTLA-4, preventing brake from engaging. T cell activates and multiplies.

Yervoy comes with a long list of possible side effects. Unlike chemo, which directly damages the body, Yervoy causes side effects by temporarily disabling that failsafe against autoimmunity. While this enables T cells to be created against tumors, it also allows the inadvertent expansion of T cells against healthy organs.

The most common side effect is diarrhea, which occurs in a third of patients. If not dealt with swiftly, it can progress to inflammation or even perforation of the intestines. Thankfully, more serious autoimmune side effects, such as attack on the thyroid gland, pituitary gland or intestines, occur in less than 10 percent of patients and can be managed with corticosteroids.

Scientists still haven't deciphered all the ways by which CTLA-4 inhibitors work.[39] "Releasing the brakes" of T cells is thought to be one of the main mechanisms. Abolishing the suppressive effects of Tregs is another. But the immense complexity and interplay between immune cells makes it likely that there are still other mechanisms behind CTLA-4 inhibitors' anticancer properties.

How PD-1 inhibitors work

After tumor-targeting T cells are created, they need to contact tumor cells in order to kill them. However, many tumors have a protein found on their surface, known as PD-L1. This protein binds to PD-1 proteins on invading T cells, thus sending the "shutdown" signal to the T cells.[40]

Many companies are developing their own antibodies that block PD-1 on T cells, such as Keytruda by Merck and Opdivo by Bristol-Myers Squibb. Others are developing antibodies that block PD-L1 proteins on the surface of tumor cells. Either strategy interrupts the shutdown signal, as shown in the following diagram:

❶ T cell "shut down" switch

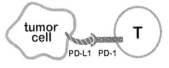

❷ PD-L1 or PD-1 antibody blocks T cell "shut down" switch

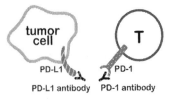

Figure 21:
Abbreviation: T=T cell

(1) Tumor cell activates T cell "off switch" when PD-L1 (on tumor) binds to PD-1 (on T cell).

(2) Both PD-1 or PD-L1 blocking antibodies can interrupt shutdown signal.

PD-1 inhibitors have fewer side effects than CTLA-4 inhibitors. This can be understood when you consider the different ways these respective inhibitors work.

As we have seen earlier, CTLA-4 inhibitors ensure tumor-killing T cells are generated in the first place (by disabling the failsafe against autoimmunity). But the temporary disabling may allow the creation of T cells against both tumors and healthy organs, leading to various autoimmune side-effects.

In contrast, PD-1 inhibitors prevent tumors from neutralizing T cells. There is less risk of autoimmunity if these T cells aren't already directed against healthy organs.

Like CTLA-4, scientists have not fully deciphered all of the ways by which PD-1 works. For example, they are still trying to understand why some tumors that lack PD-L1 can still respond to PD-1 inhibitors. In theory, tumors that lack PD-L1 cannot activate the PD-1 off switch on T cells. Without a defense mechanism to disrupt, PD-1 inhibitors should not confer benefit. But this isn't always the case, and the unexpected benefit suggests the presence of other mechanisms not yet understood.[41]

Other Checkpoint inhibitors and Immune Activators

PD-1 and CTLA-4 inhibitors were the first checkpoint inhibitors to be commercialized. But many other antibodies are being actively researched. They have esoteric names such as OX40, ICOS, 4-1BB, IDO, KIR, LAG3 and TIM-3. Some of these antibodies are checkpoint inhibitors, which prevent tumors from evading the immune system. Others directly activate immune cells to attack tumors. Scientists and drug companies are actively studying the effects of these antibodies, eager to see if they can further unleash the immune system against cancer.

When Dr. Old told us about immune checkpoints in 2010, there weren't any suitable clinical trials for me. But in recent years, the unprecedented success of CTLA-4 and PD-1 inhibitors have led to copious trials. Patients today who don't qualify for PD-1, CTLA-4 or adoptive T cell therapy trials may consider participating in trials of these other antibodies.

CHAPTER 8

Activating the Immune System with Coley's Toxins

San Diego had been home for almost 10 years—during my undergraduate and graduate school days. Even though Tijuana was just a hop away, I'd never once crossed the border.

Seen as a family-friendly destination in the 1960s, then as an international art hotspot in the '90s, Tijuana had become known as a party-town—a place for spring break jaunts and debauchery. In recent years, lawlessness, drug-related violence and high-profile stories of Americans kidnapped for ransom featured in the news. You couldn't fault us for being apprehensive about going there. But more concerning were the clinics: Did they have experience administering Coley's Toxins? Were the doctors and nurses well-trained? Were there adequate emergency services?

We found two clinics that offered Coley Fluid—the formulation of Coley's Toxins made by the Canadian company MBVax. Both were located in Playas de Tijuana: a community nestled just across the southwestern tip of the U.S. and home to many medical and dental clinics.

We visited one of the clinics. Touring the hospital where it was based, we observed corridors of locked patient rooms—about 50 rooms distributed over five floors—clearly uninhabited. We saw a single patient, there for the Gerson juice program, which the clinic administered along with Coley's. Only one physician cared for the clinic's patients—not a good sign. But the deal-breaker was the clinic director's unwillingness to administer Coley Fluid by intravenous drip (IV). The MBVax instructions called for IV infusions, but he insisted that injecting under the skin worked just as well. He had no data to back up his claim. (The MBVax protocol recommended against subcutaneous injections, as the toxins get trapped under the skin and cause a prolonged redness and irritation.)

Having ruled out that clinic, we decided to go with the Issels Treatment Center. It was based in a small, modern hospital called Oasis of Hope. They agreed to administer Coley Fluid by IV.

On a sleepy Sunday afternoon in early August 2010, we waited curbside at San Diego International Airport for the hospital van. We had two suitcases, one brimming with medical supplies, enough to keep my PICC (peripherally inserted central catheter) line—that vital entry port into my bloodstream—sterile for two months. In addition, I had a six-foot-long heating pad, folded in half, wrapped in clear plastic: my secret weapon for reducing side effects during treatment. Eddy had brought along his guitar in case the month-long stay became too boring. He also had his trusty beach chair—he'd been sleeping sitting upright in it for over a year already to circumvent severe sleep apnea, with which he was diagnosed at the end of 2008.

The van arrived late as traffic into the U.S. was heavy. We loaded up and were finally on our way. The border crossing was a sea of cars and pedestrians. But once we cleared customs, southbound travel into Mexico was fluid. Not so for the opposite direction: a stagnant river of cars snaked for a distance.

The van passed through slum areas and shantytowns, with abodes made of corrugated metal. Traveling westbound toward the Pacific Ocean, it cruised onto Highway 1D, that ran parallel to a razor-sharp barbed-wire fence that marked the border between Mexico and the U.S. We crested a hill. A short while later, the quaint seaside community of Playas de Tijuana materialized.

•。•• •°。 •• •。

The van arrived at the Oasis of Hope. It was three stories high, with a surrounding wall and sentry. Directly behind was a sleek 15-story apartment complex. Across the street to the west was the 3000-car parking lot for the Bullring by the Sea—a stadium that hosted bullfights, boxing matches, concerts and other large events.

As it was Sunday, the streets were deserted. We unloaded our things and checked into the clinic. Occupying the top floor, the Issels Treatment Center rented eight rooms from the hospital and hired its own doctors and nurses. The main therapies offered were cancer vaccines and immunotherapies. In addition, patients of Issels partook in a modified Gerson juice program provided by the hospital.

But I was there for only one thing—Coley Fluid. The Issels center had long incorporated Coley's Toxins into their program, injecting it under the skin once a week to boost the immune system. But I would be the first ever to receive it by IV, three times weekly.

The room they assigned me faced the ocean. Sliding open the vinyl vertical blinds, we discovered a glass window wall that offered a stunning view. We gazed out to take in the scenery. The sign above the six-arched entrance of the Bullring parking lot read, BIENVENIDOS.

To the left of the lot was a pub. And in the background, just below the horizon, we made out a sliver of the Pacific Ocean. The room itself was comfortable. It had two single beds, an armchair, a small round table that sat two, a wheeled hospital table and its own bathroom.

"Knock, knock!"

We turned around. A petite woman with short blond hair, probably in her early forties, beamed a beautiful smile.

"Hello there, I just want to introduce myself ... my name's Lorraine. I'm your neighbor. Welcome!"

Lorraine was from South Africa. She had arrived a little earlier with her mother, Adrienne. They had braved a forty-hour journey across the Atlantic, finally arriving in Tijuana International Airport. The cancer in her lungs made breathing difficult, causing her to pause and gulp air every few seconds. She'd learned of Issels only from the center's website. At times, during the journey, she'd wondered if the center really existed. She'd heard of gullible patients being ripped off by fake websites. But Lorraine was determined to survive her metastatic breast cancer, which had spread with a vengeance soon after radiation therapy. Her doctors back home had told her they had nothing else for her.

Later at dinner, and in the coming week, we met other cancer patients and their caregivers: Mara, a card dealer from Las Vegas, who had metastatic breast cancer, had come with her husband. Tim, a teenager from South Africa with osteosarcoma of the jaw, had been brought here by his mother. Fatima, a surgeon from Jordan, had metastatic thyroid cancer and was here with her husband, also a physician. Sarah, an insurance agent from Los Angeles, had advanced gastric cancer and was deteriorating quickly. She was accompanied by her father, a petite man in his 80s with a full head of white hair. Amir, a man in his 60s was here from Detroit with his adult son. And then there was Jimmy, the fun-loving gym owner from Tennessee, his wife by his side. Jimmy couldn't sit down at the dinner table. The radiation he'd received for his colorectal cancer had damaged his tailbone, causing spasms of pain that prevented him from sitting. Despite his pain, he had a fighting spirit, a can-do attitude and maintained a jovial sense of humor.

Each of these warriors had come for a chance to beat their advanced cancer. Most had endured surgeries, radiation and chemo. Many had painful symptoms from growing tumors or from chemoradiation. All were in the late stages of disease. A few of them had weeks to live.

I was the only one there with no concrete evidence of disease in my body.

•ₒ •• ₒ•ₒ ₒ• •ₒ

It was six-thirty, Monday morning and still dark outside. The loud rap on the door woke us. Groggy and fumbling in the dark, Eddy flipped on the lights and let the phlebotomist in. Prim and well-dressed, wearing a tie under his white coat, he was here to draw tubes of my blood. These samples would determine if I was fit to begin treatment that morning.

After he left, I lingered in bed a while longer, then descended to the ground floor dining hall with Eddy. We joined some of our new friends we'd met the day before.

"Eat a hearty breakfast," said Eddy, reminding me I'd probably have to miss lunch. From what we'd studied, once infused with Coley's Toxins, I wouldn't be able to eat again until the fever rose and fell. We had studied the MBVax protocol and figured it might take six to eight hours from the time the IV began.

Breakfast was a generous buffet of pancakes, lots of fresh fruit, scrambled eggs and oatmeal. The hospital followed a semi-vegetarian diet—eggs at breakfast and a limited amount of chicken or fish once daily. We ate our fill then rushed back to the room to meet the doctors.

Making their Monday morning rounds, Dr. Jimenez, along with his three assistants, finally got to my room. After an interview and physical exam, he declared me ready for treatment. Except for my low neutrophil count—a chronic side effect of chemotherapy—my blood work had come back normal.

Dr. Jimenez said a technician would bring the Coley Fluid, and a nurse would infuse it.

My First Infusion of Coley Fluid

Before arriving, Eddy had spoken with Ilse Marie Issels, the owner of the clinic. Her late husband, Josef Issels, M.D., a German immigrant, had founded the center. Mrs. Issels had agreed to have the technician perform the dilutions of Coley Fluid in our presence. We had requested this peculiar arrangement out of an abundance of caution.

Ever since experiencing the malfunction of a chemo infusion pump at Stanford in 2008, we had become extra cautious and were always on the lookout for potential medical mishaps. The Issels center was accustomed to performing subcutaneous injections of the toxins. When injected under the skin, a much larger amount is needed to elicit an immune response. But I was to receive it by IV—straight into my blood, where a tiny dose—one half of a microliter—could provoke a violent reaction. That the clinic had never performed IV infusions of Coley Fluid was a potential mishap in the making. A mistake during the dilution process could result in too strong a dose, and the overwhelming immune reaction could kill me—similar to what happens during septic shock.

At around 11:00 a.m., the friendly technician entered. We exchanged pleasantries and discussed the dilution strategy, which she seemed glad to do. She siphoned a tiny volume of red Coley Fluid from a vial. She then drew sterile saline into the syringe, diluting the toxins by a factor of ten. She repeated the process again, further diluting by another factor of ten, making the toxins a hundred times less potent. We watched closely, excited that after over a year of studying it, the toxins were about to course through my veins.

While performing the dilution, the technician accidentally pricked herself. Blood oozed from her finger.

She wiped the blood off and changed her glove. But then she resumed the dilution *with the contaminated needle*. The contents of that needle were going to be infused into me. No way would we let that happen.

My experience with "Red Death"—speeding into my body faster than it should have during my first round of chemo—had taught me to speak up. I respectfully requested that she restart with a fresh syringe. If I hadn't caught this breach, I could have been exposed to blood-borne diseases, such as Hepatitis or HIV.

Lesson learned: When something of concern happens in the hospital, speak up, ask questions—even if it risks offending. Medical mistakes are a leading cause of death in the U.S.[1] (Although this experience happened in Mexico, I'd already encountered malfunctioning machinery at Stanford. In the coming chapters, I experience my fair share of human error in another U.S. hospital.)

The incident greatly disturbed us. We hadn't come all the way to have basic mistakes jeopardize my safety. It made us even more vigilant.

The dilution proceeded without further problems. By the time she was done, it was close to 1 p.m.—good thing Eddy had warned me to eat a big breakfast. The technician handed the syringe to a nurse, who injected the Coley Fluid into a bag of sterile saline. As the nurse hooked up the bag to my PICC line, Eddy turned up the room thermostat to 80°F and began warming up the far-infrared heating pad that he'd spread out on my bed.[2]

I lay on the heating pad. Eddy helped me put on thick socks, gloves and a heavy woolen beanie. He then bundled me up with two blankets. Our strategy was to pre-warm my body to minimize imminent chills.

The Coley Fluid trickled through my PICC line into my bloodstream over the next 50 minutes. I felt nothing. The nurses checked in every hour to take my vitals.

Eddy began recording my vitals every 15 minutes—temperature, pulse, oxygen and blood pressure. We'd brought our own measuring devices. Aside from documenting my reaction for Dr. Old, we wanted to be extra safe, as again, this was the first time an IV infusion of Coley's Toxins had ever been done at Issels.

We continued watching for signs of chills that we'd read about from Dr. Coley's cases. Eddy added a third blanket. With the room heater going, the heating pad on medium and my body triple-bundled-up, I felt stifled and hot.

About an hour-and-a-half into the infusion, the chills began.

A sensation like a cool breeze flowed down my back and flitted from left to right. It began to intensify, a coldness radiating outwards from the center of my back. My abdomen and back muscles twitched, and I shivered.

"I'm getting the chills!" I said.

"How do you feel?"

"Umm … OK, I guess. A bit c-c-cold …" Another shiver made my teeth chatter.

"Let me crank up the heat."

Eddy set the heat pad on maximum. Within minutes, the chills vanished, leaving my body calmly simmering. We were delighted they could be tamed with predictability, just as the MBVax protocol had advised.

"Temperature's 101. Oxygen good at 99. Pulse at 100," said Eddy, reporting my vitals. "Looks like you're getting a fever!"

"Yay," I said weakly. I was starting to feel tired and hot—very hot.

Far-infrared heating pads aren't the same as conductive electric pads found in drug stores. Far-infrared radiation—also a form of invisible light from the sun—delivers heat deeper into the body. The pad itself doesn't reach high temperatures, making it safer when used in bed.

The Benefits of Fever

According to the observations of Dr. Coley and his colleagues, fever was the main measure of a "strong" immune response.[3] Patients who experienced fevers between 102-105°F were more likely to see tumors regress or achieve cures. In contrast, patients who didn't have fevers, or whose peak temperatures were lower, seemed to not benefit.

In essence, Coley's Toxins fakes a bacterial infection. Bacterial cells—including dead ones—possess certain molecules on their surface. These molecules exhibit patterns recognized by the innate immune system. Scientists believe that the innate immune system developed the ability to recognize these patterns millions of years ago.[4] When injected, this ancient recognition provokes a powerful, sometimes violent response, triggering myriad processes that send immune cells into a frenzy. These cells release cytokines (inflammatory proteins) to call for reinforcements, while raising the body's internal thermostat.[5]

In response to the thermostat change, the body produces heat, leading to fever. If the need is urgent, it tries to produce heat faster. One way it creates heat is by rapidly contracting and relaxing muscles, resulting in uncontrollable shivering commonly known as the chills. Fatigue sets in as energy is diverted to generate heat and to support immune activity.

The resulting fever stimulates further release of neutrophils from the bone marrow. Billions of fresh neutrophils enter the bloodstream, ready to attack the bacteria. Upon arriving at the site of danger, fever further augments the neutrophils' ability to spray destructive chemicals, such as hydrogen peroxide, at the bacteria.[6]

The effect of fever on the cells of the innate immune system has been best studied in natural killer (NK) cells.[7] Unlike T cells, NK cells can kill cancer without needing to be first activated. There aren't enough NK cells in our body to eradicate cancer outright, but evidence shows that NK cells can slow down cancer, thus extending life.[8] Recall from chapter 4 that NK cells can identify some cancer cells by detecting the absence of a certain protein. In addition to this mode of detection, fever helps NK cells better identify cancer by causing tumor cells to express other special proteins on their surfaces.[9,10] Known as *heat shock proteins*, these proteins stimulate NK cells, causing them to vigorously attack the cancer.

In addition to strengthening the activity of neutrophils and NK cells which belong to the innate immune system, fever also helps the adaptive immune response. First, it increases the ability of dendritic cells to engulf and consume bacteria. Next, it improves the capacity of dendritic cells to present antigen to T cells, thereby helping them train T cell armies. Finally, it also makes these T cells much more able to kill their target.[11]

Clearly, fever is a crucial response by the human body to support immune activity when it needs to repel an infection.

The Dangers of Suppressing Fever

For thousands of years, antipyretics (fever-reducing medicines such as

Tylenol and aspirin) have been used to reduce pain and discomfort for acute conditions such as the flu, gout, dental surgery, even childbirth, or chronic diseases such as arthritis and cancer.[12,13]

There are valid reasons to quell fevers, especially in patients at risk for brain damage.[14] But reducing temporary pain and discomfort may not always be the best thing for otherwise healthy patients. For example, the aches we experience during the flu are caused when immune cells secrete cytokines to call for reinforcements. By suppressing the pain, we are also suppressing these cytokines, thus dampening our immune system's response. This can prolong the flu.[15]

In many cases, the prolonged healing may only be an inconvenience. But in some cases, it can lead to secondary diseases or even death. For example, a Japanese study of children with bacterial infections showed that antipyretics led to more cases of subsequent pneumonia. The researchers suggested that antipyretics had weakened the children's immune systems, predisposing them to a worsening of their illness.[16] Another study published in 2014 by the Royal Society of London estimates that antipyretics may result in an extra 700 flu-related deaths within the U.S.[17]

Awareness of the importance of fever is increasing. Concerned about the negative effects of antipyretics, researchers at the University of Miami performed a clinical trial to objectively evaluate the impact of their use in critically ill trauma patients.[18] Over a nine-month period, they monitored patients admitted to the Trauma Intensive Care Unit, which would include victims of car accidents, life-threatening falls, burns, blasts, gun shots wounds, etc. In random fashion, they assigned patients to two groups.

Patients in group A received 650 mg of Tylenol every 6 hours if they had a temperature greater than 101.3°F. When their temperature increased above 103°F, a cooling blanket was draped over their bodies to further reduce fever. Patients in group B were not given antipyretics. Only if their fever exceeded 104°F were they given cooling blankets.

The researchers prematurely stopped the trial when an early analysis showed "an alarming trend toward increased mortality"[19] in group A. In other words, although they would have liked to accumulate more data, the researchers decided it was unethical to continue when patients in group A began contracting more infections and dying at a much higher rate. Of the

44 patients in group A, seven (16 percent) died from infections. In contrast, of the 38 patients in group B, only one (three percent) died.

Firm conclusions could not be made because the trial had been stopped. Even so, the researchers hypothesized that blunting the fever inhibited the body's natural ability to recover from infection, leading to more deaths.

Until larger studies are performed, the medical community will continue to debate the pros and cons of the aggressive quelling of fevers. Meanwhile, the consequences continue, exacting an untold effect on society, the short-term benefits of pain reduction notwithstanding.

Thankfully, some physicians are awakening to the potential dangers.[20,21] Concerned that antipyretics may weaken immunity and increase mortality in patients with sepsis (a bacterial infection of the blood), doctors at Veterans Affairs Maryland Health Care System have suggested that antipyretic therapy be withheld during early stages of sepsis, unless the body temperature exceeds 105.8°F.[22]

Given all of the above, we weren't surprised that the MBVax protocol recommended withholding antipyretics—unless my fever were to exceed 106°F. Likewise, Dr. William Coley had not attempted to suppress his patients' fevers, which could be one reason why he achieved better results than some of the later clinical trials of Coley's Toxins.

The Rise and Fall of My Fever

"You hit 102.6," said Eddy, whispering gently into my ear.

I opened my eyes. About two and a half hours after the start of infusion, my body had gained enough "momentum" to generate a strong fever—just as the protocol had described. My temperature rose rapidly. As it spiked, I became fatigued and dozed off.

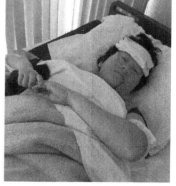

My fever exceeded the lower bound of the target range that the MBVax protocol advocated, between 102.5°F and 106°F. The company had analyzed Dr. Coley's records and concluded that success of the toxins was associated with a peak fever in this range.

Figure 22: My first Coley's Toxins infusion.

"Your face is flush red," said Eddy. "How do you feel?"

"Very tired. My back feels a little sore. And ... I think a tiny bit of aching in my hips—kind of like when I had Neupogen between chemo."

"Interesting. Maybe the toxins are causing your bone marrow to make lots of neutrophils."

"Yea, probably ... Eddy, I feel *really* hot, and dry. Maybe I should drink more of the electrolyte mix?"

Eddy had prepared a squeeze water bottle filled with an electrolyte mix—a simple solution of water, salt and sugar. The MBVax protocol described how to make it. I'd been sipping small amounts. But not too much, in case excess fluid in my stomach were to trigger nausea.

"Um, your pulse is kind of high—it's 117," said Eddy, unclipping the finger oximeter we'd brought along. "I think you might be dehydrated. Now that you've hit the target range, what say we kill the heating pad? Maybe remove the blankets?"

"OK."

Within a few minutes, I began to feel much more comfortable. (Retrospectively, we'd been too aggressive with pre-warming my body. In the following days, we'd lighten up on the pre-warming without compromising the ability to minimize chills.)

My fever continued, staying above 102°F. Aside from an intermittent dry cough, I felt quite normal, just tired. Apparently, much of my discomfort had been from the over-enthusiastic pre-warming, which had caused me to dehydrate. A nurse came in to hook up an IV saline drip to rehydrate me. She also placed an oxygen cannula into my nostrils, saying the extra oxygen would help me feel better. Eddy drenched a face towel with cold water and placed it on my forehead.

By hour four, my temperature fell to 101°F. As the bacteria in Coley's Toxins are dead, there never was any real danger of infection, and my immune system had no problem eliminating the toxins. The "red alert" was over. My body was returning to a normal state. Everything was happening just as the MBVax protocol described.

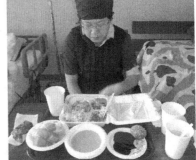

Figure 23: Dinner after Coley's Toxins treatment with high fever.

Dr. Jimenez came to check on me. He didn't have an explanation for my cough, and a recent chest X-ray showed my lungs to be clear. He seemed satisfied that the fever had gone smoothly, that I wasn't in any danger. But to be safe, he asked the nurse to bring in a machine to monitor my oxygen and pulse continuously.

By the fifth hour, my strength was returning. It was already 6 p.m. Dinner was being served downstairs. Eddy had been by my side the entire day, watching like a hawk in case of unforeseen emergencies. But now that the fever was clearly subsiding, he felt it was safe to grab dinner.

"I'll bring dinner up to you," he said, rushing off.

About fifteen minutes later, he returned—with a trayful of happiness. Setting it on the wheeled hospital table, he drew a chair and helped me up from bed. I was hungry. The fever had drained my energy. I was ready to replenish myself.

My eyes beheld a sumptuous assortment of colorful foods held in Styrofoam containers. The main dish was rice and pan-fried fish, with mixed carrot and beans and a side of salsa. But more attractive were the sides: a bowl of squash soup; a plate of red beets, banana chips and an oatmeal muffin; a heaping bowlful of juicy pineapple and papaya cubes; a fruit-and-nut cake; and a cup of thick mango juice.

The sun began to set, casting a deep orange hue and long shadows over the Bullring parking lot across the street. We'd done it—we'd completed my very first Coley Fluid infusion without any major side effects. It would be the first of over two hundred in the years to come.

Five Weeks of Fever

And so, my Coley's Toxins therapy had begun. I had fevers every Monday, Wednesday and Friday. Eddy would sometimes play the old song "Fever" by Peggy Lee on his laptop whenever my temperature started rising: *"Fever! In the morning, Fever all through the night ..."*

The fevers were predictable. They followed the same pattern of my first infusion—a slow rise, followed by an accelerating spike, marked by onset of fatigue, slight chills, and sometimes, a tinge of pelvic ache, then the robust peak, which would persist for an hour or two, accompanied by a sporadic dry cough and ending with a gradual return to normalcy. Five to six hours into treatment, I'd be antsy to get up, hungry for food and companionship. I so looked forward to joining my newfound friends at dinner downstairs.

We worked hard to achieve a peak fever above 102.5°F, which we succeeded in attaining for the most part. Dr. Coley and his colleagues had used the maximum attained temperature to guide their injections. The body quickly becomes tolerant to the toxins, so they often had to increase dosage, sometimes rapidly, until the injections once again elicited strong fever. Likewise, when my peak temperature began to languish, or when my fevers seemed to subside sooner, we knew it was time to increase dosage. Over a five-week period, I had a total of 15 infusions.

IV	Date	Dosage (mcL)	Max temp (°F)
1	8/09/2010	0.50	102.6
2	8/11/2010	0.50	103.5
3	8/13/2010	0.50	102.6
4	8/16/2010	0.50	102.9
5	8/18/2010	0.75	102.7
6	8/20/2010	0.75	102.7
7	8/23/2010	2.00	102.5
8	8/25/2010	2.00	102.3
9	8/27/2010	3.00	102.4
10	8/30/2010	4.00	101.9
11	8/31/2010	6.00	102.7
12	9/02/2010	9.00	104.0
13	9/04/2010	9.00	103.1
14	9/06/2010	9.00	103.6
15	9/09/2010	12.00	102.7

Table 2: Coley Fluid Infusions in Tijuana, with infusion dates, amount infused and peak fever.

During the first week of treatment, the doctors checked on me two to three times a day. By the second week, they saw me just once. For most of the day, we were left to ourselves, except for a nurse who'd check vitals every hour or occasionally hook up a bag of saline to keep me hydrated.

Eddy was my protector and companion, eagle-eyed, faithfully taking my vitals every 15 minutes. This way, he could closely track my fever and page the doctor if any unanticipated trouble brewed. But that need never arose.

The fevers became predictable, even mundane. We now better understood one reason why radiation therapy had supplanted Coley's Toxins: most doctors and patients would probably prefer the quick radiation sessions over the arduous Coley fevers—a matter of practicality and logistics. The young Dr. Gruver had injected his mother for three years, tending to her for hours. But not every patient has a loving son for a doctor. The Mayo brothers (of the Mayo Clinic in Minnesota) had become advocates of the toxins.[23] But they couldn't handle the burdensome, long-term injections. Instead, they instructed the patient's referring hometown physician to continue the injections after the patient had returned home.[24] In short, Coley's Toxins was hard work.

Even though the fevers had become mundane, we had visitors to help break the boredom. My mom, my uncle, and his wife, came to visit us. My uncle was eager to explore the environs and sample the taco shop down the street. Eddy went with him, leaving me to catch up with mom and my aunt.

From our window, we'd watch armed convoys of police, bearing machine guns, clad in black, faces shrouded to protect their identities. We wondered what they were up to. Perhaps a show of power to stave off gang violence? Or maybe a warning to drug traffickers? They served as a reminder that we were in Tijuana, and perhaps not to venture out at night, beyond the walls of the hospital.

Friday evenings were boisterous. Music blared from the bar across the street. Some weekend evenings, throngs of visitors would pack into the Bullring for a concert or show. After the event, chaos would erupt as six lanes of traffic exited the lot. On occasion, the room would pulse with sound for a good 15 minutes, as hundreds of motorcycles strung in convoy rumbled past.

But for the most part, though, the oasis was peaceful, filled with warmth, friendship and fellowship among us patients.

Final Goodbyes

El Yogurt Place had become a favorite destination for Issels patients. The quaint restaurant nestled amid lush vegetation about a thousand feet north of the hospital—close enough for a pleasant stroll—and past the graffiti-stained eastern wall of the Bullring. It was inviting and serene, offering stained glass lamp shades and a treetop view of large residences, juxtaposed with a glimpse of the barbed-wire border fence between the U.S. and Mexico.

Hummingbirds flitted by the expansive windows as we sat, enjoying our last meal together with our friends. They had all completed treatment and were about to return home. We were also returning to San Jose for the weekend, as it was time for a CT scan at Stanford. We planned to come back to Tijuana in a few days to resume the Coley Fluid infusions. Life in the hospital would be so different without our friends.

Jimmy and his wife, Pam, loved to frequent El Yogurt. They were a fun-loving couple, probably in their late 50s, who never once let his difficult prognosis dampen their spirits. On the weekends, they'd call up their favorite taxi driver, who'd take them to their second favorite spot—the local casino. Lorraine, the South African breast cancer patient with an indomitable spirit, and her mom, Adrienne, often came as well. So did Mara, the card dealer from Vegas, and her husband, Jeremy. The last time I was here, I'd had come for lunch with Mara and had eaten the ostrich steak with sautéed onions and asparagus.

We sat in a large, curved booth, laughing at Jimmy's jokes, enjoying the meat and all the butter we wanted. We never had butter at the hospital—dairy products were banned as part of the anticancer diet. We burst out laughing as we recalled how, a week ago at the cafeteria, Jimmy had whipped out three individually-wrapped pats of butter, which he had smuggled in from El Yogurt Place, eliciting oohs and ahs from every butter-deprived person around the table. As I looked around at each of our friends, I was thankful for the opportunity to have crossed paths with these very special souls.

We'd been ward-mates for only a few weeks, but the camaraderie we had developed was enduring. We'd shared meals; taken walks down to the beach together; visited each other's rooms, sat and listened to life stories: who we were, what was important to us, why—or for whom—we were fighting to survive. We savored these sweet moments of laughter, encouragement and communion. We were a conference of human beings, from different parts of the world, bonded together in a quest to survive, treasuring the companionship of those who understood our plight.

The next day, we bid our dear friends goodbye. Eddy and I had gone there for Coley Fluid, but we'd received more than that. We'd witnessed spouses tenderly caring for their beloved, adult children caring for parents and elderly parents caring for adult children. Our friends with cancer were all approaching death. But all of them had chosen not to give up. Having witnessed their unbroken determination, we were roused to fight even harder.

A Mysterious Fever

Back in California, my scans showed stability. The three tiny cysts were still small and therefore not a concern. The axillary lymph nodes were stable and shrinking. So we celebrated—rejoicing the absence of new tumors, the stability of existing lesions, and that my initiation into Coley's Toxins had gone smoothly.

First, we attended a picnic with former research colleagues from Stanford. Glad to see them, I recounted our adventures and my experience with the toxins. Later that evening, we met up with my extended family, eagerly sharing tales of Tijuana over a meat-laden potluck—a welcome break after five weeks of involuntary pseudo-vegetarianism.

After dinner, I suddenly started to feel cold. Thinking that the thermostat had perhaps been turned down, I asked my uncle what it was set to. *Sixty-eight degrees? Strange ... I shouldn't be feeling cold.* I donned a jacket and waited a while, but the cold persisted.

Suddenly, I began to shiver. *OK, this is weird.*

I had to lie down on the couch. I asked my aunt for a large comforter and wrapped myself in it, but the chills only intensified. And then my teeth began to chatter. Within minutes, my body began to shake intensely.

These symptoms were all too familiar. They were exactly what I'd experienced during the chill phase of a Coley's Toxins-induced fever. But my last treatment had been three days prior. *This should not be happening.*

Eddy asked my aunt for a thermometer. Reading the mercury, he said I had a fever of 102°F.

Baffled, Eddy bundled me into the car, draped his light fall jacket over mine and cranked up the heat to maximum. We drove down the 280 freeway to my parents' home in San Jose, hoping the fever would subside. Instead, the mysterious fever continued deep into the night ...

CHAPTER 9

The Violence of the Immune System

THE CHILLS WERE INTENSIFYING. My teeth chattered uncontrollably. My thighs ached as they trembled with force.

"Temperature's 103," said Eddy, piling a fourth blanket over me.

I felt cold. Ice cold. The far-infrared heating pad sandwiched between my body and the mattress was cranked to the max. My body absorbed all the external heat the pad could feed it, in an urgent attempt to generate fever.

We'd arrived home from the family potluck at around 9 p.m. Now, it was after midnight.

Having gone through five weeks of Coley infusions in Mexico, we'd been conditioned to embrace fever. Our goal in Tijuana was to provoke my immune system into fever, and in the process extirpate microscopic remnants of cancer. With this in mind, we withheld the fever-reducing drugs.

We wondered if the perplexing pyrexia might be a "late effect" of my last Coley infusion, received three days earlier. We hadn't encountered a case of delayed reaction in all of our research. In Tijuana, each infusion had generated a fever within an hour or two; by hour six, I'd be back to normal. Then again, I had an infusion every two or three days. Any "late effect" could have been masked by the infusion that followed.

Had I caught a virus? Perhaps on the plane ride from San Diego? Planes are incubators of infectious viruses, such as the flu. But the flu usually announced itself with a runny nose or sore throat—never with a fever.

The chills continued unabated. By 2 a.m. my temperature hit 104°F. The dry cough I experienced in Tijuana returned. Eddy suggested I try one tablet of Motrin, a common anti-inflammatory available in drug stores. He suspected that a surge of neutrophils in my lungs was causing the cough, and wanted to see if Motrin would stop it.[1] The cough improved. Shortly after, the chills relented, the fever subsided and, exhausted, we fell asleep.

The next morning, I felt better. The fever still simmered at 100°F.

The first thing we did was to call the clinic in Tijuana. The physician we spoke with was confident the fever represented a delayed reaction.

"Take Tylenol," she said.

But we weren't persuaded. She didn't offer a convincing reason why Coley's Toxins would cause a delayed fever. To blindly believe a convenient explanation could prove dangerous. What if a *real* infection lurked? What if I had sepsis—a potentially lethal immune response to live bacteria in my blood?

The symptoms of sepsis are similar to that of Coley's Toxins. After all, both are caused by bacteria—alive in the former, dead in the latter. Tylenol would only mask the symptoms, leading to belated treatment—which could prove fatal.

We were supposed to fly back to San Diego later that day to resume treatment in Tijuana. But given the unexplained fever, we cancelled the flight.

By dinnertime, I again felt cold. My appetite vanished.

"Temperature's 102," said Eddy, as he helped me into bed, turning on the heating pad and piling blankets over me. The heat would help my immune system fight an infection—just in case one lurked within me.

Despite these aids, I once again felt cold. The chills returned in force. My thighs and abdomen grew sore from the tremors. My teeth chattered, temperature skyrocketed, and by 8 p.m., it reached 104.6°F. It hovered above 104°F for a couple of hours, then dipped to 103°F. By 11 p.m., it moderated to 102°F.

This second fever spike made a delayed reaction seem even less likely.

As it was late, we were tempted to do what we'd done the previous night—take a Motrin, sleep it off, then see how I felt in the morning. But sepsis was serious. I'd never experienced it, only read about it. People died from it. Lucky patients that survive often end up with oxygen-starved limbs amputated.[2] If I had sepsis, I needed immediate treatment.

As we debated whether to risk sleeping it off, our indecision was cured by the next temperature reading—105.9°F.

"If this is a delayed reaction to Coley's Toxins, it should be getting better, not worse. You may have sepsis. We need to go to the ER," said Eddy.

I agreed. We dressed quickly. Eddy gave me a dose of Tylenol so I could make it to the emergency room without the shakes. He kept asking simple math problems to check my cognition, worried I might fall.

"Yes, I know what two plus two is!" I said in irritation, even as I herded my bleary-eyed parents and brother into the car.

The Girl Who Cried Sepsis

In the emergency room at Stanford Hospital, we explained my medical history, described my symptoms and voiced our concern about sepsis.

The nurse took my vitals: Pulse 115. Temperature 99.1°F. Respiratory rate 28. Oxygen 93%. Blood pressure 102/48.

She asked for a urine sample, drew tubes of blood and ordered a culture. If there were bacteria infesting my blood, they would feed on the culture medium, multiply and become detectable.[3] But the process could take up to a day or two.

The doctor wasn't convinced I had an infection, even though my vitals matched the criteria for sepsis.[4] Was it because my temperature had abated to 99°F—a consequence of taking Tylenol? I told her my fever had reached 105.9°F ... But maybe going to Mexico for an obscure treatment had compromised my credibility? Or maybe because I was lucid and sitting upright? Perhaps she expected me to be in a worse condition since my first fever had spiked almost 30 hours earlier—an eternity for a disease where each hour delay can decrease survival by 7.6 percent.[5]

My urine came back as normal. My white blood cell count was 11.3, just over the upper limit of normal, 11.0. The near-normal white count was deceiving. As chemo had permanently reduced my white count to 3.0, the much-elevated level of 11.3 signaled that my body was fighting an active bacterial infection. But the doctor—unfamiliar with my history—may not have perceived this nuance.

An hour passed. A technician wheeled in a machine to X-ray my lungs. A change of shift occurred, and a new doctor came by. Attentive and patient, he listened to my story. He agreed to treat me empirically—meaning he'd start the antibiotics even without clear evidence of infection.

By 1:30 a.m., they'd hooked me up to numerous IVs. Antibiotics coursed through my veins. Fever-reducing drugs were infused. Benadryl was given to avert an allergic reaction to the antibiotics. Then, they extracted my PICC line, as it was the likeliest nest for bacteria.

Suddenly, my blood pressure plummeted. At that point I had either fallen asleep or was unconscious—oblivious to the commotion. Eddy would recount what had transpired: A small army of staff rushed in to stabilize me. They plied me with aggressive infusions of supporting fluids.

Turning to Eddy, the doctor said he was concerned my blood pressure had plummeted to 80/42. The sudden drop was an ominous sign of septic shock—a medical emergency. It happens when cells of the innate immune system overreact to infection, producing uncontrolled amounts of signaling molecules to recruit other immune cells. The recruits emit even more signals, and a vicious cycle is born—the cytokine storm. Recall that Dr. Steven Rosenberg's CAR-T patient died when the modified T cells she received triggered a cytokine storm. This is one major way sepsis can kill.[6]

"Rene's normal blood pressure is around 100/60," said Eddy, in response to the doctor's concern about the blood pressure. "During chemo, it sometimes dropped as low as 90/60."

"That's interesting to know. I'm more concerned about the diastolic—the lower number, which is at 42," said the doctor.[7] "But overall, your wife doesn't *look* like she's in septic shock—patients usually appear sicker. All we can do is support her body. The rest will depend on how her body handles it. ...."

> The risk of death from sepsis is staggering. *Between 28 and 50 percent of patients with sepsis die.*[8] An estimated half of all hospital deaths are caused by sepsis.[9] In 2008, 1.1 million people were diagnosed with it in the U.S.[10] More patients die from sepsis than from prostate cancer, breast cancer and AIDS combined.[11]

Barely an hour later, I roused, weak and tired. But considering I'd been up most of the night, I felt quite normal.

Eddy was relieved to see me alert. Deep within, he believed I had sepsis, and understood the dire implications of the blood pressure plunge. The up-to-fifty-percent probability of death was comparable to that of my cancer—except with cancer, I'd live longer!

It was almost 6 a.m. Eddy was dozing off, his body precariously balanced on the small chair by my bed. Between naps, I whiled away the time eavesdropping on my neighbors, trying to guess their ailments from their conversations with doctors. Five of us patients, separated by curtains, were crammed into the small and busy room.

As the hours passed, my vitals strengthened. The staff watched me closely, but nothing else alarming happened. By noon, they were ready to transfer me out. Because I'd received chemoradiation at Stanford two years ago, they sent me to the chemo ward where the oncology team could monitor my recovery.

The chemo ward brought back memories. I remembered having so much hope that chemo would secure my future. I'd been a trooper. I'd done everything the nurses and doctors instructed. I'd grown attached to the ward and some of the nurses.

After I'd completed chemo, I made little crafts on every major holiday—paper roses for Valentine's Day, fuzzy bunnies and chicks for Easter, paper Christmas trees—then made my rounds, offering them to patients undergoing chemo and their nurses. It was my way of thanking the staff and cheering on a fellow human being in suffering. The little note of encouragement I attached to the craft was my way of saying, "Hang in there. You can make it, too."

It's been two years since chemo. I'm still alive. Now, I've had 15 Coley infusions, followed by a powerful live infection. I smiled as I remembered Mr. Fred Stein—the patient who'd sparked Dr. Coley's lifelong obsession. Mr. Stein's sarcoma had disappeared after a live bacterial infection. Maybe this live infection would also destroy the inscrutable cancer within me?

The blood culture returned. We were right. I *did* have sepsis. The doctor said it was caused by "high grade bacteremia"—my blood teemed with *Pseudomonas,* a bacterium that commonly infects hospital patients. Normally lurking in inadequately chlorinated pools and causing ear infections in children, Pseudomonas has become a notorious problem in hospitals. Rampant overuse of antibiotics has caused it to mutate, creating resistant strains. Up to eight percent of patients hospitalized with antibiotic-resistant Pseudomonas die.[12]

Later, we obtained medical records of the ER visit. Even as the doctors pumped me with antibiotics, they'd written: "low suspicion for sepsis." Somehow, my body seemed to have tolerated the teeming bacteria and 30 hours of fevers—so much so that the doctors initially doubted I had sepsis. Perhaps the 15 infusions of dead bacteria had prepared my body to better handle a live infection?

Later, Eddy called Dr. Old to let him know what had happened. He wasn't surprised my body had tolerated the sepsis. Experiments showed that mice injected with bacterial toxins were protected when subsequently infected with live bacteria.[13,14] He suspected the 15 infusions of Coley's Toxins had similarly protected me.

Tracing the Source of Sepsis

The infectious disease specialist came to my room. She said the Pseudomonas had colonized my PICC line, latching itself onto the inner surface. She explained that the on-again, off-again fever occurred when the bacteria periodically shed from my PICC line, entered my blood and provoked an immune response.

The strain of Pseudomonas in my blood had been tested against various antibiotics. They all worked, easily killing it, meaning it wasn't resistant at all.

"Even though susceptible to antibiotics, the bacteria had bred into a thick layer of *biofilm*, making it harder to eradicate. That's why we had to remove your PICC line," said the specialist.

But how had the Pseudomonas gotten into my PICC line? Perhaps the Coley Fluid was contaminated with live bacteria? Or maybe it was the saline with which the nurses used to flush the line (a practice normally done before and after each infusion)?

The only other possible source of infection was the recent head MRI I'd received at Stanford upon returning from Mexico. The technician had injected gadolinium contrast (a substance that enhances MRI images) through my PICC line.

That my bacteria weren't resistant to antibiotics hinted the infection had happened in Tijuana, where abuse of expensive antibiotics would be less rampant in cost-conscious clinics. Furthermore, the Stanford MRI had occurred just one day before my first fever—not likely enough time for an infection to brew.

We immediately thought of our new friends who had just left the Mexican clinic, concerned they may have been infected. They all had advanced cancer, their bodies weakened by recent chemoradiation. Sepsis could easily kill them.

We quickly emailed them, urging them to be vigilant for the warning signs. It turned out that Jimmy, the affable gym owner from Tennessee, was literally in the early throes of sepsis! His wife, Pam, emailed us back, saying they'd just returned from the ER, where Jimmy had spiked a temperature of 102.7°F. She immediately called Jimmy's oncologist and read out our email to him over the phone. The oncologist instructed them to return to the ER for a blood culture. The culture confirmed infection. Like me, Jimmy had Pseudomonas in his blood—also easily killed with antibiotics.

With early intervention, Jimmy recovered. In time, we learned that none of the other Issels patients had been infected. They had all received Coley Fluid, which suggested it wasn't the source of infection. Still, we reported the incident to MBVax, the Canadian manufacturer. The company immediately began an investigation, eventually finding no problems with their formulation.

We suspected the Pseudomonas had originated in Tijuana. I vividly recalled how the technician had pricked her finger and intended to reuse the contaminated needle. Perhaps a similar error had occurred when the nurses prepared fluids to be infused into me and Jimmy?

Errors of contamination also happen in the U.S. I would later see such negligence committed by my nurse in a Detroit hospital: About to connect IV tubing to my PICC line, she accidentally dropped the end of the tubing onto the bed. The sheets hadn't been washed for three days. Instead of using a fresh alcohol swab, she reused a dried-out one to wipe the tubing end, then inserted the likely still-contaminated end into my PICC port, potentially transferring bacteria into my blood. Another time, a nurse, having only one free hand, used her mouth to unscrew the cap off a sterile syringe. She then connected the screwed tip of the syringe to my PICC port to flush it, potentially transferring bacteria from her mouth into my body. I would eventually find out that Heather—the other Stanford scientist with synovial sarcoma—had contracted sepsis during treatment. Hers originated at Stanford Hospital.[15]

Whatever the cause of infection, I couldn't risk another one. We decided against returning to Tijuana. Now that I'd begun Coley's Toxins, I could legally bring a small amount of Coley Fluid back to the U.S. for personal use. It'd be considered a continuation of treatment begun abroad for a serious disease.[16]

•₀ •• •₀ •• •₀

The emergency was over. We sat on the couch in the living room, watching Friday night TV, enjoying Chinese take-out, eggplant with spicy garlic sauce, beef and broccoli, Kung Pao chicken and steamed rice. Notwithstanding the Americanized names, the cooking was authentic and the food was delicious.

The portable antibiotic pump lay on the couch by my side, attached to the newly installed PICC line threaded through my arm into my heart. Every six hours, the pump injected a large dose of antibiotics into my bloodstream. In between, it fed me smaller amounts. This would continue for two weeks to eradicate any lingering Pseudomonas.

As we reflected on the excitement of the past week, we realized how tricky it can be to distinguish an infection-induced fever from an immunotherapy-related fever. We resolved to pay close attention to future symptoms, especially those that come after unfamiliar treatment.

> In the case of Coley Fluid infusions, the fevers predictably subsided within a few hours. This may not be the case for other immunotherapies. Therefore, it's key to work with experienced physicians who understand how the immunotherapy works, and know what to look out for.

Dropped

Patients who pursue unproven therapies are sometimes dropped by their conventional doctors. One of our friends at Issels, Mara, shared how her oncologist in Las Vegas dropped her after she returned from Mexico, refusing to order further scans, blood tests or treatment. We'd read similar stories from online discussion forums. Little did we know that I was soon to experience this myself.

Two weeks after being discharged for sepsis, I returned to Stanford Cancer Center to see my sarcoma oncologist, Dr. Ganjoo. In that visit, she expressed discomfort that I had gone to Tijuana for unproven treatment. She described how she'd recently watched a documentary of patients who had gone to Mexico for treatments that lacked scientific basis. While we understood her concerns, they said nothing of the intense research and careful planning we'd put into Coley's Toxins, nor of the support and approval we'd received from Dr. Old.

We tried to explain the scientific validity of Coley's Toxins, how it was once used by leading American surgeons, our rationale for pursuing it, the credentials of Dr. Old, and that Mexico was the only place we could get it—despite our initial reservations about going there. But unfortunately, her impression had already been formed.

Dr. Ganjoo expressed that she didn't feel comfortable continuing to see me. She suggested I look for another oncologist. We left the clinic stunned.

In records later obtained, she wrote, "Patient is getting the 30-day notice to find another physician."

I was shaken. But I'd survived the ravages of surgery, radiation and chemo, and had endured fevers and shakes and sepsis. This minor setback would not break my spirit, nor would it deter me from pursuing what I believed was scientifically sound and could make a difference in my survival.

At Stanford, I continued to see my surgeon, Dr. Kaplan, and my radiation oncologist, Dr. Le. These physicians had treated me in 2008, and they knew the seriousness with which I approached my medical treatment. They continued ordering my scans.

Graves' Disease

It was Christmas of 2010. We were again at my uncle's for food and fun. Three months earlier, the sudden chills had occurred here, marking the beginnings of sepsis. My cousins were downstairs in the den, playing ping pong. Drawn to the laughter and merriment, I moved toward the spiral stairs. Holding tightly to the railing, I took one step down. Then another. And another.

"Surprised you made it down by yourself," said Eddy. "Here, take a seat and watch the guys."

I was glad for the respite. My thighs were tired from negotiating the 16 steps.

After the sepsis, I had completed another two weeks of home antibiotics. Every week for the next month, I visited my primary doctor, Dr. Agah. He had expertise in infectious diseases and was devoted to my full recovery from Pseudomonas. Four weeks passed, and I grew stronger. And then, on October 25, something out of the ordinary happened.

"Your pulse is 99," said Dr. Agah. "Let's take it again after you sit quietly for a while."

"Still 100. I'm ordering a full complement of thyroid blood tests. Go downstairs and get them drawn right now."

Dr. Agah was right. The tests showed I had high levels of thyroid hormones circulating my body. They also indicated the cause as Graves' disease—an autoimmune reaction to my thyroid gland.

The attack on my thyroid by immune cells was provoking it to generate large amounts of hormones. Thyroid hormones control our metabolism— the ability of our bodies to break down and convert food into energy. They also regulate vital aspects such as breathing, heart rate, body temperature, muscle growth, muscle function, nerve function and much more.

The high levels caused my metabolism to go into overdrive. My heartbeat reached 100 beats per minute at rest. I developed diarrhea. I fatigued easily. My muscles began to waste. By Christmas, my thighs were so feeble that I couldn't get up from the sofa; Eddy had to pull me up. The relentless assault on my thyroid made the gland swell from the influx of immune cells, making it difficult to swallow.

Autoimmune diseases like Graves' disease affect up to 23.5 million Americans and are a leading cause of death among young and middle-aged women.[17] There are more than 80 types of autoimmune diseases affecting disparate parts of the body. Some of these are: *rheumatoid arthritis*, where the immune system attacks joints and surrounding tissue; *inflammatory bowel disease*, where the digestive tract is attacked, resulting in diarrhea, pain, fatigue and weight loss; *systemic lupus erythematosus*, where the skin, joints, kidneys, brain and other organs are attacked; and *psoriasis*, which causes buildup of dry and itchy patches of red skin, often with silver-colored scales.

The root causes of autoimmunity are still largely unknown. But all of these diseases reflect a misguided immune system. T cells lock onto antigens found in healthy tissues. Safety mechanisms of tolerance that guard against unintended autoimmunity—such as immune checkpoints and Tregs (described in chapter 7)—are silenced. With these suppressive mechanisms out of the way, T cells freely attack healthy organs, causing unintended damage.

But what had caused the misguided attack against my thyroid? We believe the likeliest explanation was the intense radiation I'd received in 2008 to my jaw and neck. Radiation therapy is a well-documented trigger of Graves' disease. It may have killed some cells in my thyroid gland.[18] The cell death resulted in the creation of T cells against thyroid antigens. The Coley Fluid infusions could have removed mechanisms of tolerance, thus allowing T cells to attack my thyroid. Similarly, patients receiving other immunotherapies like checkpoint inhibitors may also experience attack on healthy organs.[19,20]

This immune onslaught was what we needed to create against my cancer. At its full fury, the immune system is capable of rejecting whole organs—transplanted livers weighing up to three pounds are repulsed unless powerful immunosuppressive steroids are given. As Dr. Old once put it, I needed to "create an allergy toward my cancer." Only now, it was directed toward my thyroid.

A Cautious Decision

From November through January, we consulted three endocrinologists. Each had a preferred method for treating Graves' disease. The first two recommended destroying my thyroid with radioactive iodine. The iodine, laced with radiation, circulates in the blood and accumulates in the thyroid, slowly killing it. The third recommended antithyroid drugs, oral medicines that suppress the immune system, thus reducing the immune assault on the thyroid.

By now, we'd learned the importance of thinking through the consequences of medical choices. The endocrinologists focused only on my thyroid. They had no experience with my cancer, nor did they demonstrate the desire to explore the ramifications of thyroid treatment on my cancer. My recovery from sepsis had delayed the return to Coley's Toxins for months. What if the treatment for Graves' introduced even more delay?

I couldn't afford that; it was now two years after chemotherapy—the typical time my cancer would rebound.

Some of the endocrinologists urged us to take the treatments they offered. But we resisted the temptation to act on impulse. To buy time for research, I consumed *L-carnitine*, a common supplement that bodybuilders take; Eddy had learned it could suppress the harmful effects of excess thyroid hormones.[21] The supplement reversed my diarrhea, fatigue and muscle weakness.

We discovered that both radioactive iodine and antithyroid drugs can take *months or even years* to work. One study of radioactive iodine showed that after six months, only 70 percent of patients had normalized levels of thyroid hormones; it took 3 years before 90 percent were cured.[22] Another study showed it can take up to three months for antithyroid drugs to fully work.[23] None of the endocrinologists had mentioned how long these treatments would take to work. Doctors often prescribe solutions, then evaluate how patients respond, adjusting medications over weeks or months. While otherwise-healthy patients could afford an open-ended iterative process, I could not.

Delving further into medical studies, we learned that both approaches—radioactive iodine and antithyroid drugs—can suppress the immune system.[24,25,26] My immune system was already permanently handicapped from chemoradiation. Any further suppression would sabotage efforts to activate it against cancer. The endocrinologists we consulted didn't think the immunosuppression would jeopardize my cancer. But they had no expertise in the treatment of my cancer, let alone in immunotherapy.

In addition to the potential delay and immunosuppression, there were other serious ramifications. For example, even if antithyroid drugs worked for me, I would have to stop them to resume cancer immunotherapy (because they suppress the immune system and thereby counteract immunotherapy). Upon stopping antithyroid drugs, up to 40 percent of patients relapse.[27] If Graves' disease were to recur in the middle of Coley Fluid infusions, I would run the risk of a life-threatening situation called a thyroid storm. A melanoma patient experienced a thyroid storm after receiving Yervoy.[28] These tempests release astronomic levels of thyroid hormones that kill up to half of patients.[29]

Through our own research, we learned of a third solution—surgical removal of my thyroid gland. We were surprised none of the endocrinologists had suggested it. Surgery was a safe and established treatment for Graves' disease. Surgery would conclusively eliminate the source of excess hormones, without damaging my immune system. Surgery would allow me to return to fighting my cancer immediately, unlike the less predictable results of antithyroid drugs or radioactive iodine. Surgery would preclude the risk of a thyroid storm. I would have to take thyroid replacement pills for the rest of my life, but that would also be the case with radioactive iodine.

We discussed the option of surgery with a fourth endocrinologist, a former professor at the University of California, San Francisco who had decades of experience treating thyroid diseases. He concurred with our reasoning and supported our decision, saying "once you're allergic to a strawberry, you're always allergic to it." This out-of-the-box thinker understood the greater urgency of my cancer. He agreed that the removal of my thyroid would free me to deal with the more pressing threat.

Lesson learned: Cancer patients who experience other medical problems have to carefully consider how the recommended solutions to those problems will impact their cancer therapy. Solutions that weaken the immune system or introduce lengthy delays or uncertainty may jeopardize their cancer therapy. In that case, patients may consider other alternatives that aren't typically recommended. It may make sense to "sacrifice a pawn" in the greater context of surviving the cancer chess game.

We consulted three thyroid surgeons, deciding on one—a pioneer in the field of minimally invasive, outpatient thyroid surgery. Eddy had identified Dr. Terris by studying medical papers of thyroid surgery techniques. Instead of the traditional three-to-four-inch neck incision to remove the thyroid, Dr. Terris' technique required a one-inch incision; less cutting meant quicker recovery. Moreover, his technique allowed patients to return home immediately after surgery, instead of recovering at the hospital.[30] Finally, the procedure didn't require general anesthesia, which meant less suppression of the immune system.

Deciding that the benefits were worth the effort, we flew to Georgia for the outpatient procedure. By now, we had learned to look past the inconveniences of travel.

Losing My Thyroid

Brimming with curiosity, I was excited I'd be awake during surgery. Never before had I been sentient while being operated on. Eddy spent the night before compiling soothing melodies on an iPod. They would drown out the clanging medical devices or the sizzling of cauterized flesh.

On a cold and wet February morning in 2011, we drove to the Medical College of Georgia—once headquarters for Confederate surgeons during the Civil War.[31] I checked in for surgery. The anesthesiologist wheeled me into the operating room. We'd met with Dr. Dubin the day before. He'd agreed to use certain anesthesia drugs thought to be less immunosuppressive. With earbuds in, and tranquilizing tunes playing on my iPod, I was ready for the procedure.

Suddenly, I realized it was over. Perplexed, I couldn't recall the operation. Nor did I remember listening to the songs Eddy had lovingly compiled.

The surgeon came by. He told me I'd done very well. He said I had stayed calm throughout, and conversed with him at key points during the procedure when he needed to verify my vocal cords were still functioning. But why couldn't I remember any of it?

It was then that I discovered that "being awake" during surgery doesn't mean you'll *remember* being awake. (It's common practice to give patients drugs that suppress memory.) We were later told that erasing memory decreases the stress response, which helps the body to heal after surgery.[32]

Preparing to Resume Coley's Toxins

The minimally invasive surgery was a complete success. I rested in the hotel the remainder of the day, then gallivanted around a nearby mall the next. For a few days, the front of my neck was swollen. It was hard to swallow and I could only whisper. My voice returned in two days, but sounded robotic. Within weeks, the one-inch incision was barely noticeable, the high levels of thyroid hormones plummeted, and my voice returned to normal.

With the gland gone, I could now control my thyroid hormone levels, simply by consuming the appropriate amount of synthetic hormones. Our efforts had paid off. We'd avoided the uncertainties of antithyroid drugs and radioactive iodine. We could now resume immunotherapy, with no risk of a thyroid storm.

Our original goal had been to complete six uninterrupted months of Coley's Toxins—aiming to replicate one of Dr. Coley's "best practices." But after only five weeks in Mexico, we'd lost seven months to sepsis and Graves'. There was no time to lose.

Even though we had exonerated Coley Fluid as the cause of sepsis, Eddy and I wanted to be doubly sure. Seizing control of mom's oven for a week, we set up an experiment to test the Coley Fluid for live bacteria. We ordered agar plates—petri dishes with jelly-like culture medium that served as food for bacteria. Donning sterile gloves and face masks to avoid contamination, we squirted some Coley Fluid onto three plates. As with all science experiments, we set up controls: three more plates received sterile water; three others received a foolproof source of bacteria. (I'll leave it to your imagination to figure out what we used!)

The experiment showed the following: The plates that received the foolproof source grew opaque spots, signifying teeming colonies. In contrast, the plates that received sterile water or Coley Fluid didn't grow bacteria. This implied that the Coley Fluid was safe from contamination.

In the labs of the University of California, San Diego and Stanford, I had plated bacteria thousands of times over a decade of research. But now, I was plating bacteria for my survival. We tested every vial of Coley Fluid in this manner, before eventually using them for intravenous infusions. None of those future infusions resulted in sepsis, and would confirm the Coley Fluid was sterile.

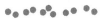

Beginning in mid-April 2011, I completed ten uneventful Coley infusions at home, starting with the lowest possible dose, carefully ramping up until the fevers reached 103°F.

On May 5, 2011, we went to Stanford for a routine head MRI. We'd just returned from a late lunch when the phone rang. It was Dr. Le, my radiation oncologist. We knew something was wrong the moment she identified herself, because my doctors never called on the day of the scan.

Dr. Le said the MRI showed a bright spot in the area of my primary tumor. It signified a local recurrence—the cancer had returned in my head.

Dr. Le urged me to see my surgeon, Dr. Kaplan. Immediately.

CHAPTER 10

Waiting for Immunotherapy to Work

My HEART POUNDED as Eddy loaded the MRI images onto his laptop. We'd obtained a CD of the images earlier that morning, before Dr. Le's call.

The loading completed. A ghastly frontal image of my skull materialized—a gray apparition in a sea of black.

Eddy switched the computer program to view cross-sectional images of my head. Think of the head as a whole ham, and the MRI images as horizontal slices of meat, each five millimeters thick. Starting from the top of my skull, he flitted through the slices, arriving at the level of my nostrils. Planted within the area where my original tumor once existed, abutting my right jawbone, was a bright shining mass one centimeter wide.

Dismayed, we compared the MRI against the previous scan taken in February, one week after I'd returned home from thyroid surgery in Georgia. Even though the February report had made no mention of the mass, it had already been present then, but smaller, at half a centimeter.

The nature of the mass was indisputable. It resided right where the original tumor was found, doubling in size over three months. Unlike the bilateral armpit lymph nodes that later shrunk, and the equivocal lung cysts that remained small, its location and growth rate left little room for doubt.

Tears of disappointment trickled down my cheeks as my mind grappled with the implications of this recurrence. Two-and-a-half years ago, after completing first-line therapy, we'd forsaken a normal life to prevent this day from happening. Those years of effort—the experimentation with alternative medicines, the NY-ESO-1 vaccine, the Coley's Toxins—seemed helpless to alter my future. My cancer had returned *right on time*, just as the MD Anderson oncologist had predicted, erasing hope of my becoming an "outlier"—that rare survivor whose outcome defies the survival curves.

If I was going to die despite all that effort, maybe I should've listened to Dr. Jacobs—gone back to a normal life. Not tried so hard? At least I'd have experienced two-plus years of semi-normal life? Maybe even had kids? That way, Eddy would have someone to remember me by?

Analyzing Your Own Scans

Oncologists rely on diagnostic radiologists to analyze scans for tumor growth. But diagnostic radiology, like other fields of medicine, is dependent on the skill and experience of the radiologist scrutinizing the scan. Smaller tumors may sometimes be missed by radiologists. Such recurrences go undetected until spotted on subsequent scans. In my case, the recurrent head tumor was first reported in May, even though already visible three months earlier. While nuanced interpretation of scans should be left to radiologists, proactive patients can still check for obvious recurrences or tumor growth using powerful, free software like *Osirix*.

The tumor had recurred at the primary site. This cradle of malignancy had been scorched with the maximum dose of radiation, then poisoned with chemotherapy. And yet, the shrouded seeds of leftover cancer had survived. Their obstinacy implied they'd become resistant to chemoradiation. Having ruled out high-dose ifosfamide, and immunotherapy seeming to have failed, surgery was my last line of defense.

A week later, we saw Dr. Kaplan, the surgeon who'd removed my original tumor over three-and-a-half years earlier. He recommended a conservative resection: cut out the tumor along with a surrounding margin of flesh. If the surrounding tissue was found to be contaminated with cancer, we could then consider another more extensive surgery.

Despite the diminutive, one-centimeter mass, we felt uneasy about a limited surgery. After three years of studying my disease, we feared a limited resection would fail to remove the unseen tentacles—those famous feelers that radiate from sarcomas and spread along muscles, forcing surgeons to amputate whole limbs. Failure to remove all of the invisible extensions would leave many sons of sarcoma.

Those progeny would besiege my surgical wound. Fueled by growth factors meant for promoting the healing of tissues, the fledgling tumors might grow even faster than if their parent hadn't been removed in the first place.[1]

The ring of tumors would then expand, eventually merging into a monstrosity of malignancy, ensnaring vital structures such as the carotid artery, eye, throat, brain. This doomed scenario is known as the loss of *local control*, and patients with sarcoma in this area of the head often die from it—not from the spread of their cancer.[2]

I knelt on the floor by the bed. In despair, I buried my head in my blanket, my energy drained. Our attempt at a cure had seemed straightforward: create T cells against my cancer; use Coley Fluid to take out tumor defenses; watch tumors vanish; return to normal life. But this recurrence put us back to square one—only, the stakes were now much higher, the timing urgent, and the coming sacrifices greater.

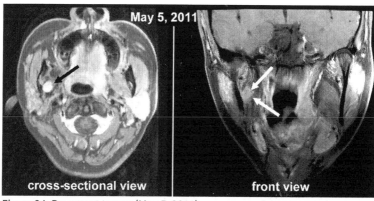

Figure 24: Recurrent tumor (May 5, 2011)

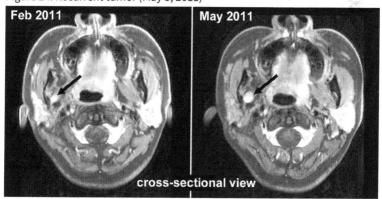

Figure 25: Feb 2011 and May 2011 MRI images reveal tumor growth over 3 months

Accepting Reality, Letting Go of Children

We'd indefinitely postponed starting a family. My future was uncertain; our efforts at finding a cure were all-consuming. But while receiving Coley

Fluid in Tijuana, I began daring to dream we'd succeed and soon be able to return to a normal life. One afternoon, as my toxin-induced fever abated, I merrily chirped out names of our future child to Eddy.

"I've got it! If it's a girl, we'll call her Lora ... L-O-R-A, for Lloyd Old, Ravin Agah," I said, pre-dedicating our future daughter's name to the two physicians who had imbued the strongest hope in us. We were indebted to the numerous medical professionals who'd cared for me over the three years since diagnosis, including behind-the-scenes anesthesiologists, radiologists and pathologists. But these two doctors were our constant companions, running alongside us in this marathon of survival.

"You sure you don't wanna name her Kim?" Eddy asked, grinning. (Combining "Kim" with our last name "Chee" forms "Kim Chee," the name of a popular fermented Korean side dish, which would undoubtedly lead to merciless teasing.)

As a child, I looked after my two younger brothers. I'd sit with one on each side, reading to them, letting them lean on my shoulders as they dozed off. As a teenager, friends told me I'd someday make a good mom. I'd always loved children and found myself quite natural with them. I loved helping out at the church nursery with the youngest babies and was unbothered by their cries.

After Eddy and I got married, I knew he'd make a wonderful father. He had good values and a generous dose of playfulness. But how could we now think of children when our backbreaking efforts had failed to prevent even a smattering of cells from regrowing?

No longer were we combating microscopic cancer. Now, I had a fast-growing, visible tumor spewing malignant cells. That single bright spot on the scan—about the size of a blueberry—erased our dreams of a family.

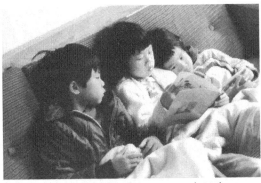

Figure 26: Reading to my brothers (1985)

Hope (May 25 MRI)

We trusted Dr. Kaplan and his surgical skills. He'd saved my life three years earlier. But we resisted the overpowering urge to cut out the lesion, and instead planned a return visit to MD Anderson (MDA) to consult a medical oncologist for a bigger picture on how to best treat my recurrent cancer.

Dr. Benjamin, the experienced oncologist we'd once seen, was out on leave. I was scheduled to see another oncologist, Dr. Patel. By the time of the appointment, the tumor would have had three weeks to grow. Petrified, we forged ahead with more Coley infusions, squeezing in eleven fevers, praying they would keep my tumor in check.

On May 26, 2011, we saw Dr. Patel. The head MRI that I'd taken the day before affirmed the presence of tumor—still about the same size as it was on May 5. *About the same size? Shouldn't it be slightly bigger now that three weeks had passed? Could it be that the Coley infusions had halted my tumor?*

Eloquent and accommodating, Dr. Patel confirmed what my Stanford radiation oncologist had advised—that repeat radiation would be ineffective and dangerous. Dr. Patel had also ordered a full-body PET, a scan that detects metabolic activity of tumors, scheduled for the following morning. He said if my jaw tumor alone was active on the PET, he'd recommend surgery. However, if the lung lesions also looked active, that would mean my cancer had spread, in which case I'd need chemo, namely, high-dose ifosfamide.

We asked Dr. Patel what the odds were that my cancer would keep returning even after more surgery or chemo.

"Unfortunately, you're not going to like the answer," he said.

Given that the tumor had survived prior chemoradiation, the odds were "high"—meaning anywhere from 50 to 90 percent (In a later visit, Dr. Benjamin would narrow the odds of further recurrence to over 80 percent). The lack of data made precise prognostication impossible. But Dr. Patel said that sarcomas that return within the first two years after first-line treatment are the ones that keep coming back.

In other words, *a cure was now improbable*—it was a matter of time before I would die.

The next morning, I went for the PET scan, grabbed lunch, then saw the head and neck surgeon Dr. Patel had referred us to.

"Hi, I'm Dr. Hanna. Wow ... impressive story—high grade sarcoma since 2008," said Dr. Hanna as he entered the room. He was pleasant and kind and spoke slowly and clearly.

"I don't know what's going on with you ... I can't tell," he said. "Your PET this morning was negative. Nothing showed up on it."

Nothing? Did he say nothing *lit up?*

Further elaborating on the PET, Dr. Hanna said, "Sometimes, very slow-growing tumors won't show up. But you had a confirmed high-grade sarcoma; a recurrence of your tumor should show up on PET."

The PET scan measures how fast tumors guzzle glucose from the blood. Aggressive tumors like synovial sarcoma should register. But neither my head tumor nor my lung lesions had, which stymied Dr. Hanna.

As I listened to Dr. Hanna, an excitement welled up within me. *Perhaps the eleven recent Coley infusions had worked!*

Dr. Hanna spent the next hour looking through the MRI images with us—all the way back to my primary tumor in 2008. Despite the negative PET, he felt that the lesion probably represented a recurrence.

Bringing the consult to a close, he said I had three options: wait and rescan in two months, perform a needle biopsy or operate immediately.

The rationale for waiting two months was to watch for continued tumor growth, which would confirm malignancy. As my tumor hadn't lit up on PET, Dr. Hanna felt it was slow-growing, so the risk of it becoming inoperable in two months was low.

A needle biopsy could also confirm malignancy, justifying surgery. Sarcoma surgeries are often done *en bloc*: the surgeon gives wide berth to the tumor, removing large chunks of attached muscle and bone in one fell swoop. This approach offers the best hope of removing all the microscopic extensions around the tumor without disturbing it. But, with major side effects and the possible diminishing of quality of life, en bloc procedures call for proof of cancer, which a biopsy would satisfy.

The third option: immediate surgery. Surgery would be extensive, requiring amputation of my right jaw bone (the tumor looked to have infiltrated it). To reduce long-term pain, Dr. Hanna would also remove my jaw joint. He would have to remove surrounding muscles, causing my lower jaw to skew right, and my upper and lower teeth to misalign, affecting speech and chewing. These would further compromise my ability to eat from the lack of saliva caused by radiation in 2008. For cosmetic reasons, a plastic surgeon would transfer flesh from my leg to pad the gaping hole. But scar tissue would develop, permanently making it difficult to open my mouth more than a centimeter or two. I'd be hospitalized for two weeks. Overall healing could take another six.

"Personally, I think there's a tumor ... and I think it's been there for a while. I think your tumor was inactivated or slowed down by the vaccine. But now that you're off the vaccine, it's slowly starting to activate," he said. He further qualified his thoughts as a best-guess hunch.

We were surprised Dr. Hanna felt my NY-ESO-1 vaccine had conferred benefit. Most of the conventional doctors we'd seen had been, at best, neutral toward our immunotherapy efforts. *Perhaps the MRI images were compelling enough ...*

A Dying Tumor?

"One last question please," I said. "What do you think about the *cystic* nature of my jaw tumor?" Dr. Patel had mentioned that my tumor had hollowed out and was now filled with fluid. He explained this can happen when chemotherapy kills a tumor, or when part of a fast-growing tumor spontaneously dies as it outgrows its blood supply.

"Most cancers, when they have any *necrosis* in them, will contain some fluid," said Dr. Hanna. (Necrosis refers to the death of cells within a tumor.)

"Necrosis happens when they outstrip their blood supply, right?" said Eddy. Dr. Hanna nodded.

"But will the tumor outstrip its blood supply even at such a small size?" I asked.

From what we'd read, spontaneous necrosis usually occurred in larger tumors. But mine was still small, one centimeter wide. And 20 days earlier, the tumor was about the same size, yet had shown no necrosis. Why would it suddenly happen now?

Eddy and I suspected the necrosis was caused by the Coley infusions I'd done in the 20 days in between the Stanford and MDA MRIs. Two days before the MDA MRI, I'd completed four straight days of Coley infusions in a hotel room in Houston.

The occurrences of tumor necrosis in Dr. Coley's case reports also supported our belief. Furthermore, modern experiments showed that bacterial toxins can cause tumors to necrose.[3] But with no proof of our hypothesis, we kept these thoughts to ourselves.

Dr. Hanna had no further comment on the necrosis. He encouraged us to focus on the three options, stating that he favored biopsy, as he preferred to have proof of malignancy before operating. We thanked him, saying we'd discuss the options, and get back to him.

Leaving the appointment, we brimmed with cautious optimism. The following day, we obtained a CD of the MRI. Comparing it against the 20-day-old Stanford MRI, we marveled at the distinction between tumor core and rim. The implied necrosis beaconed a ray of hope.

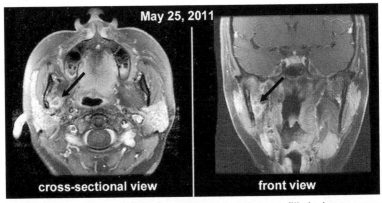

Figure 27: MD Anderson MRI shows "hollowed-out" tumor (likely due to necrosis).

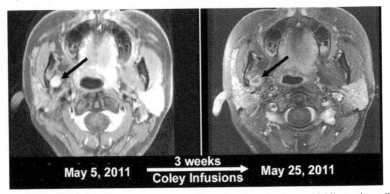

Figure 28: After 20 days of intensive Coley infusions, my tumor "hollowed-out."

Debating The Options

Back at the kitchen table in San Jose, we debated the choices.

We disliked the idea of doing nothing for two months. Unlike Dr. Hanna, we believed I had a fast-growing tumor—and that Coley Fluid had halted its growth. But what if the Coley Fluid were to stop working? Sarcomas can suddenly accelerate, and the precarious location could render it inoperable. Bessie Dashiell's knuckle tumor, the size of half an olive, had spread and annexed her body within three months.[4]

We also disliked the idea of a needle biopsy. We'd heard stories from other patients of sarcomas spreading along biopsy needle tracks. The shaft created by even a fine needle could be a gaping multi-lane tunnel into which microscopic cells could pour. Recognizing the danger, some oncologists even advocate surgical removal of the needle track after a positive biopsy.[5] Since we were convinced that the lesion was cancerous, the risks of a biopsy outweighed the need.

An extensive surgery was the best option of the three. I loathed the idea of losing my jaw bone, but surgery had a small chance of curing me—unless there were other invisible tumors lurking. Earlier, Dr. Patel had said that my chances of survival depended on whether my recurrent tumor was an isolated focus of cancer cells or a harbinger of diffuse cancer. If many micro-tumors were waiting to grow, no form of surgery could cure me.

After days of exhausting debate, we concluded it was wishful thinking to hope that I had a single tumor. We based this conclusion on the medical studies and on the odds Dr. Patel had given. Since surgery was unlikely to cure me, my best chance at survival was to keep leveraging immunotherapy to eradicate the micro-tumors in my head.

We believed Coley fluid was the best tool available to achieve this goal. There were already signs it was working: the negative PET, the necrosis, the stable tumor size. And there were virtually no side effects beyond transient fever. If Coley Fluid had necrosed a one centimeter tumor, perhaps it could more easily destroy microscopic cancer? Just as chemo is used to pre-shrink tumors, we could use Coley's Toxins to first eradicate those micro-tumors, thereby maximizing the results of subsequent surgery.

Six Months of Coley's Toxins

The strategy of using immunotherapy to improve the odds of surgery had a precedent: Dr. William Coley adopted the same strategy over a century ago, injecting patients before and after surgery for a total of six months or more. In an era before chemoradiation, he used the toxins to shrink tentacles and eliminate invisible micro-tumors before cutting out large sarcomas. Another surgeon in Belgium, Henri Matagne, also used this strategy to achieve "a percentage of cures much higher than ordinary surgical treatment alone."[6]

Having decided on this strategy, our next step was to implement it. We had already achieved five weeks of Coley infusions. Our goal now was to reach six continuous months.

Direct injection into tumors was one of Dr. Coley's "best practices." Recall from chapter 5 our theory that injections of Coley's Toxins into tumors would cause a sudden surge of innate immune cells. These immune cells would kill some tumor, leading to the creation of T cells against various tumor antigens.

For this reason, we contemplated injecting Coley Fluid into my tumor. Unfortunately, there was no practical way to safely get a needle into it, as the tumor was shielded by my jaw bone. And subcutaneous injections under the skin were not recommended by MBVax (the company that made Coley Fluid). The best we could do was continue with intravenous infusions.

Day after day, Eddy and I slogged through the infusions. Given the dismal prognosis, we had a new resolve; the fevers didn't feel daunting. The mental image of tumors regrowing in my head—like a multi-headed hydra arising from its invisible tentacles—was terrifying enough an incentive. We achieved a rhythm: three to four consecutive days of infusions and fevers, two days of rest. Most fevers exceeded 102.5°F. For the next six months, I would repeat this cycle week after week.

Evaluating treatment

It was crucial to measure the effect of Coley Fluid on my tumor. If Coley Fluid stopped working, we needed to know at once so we could switch strategy. But there were no blood tests to measure the extent of sarcoma in my body. So, Dr. Old suggested we measure blood levels of certain proteins secreted by immune cells. One of these proteins is *interferon gamma*, which increases when the immune system is activated, such as during viral infection.

One midweek afternoon, moments after my Coley fever had peaked, we rushed to a nearby clinic to capture the level of interferon gamma. Despite running a fever of 102°F and feeling fatigued, I managed to hobble into the car with Eddy's help. He drove me down to the clinic for the blood draw, then rushed me back home. I hobbled back into bed. We'd have to wait a few weeks for results.

Scans are the gold standard for measuring tumor growth. Sometimes when a patient is on active treatment, an oncologist may order monthly scans. This way, if therapy fails, treatment can be quickly switched.

As the Coley Fluid was self-administered, no single doctor was ordering scans to closely monitor the progress of my treatment. The oncologist at my local clinic who'd administered the NY-ESO-1 vaccine in 2010 was willing to order scans. But to minimize further confusion, we tried to limit the scans to Stanford or MDA. Somehow, we managed to arrange for monthly scans, alternately from Stanford and MDA.

It was an awkward situation—my care highly fragmented. The doctors who'd treated my original tumor in 2008 were at Stanford, but I no longer had a sarcoma oncologist there. I'd consulted at MDA twice, but had never been treated there; each time I flew to Houston, they'd run a new set of scans. My Coley Fluid infusions were a continuation of treatment begun in Mexico, but my primary physician was ordering weekly blood tests to ensure my safety. Finally, Dr. Old was tracking my progress, doing his best to guide our decision-making, as he was the only one who understood the science.

We had to make the best of this uneasy arrangement. In 2011, immunotherapy was still "experimental." (Yervoy had just been approved in March, but it was still largely viewed as a treatment for melanoma.) To expect my doctors at Stanford and MDA to drive my monitoring needs was unrealistic. I had to take what I could get.

The Smell of Victory (June 30 MRI)

We continued with the Coley fevers. Aside from the monthly MRIs, we were waging a blind war against my tumor, with no way to evaluate moment-by-moment victories or losses. As it had been with Dr. Coley, fever was our only guide.

I kept hitting fevers above 103°F, three, four, sometimes five days consecutively. It was grueling for both Eddy and me; each infusion required a full day's effort. Thankfully, mom prepared all our meals.

While I fevered, Eddy monitored. For endless hours, he sat by my bed, taking my vitals every fifteen minutes and recording them in a spreadsheet. He plied me with blankets and cranked up the heating pad to reduce chills. He kept me hydrated with electrolyte mix. Once a week, he obsessively sterilized my PICC line (through which I received the Coley infusions) to prevent sepsis.

Dr. Old was fascinated I was reliving a forgotten part of American medical history. He implored us to document my experience. We talked frequently by phone, almost weekly. He advised us to cut back the fevers to three times a week, concerned that too much of the toxins might weaken my body.[7]

The next MRI was taken on June 30 at Stanford. With bated breath, we loaded the images onto Eddy's laptop, eager to find out the results of our hard work of generating fevers.

Elation erupted. My tumor seemed to have shriveled!

We hugged each other, crying tears of joy.

Measuring, re-measuring, then measuring again, we estimated a fifty percent shrinkage since May.

We were possessed with exhilarating thoughts: Had we achieved immune control of my tumor? Could my T-cells now hunt down all cancer in my body? *Was a cure within reach?*

The next day, we spoke with Dr. Old. Recently diagnosed with prostate cancer, he was busy dealing with his own medical care. Even so, he made time to call us, his voice strong and bright and eager to hear more about the tumor shrinkage Eddy had reported in an email.

"That's an incredible level of interferon gamma," said Dr. Old, excited at the high levels in my blood (measured the day I hobbled into the clinic). Normal values are between 0 and 5 pg/mL—mine was at 41.

"When I saw that Gamma reading, I suspected we'd see stabilization or decrease in your tumor," said Dr. Old.

Dr. Old then described the importance of interferon gamma, enumerating its benefits, such as its ability to make tumors more recognizable to the immune system and making macrophages and T cells better able to kill tumors.

Intoxicated by this victory of tumor shrinkage, we forged ahead with euphoric optimism, the smell of victory perhaps a scan or two away.

Regrowth? (August 1 MRI)

On August 1, we returned to MD Anderson, brimming with confidence, finally letting our guard down a little. I had completed 33 fevers since my visit in May.

Leading up to the appointment, we'd stopped Coley Fluid for ten days, thinking to minimize the risk of tumor flare (the enlargement of tumors due to the surge of immune cells). Overconfident, we wanted the MDA physicians to see our grand achievement—that we'd succeeded in shrinking an invincible sarcoma with Coley's Toxins. We visualized their amazement, and imagined them wanting to know how I'd achieved the impossible without side effects. Most of all, we were eager to see how much further my tumor would have shrunk. Tumor flare would jeopardize the interpretation of the scans, which is why we stopped Coley Fluid.

An hour before our appointment with Dr. Benjamin, we obtained a CD of the MRI. Scarfing down our lunch, we compared the images against previous scans.

Our elation gave way to dismay.

The MRI showed my tumor had regrown to its May size.

It had become full-looking once more.

The sudden reversal jolted us out of our jubilance. We believed we "had this in the bag"—that, if we kept hitting high fevers, my tumor would surely vanish. This reversal sent us careening down an emotional roller-coaster: *Was the enlargement a manifestation of tumor flare—in which case, the next scan would once again show shrinkage? Or had Coley's Toxins stopped working, and the tumor was now regrowing? Maybe that ten-day break had allowed it to regrow?*

In a twist of irony, the MRI report showed that the senior radiologist didn't think my tumor had shrunk or regrown. Ignoring the Stanford scan from June 30 (that showed shrinkage), he had compared the current scan to the May 25 MRI. This is what he wrote in his report:

"...my sense is that the disease is stable. The question arises as to whether this is an active tumor versus potentially some type of post-treatment effect.

The presence of actual mass-like enhancement certainly suggests persistent disease and that remains my sense despite considerable stability of this finding."

"From May to August, there's no change in your tumor," said Dr. Benjamin, referring to the MRI report. He went on to explain that once sarcomas grow, they don't stop expanding, as mine had. Either the lesion in my head wasn't cancer, or immunotherapy had stabilized it.

Back in the hotel room, a fifteen-minute drive from MDA, we restarted the Coley Fluid infusions, disappointed that the MDA radiologist hadn't performed a more nuanced analysis of my tumor. Nor had he commented on the rapid regrowth over the past month. But these were the days before the greater oncology community was cognizant of the unconventional ways that tumors respond to immunotherapy (as compared to chemoradiation).

"We shouldn't have stopped for those ten days," said Eddy, as he hooked me up to the saline bag containing diluted Coley Fluid, dangling from a portable IV pole. "Maybe that was our mistake. Dr. Coley warned against stopping too soon ..."

Three days later, we again saw Dr. Hanna, the head and neck surgeon. Like Dr. Benjamin, he, too, felt that my tumor had stabilized over the three months, based on the MRIs. He suggested holding off on surgery.

In essence, our MDA consultants had effectively confirmed that Coley Fluid had arrested my high grade recurrent sarcoma for three months. Votrient would soon be hailed as the first new drug approved for sarcoma in decades. The FDA would green-light it based on its ability to arrest tumor growth by an average of 4.6 months (even though it didn't extend the overall life-span of patients).[8] In return for the temporary delay in tumor growth, patients on Votrient experienced a long list of side effects which included significant fatigue; liver damage; lowered blood counts; pain and swelling in the hands and feet; and even death.[9] In contrast, Coley Fluid had given me almost the same amount of delay in tumor growth—but with no side effects.

The significant "stability" of my tumor had led my doctors to question the recurrence of my cancer. We remembered Dr. Coley's skeptics. Incredulous that his toxins could reverse invincible sarcomas, they explained away his successes by disputing the diagnoses of his patients.[10]

Even though our MDA consultants had said my tumor was stable, we had no doubt that I had an aggressive, fast-rebounding tumor. The illusion of stability was only because they had not looked at all of my scans. Trying not to panic, we remembered how Dr. Coley experienced temporary setbacks, later to salvage the situation by using stronger doses or more frequent injections. Perhaps the ten-day break had given my tumor a chance to regrow? Perhaps resuming the toxins more aggressively would shrink it once again?

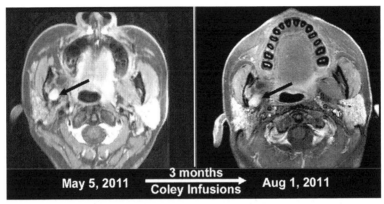

Figure 29: Comparison between 5/5/2011 and 8/1/2011 MRIs gives **false impression** of stability over a three-month period.

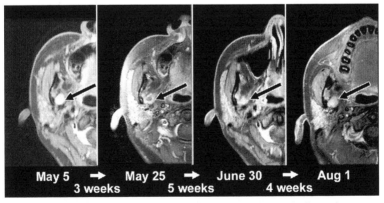

Figure 30: Monthly MRIs reveal tumor changes: By May 25, it hollowed out. By June 30, it shrunk to 0.5 cm. By August 1, it regrew to 1.1 cm.

Back again in the hotel room, we started another infusion. As my fever peaked and ebbed, I was overcome with a sense of weariness. By now, I'd completed 54 fevers over a span of four months, with many exceeding 104°F.

Despite the hard work, Coley Fluid had postponed my death *with no side effects*. Yes, it required lugging bulky medical supplies wherever we went: IV tubing, bags of saline, alcohol swabs, syringes and a mishmash of fifty different parts for keeping my PICC line sterile. Yes, it stole hours from our days and precluded us returning to work and normal life. But I was still alive! And aside from the lingering fatigue from chemo, I felt normal. I determined not to stop fevering—until it was clear that Coley Fluid no longer worked.

As my fever subsided, the phone rang. It was Dr. Old, calling in response to another email update from Eddy. This time, his voice was weak from the pain of his advancing cancer.

"The stability you got from May ... that's a good duration ... that's what you get from Yervoy. I wouldn't call that discouraging," said Dr. Old, seeking to cheer us. "I would see this as further validation of continuing the toxins ... without question."

Eddy and I began to tear up as we listened to Dr. Old's halting speech. We visualized the pain he was enduring. Despite his misery, our brave and noble mentor instead sought to comfort and encourage us.

Noting the possibility of tumor flare, Dr. Old suggested it was reasonable to wait another month before concluding that my cancer was progressing. For as long as my tumor remained stable, he felt I should continue with Coley's, then transition to PD-1 inhibitor clinical trials once they became available.

Tumor Flare or Tumor Growth?

Did the regrowth in August represent immune cells attacking dying cancer? Or was my tumor actually enlarging? Unfortunately, the scans couldn't answer the question.

Recall from chapter 7 that Mr. Telford—the melanoma patient to whom Dr. Jedd Wolchok had given Yervoy in 2006—experienced initial growth of his liver and kidney tumors at 12 weeks. Perhaps that growth was a result of tumor flare? Thankfully, Dr. Wolchok had waited another two months instead of giving up, enabling him to catch the belated tumor shrinkage. Mr. Telford's experience demonstrates the importance of giving immunotherapy time to work.

We would later befriend a sarcoma patient, Jake, and his wife. Jake had exhausted all conventional therapy. His cancer was advancing in his lungs. The FDA had approved the PD-1 inhibitor, Opdivo, for melanoma. And clinical trials for sarcoma had begun. We referred Jake to a physician in Los Angeles who'd administered Opdivo to hundreds of patients. But he decided to enroll in a clinical trial in Tulsa, Oklahoma.

Nine weeks after receiving Opdivo, a scan showed slight growth of his lung tumors. The inexperienced Tulsa doctors booted him off the trial, believing the treatment had failed. Jake re-engaged the veteran doctor in Los Angeles who advised him to re-scan three weeks later. That later scan showed all of his lung tumors had either shrunk or stabilized. Like Mr. Telford's, Jake's experience demonstrates the importance of not jumping to premature conclusions without giving enough time for immunotherapy to work.

Still, to hope that the regrowth in my head would soon be followed by shrinkage was a gamble. If my tumor continued its one-month doubling rate, it would measure two centimeters by the next scan, risking inoperability. Were we playing with fire? Was it now time for surgery? Or should we first try to recreate the shrinkage we'd achieved earlier with Coley's Toxins?

After much debate, we decided to give it another month. Waiting for the next scan was terrifying.

An Unbiased Analysis

With nervous resolve, we continued the Coley infusions. Meanwhile, we sought clarity on the MRIs. The analyses we'd gotten from MDA and Stanford were incomplete. That my Coley Fluid wasn't administered by either institution—and that both institutions only looked at their own scans—confused the issue. But that was the reality of my fragmented care.

We'd not come this far to be confounded by logistics. Those monthly scans contained objective information crucial to decision-making. From the sarcoma internet forum, Eddy had learned of a consultation service that offered advice from doctors at the Dana-Farber Cancer Institute—the top cancer center in New England. The service provided expert medical opinions remotely to patients around the world. Realizing that their radiologists routinely analyzed MRI images from external institutions, we paid for all my MRIs to be cohesively reviewed.

"6/30/2011: Lesion is much smaller measuring only 5 x 4 mm ... with minimal enhancement," wrote the radiologist, confirming our amateur assessment that my tumor had shrunk in June.

"However on the most recent study done on 8/1/2011, lesion has increased in size to 11 x 8 mm ... very similar to study dated 5/5/2011," he wrote, further confirming the regrowth.

Having an experienced radiologist verify that Coley Fluid had indeed shrunk my tumor in June gave us a sliver of hope. Perhaps if we increased dosage or eschewed ten-day breaks, we could once again shrink the tumor?

The September MRI

I completed another 16 fevers. Petrified by the doubling of my tumor, we ratcheted up the toxin dosage, which caused me to hit a fever of 105.9°F. This was the one time I experienced an unexpected side effect—babbling. For about 10 minutes, I babbled semi-coherently, as Eddy ran to grab an ice pack. Wrapping it in a small towel, he placed it on my head. He also ran to grab Tylenol, ready to kill the fever if it worsened. But the cold helped, my temperature stabilized and I regained full alertness.

As the weeks passed, I began to experience disturbing symptoms. It became increasingly difficult to open my mouth—hardly wide enough to insert a toothbrush. I experienced night sweats. My appetite vanished. These symptoms greatly troubled us. We knew they portended bad news. But we'd chosen our path.

It was September 1, 2011, time for the scan—this time at Stanford.

Huddled in our bedroom, shades down, laptop open, the screen dark, Eddy deftly scrolled to the relevant image.

Lying next to my jawbone sat the lesion.

It hadn't gone away.

It hadn't shrunk.

It measured 1.5 cm across—50 percent larger than a month ago—and now comprised two "lobes."

It pushed against neighboring structures—the jawbone to the right, the salivary gland to the rear, the throat to the left—and eroded the muscle in which it was growing.

It was jostling for more space in my head.

CHAPTER 11

Combining Immunotherapy for Better Results

IN THE SURGERY STAGING AREA in the basement of the Detroit Medical Center, I sat propped up in a hospital bed. I was being prepped for a procedure known as *cryoablation*. The procedure would be performed by a specialist known as an *interventional radiologist*. These are radiologists who go beyond reading scans—they take action to help solve medical problems.

Peter Littrup, M.D., would soon insert special needles—1.7 mm thick and 23 cm long—straight through my face to reach my jaw tumor. A machine would pass argon gas through the hollow needles, bringing the tips down to a chilling -180°C (-292°F). The extreme cold would form an ice ball, killing any living cells within it, including the tumor. The ice ball would be left to thaw, and the freeze cycle repeated. Three cycles would destroy my tumor.

Dr. Littrup had presented my case to the tumor board. A head and neck surgeon cautioned that the cryoablation could cause intense inflammation and swelling, compromising my ability to breathe. Dr. Littrup offered steroids to reduce the swelling, but I declined, seeking to avoid inadvertent suppression of my immune system.

Cryoablation had an important advantage over surgery. Not only could it directly destroy my tumor, but it could teach my immune system to attack cancer in other parts of my body. This is known as the *abscopal effect*.

So important was the abscopal effect that, if necessary, I was willing to undergo a tracheostomy—an incision through my neck and windpipe would be made to create an artificial airway, should my throat swell shut. They didn't think it would come down to that. But for safety, an uncomfortable breathing tube was placed down my throat.

The anesthesia dripped into my bloodstream. I felt groggy. I let go, entrusting my welfare into the hands of my physicians for a procedure I'd never experienced.

The procedure was over. Guided by a CT scanner, Dr. Littrup had inserted four needles straight through my cheek, reaching deep into the back of my jaw. He took care not to damage critical nerves and blood vessels in my head. The needles shaped an ice ball that not only encompassed my 1.7 cm tumor, but also the adjacent jawbone. Cryoablation did what surgery couldn't; it killed the cancer in the bone, eliminating the need for amputation of my jaw. Altogether, the procedure had taken two hours.

The next 16 hours were pure hell—not from the cryo, but from the discomfort of the breathing tube. The anesthesiologist had promised to keep me sedated to minimize gagging caused by the tube. But she disappeared and the ICU staff refused me sedation. Not believing our recounting of a similar experience with a breathing tube in 2008, they insisted I was suffering from post-operative nausea and instead prescribed anti-nausea medication.

At midnight, a nurse tried to jam a nasal tube down my nose for oral medications. Unable to speak because of the breathing tube in my throat, I whimpered in pain. Tears streamed down my cheeks. As he retracted the tube, it was lined with blood. I spent most of the night coughing and gagging, unable to speak or to convince the doctors to give me the sedative.

The next morning, a doctor dropped by. He relented and prescribed the sedative. The gagging and coughing finally abated.

Hours later, a team of doctors came to insert the nasal tube. Using proper tools and technique, it went in smoothly. No bleeding this time.

I stared at the mirror. It took a moment to get over the grotesque tubes emanating from my nose and mouth. A single Band-Aid covered the holes on my cheek through which Dr. Littrup had inserted his needles. The right side of my face ballooned like a chipmunk's, a result of intense inflammation caused by the destruction of tissue that had been unleashed in my head.

Billions of immune cells were swarming the area, drawn to the ball of dead tumor.

Debating Cryoablation Versus Surgery

"What would you do if you were in this situation," Eddy asked Monica, as we

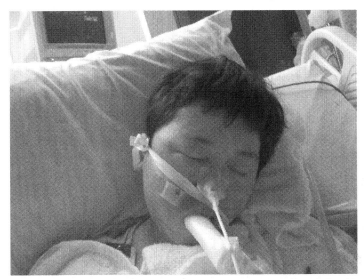

Figure 31: In the ICU after cryoablation. Translucent breathing tube parallels white rolled-up gauze which prevented me from biting down on breathing tube. Thin nasal tube threaded through my nose supplied liquid medications. Small bandage covered puncture sites. Right cheek swollen from acute inflammation.

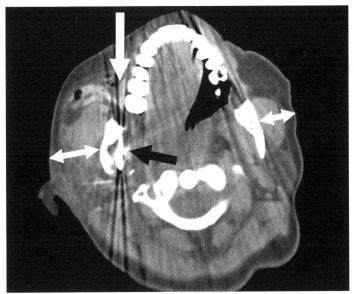

Figure 32: CT image of cryoablation. White single arrow: direction in which cryoablation needle was inserted. Black single arrow: tip of one of four needles. White double arrows: comparison of right cheek (intensely swollen and inflamed) with left cheek (not cryoablated). (Note: image is horizontally inverse. Right cheek appears on the left.)

sat in the living room at my parents' home, the weekend before my cryoablation procedure. Monica was a colleague from Professor Lucy Shapiro's research lab. Over the years, we'd grown to value her balanced perspective.

"Hmm ... that's a hard one," she said, pausing to ponder the alternative.

We'd recounted the low likelihood that the bright mass on MRI was the only focus of cancer. We also recounted the potential negatives of surgery, how it could delay my return to immunotherapy, accelerate existing disease (by triggering growth-promoting substances), and impact my quality of life (from pain or inability to chew food).

We told Monica about cryoablation, how it was also a form of immunotherapy. Since 1972, scientists have observed that freezing one tumor teaches the immune system to attack others, sometimes causing distant untreated tumors to vanish mysteriously.[1,2,3,4]

"We know what results to expect from surgery, but tell me more how this abscopal effect works?" asked Monica.

"The key is frozen tumor is left in the body. Immune cells such as dendritic cells come to garbage-collect the dead tumor cells. In the process, the immune system is awakened to cancer, creating T cells that can attack my cancer," I said.

"Maybe my tumor had escaped Coley's because it no longer expressed NY-ESO-1—that single target Dr. Old had vaccinated me against. Cryoablation might salvage the situation, acting like a broader vaccine, inoculating me against the plurality of antigens found in my tumor."

Continuing to explain the other advantages of cryoablation, I described how it doesn't change the way tumor proteins look, unlike heat-based ablation. Preserving these antigens was crucial. Otherwise, immune cells can't be taught to go after similarly looking remote tumors.

"Think of freezing and then defrosting a piece of meat—how the thawed meat still resembles fresh meat," I said. "In contrast, when you cook an egg—you denature it ... The proteins don't look the same anymore."

"Another advantage is freezing causes acute inflammation. Think of the pain and redness that accompanies frostbite ... that's inflammation—it represents immune cells rushing in to heal and clean out dead tissue," I said.[5] "The violent cell death creates danger signals, like when bacteria infect a wound.[6] The inflammation and danger signals help awaken the immune system to the cancer."

"Don't forget how non-invasive cryo can be," said Eddy, reminding me that the recovery time is much shorter than surgery. Usually, cryoablation is an outpatient procedure, often done under local anesthesia. As the needles are slender, no large cuts are needed, and, once retracted, minimal bleeding occurs. When done, the interventional radiologist slaps on a small adhesive bandage over the puncture wound, monitors the patient for an hour or two, then sends the patient home.

"If you choose cryo over surgery, you'll be able to resume Coley's or other immunotherapies much sooner," said Eddy.

"So, from what I'm hearing, cryo has all these advantages—the ability to vaccinate against whole tumors, faster healing, shorter interruption to immunotherapy. But how about the disadvantages?" asked Monica.

"The main disadvantage is there's no way to verify that you've gotten it all—that is, if the ice ball has encompassed all of the tumor's microscopic extensions," I said. "In contrast, during surgery, the surgeon gets to check margins … He sends samples from the cut edge to a pathologist who looks for microscopic tumor. If none is found, the surgeon is reasonably confident that he's gotten the microscopic extensions. But with cryo, you're making a best-guess," I said.

"But does the ability to inspect margins really matter in this situation?" said Eddy. "If surgery can't get all other invisible tumors, it won't matter if cryo fails to get the microscopic tentacles in the margins of the visible tumor. So, the more important question is whether there are other unseen tumors besides this one."

Deep in thought, Monica weighed the pros and cons of surgery versus cryoablation. As the sun set, the room grew dark, and she gave us her verdict.

"Given all that I've heard, I think I'd choose cryo. The odds for a surgical cure are low, as corroborated by your MD Anderson oncologists. So I'd want the faster healing, the fewer side effects and the potential immune effects of cryo," said Monica.

Defying My Doctors

Decisions that determine one's fate are difficult to face. This was why, at the start of my cancer diagnosis, I'd instantly accepted my doctor's recommendations without doing more research. The specter of death compelled me to believe that the accomplished person in the white coat sitting across me—the one with academic accolades from prestigious institutions—held the keys to my survival.

Doctors, no matter how experienced, knowledgeable and compassionate, can only speak to their area of expertise. A sage medical oncologist like Dr. Benjamin can assess my survival odds after surgery or chemo. An expert surgeon like Dr. Kaplan at Stanford or Dr. Hanna at MDA can craft the best surgical approach. An experienced radiologist can describe the tumor down to the millimeter, listing structures it's invaded. And the rare cancer immunologist like Dr. Old can help me choose immunotherapies.

On September 1, 2011, 12 days before the cryoablation—when the MRI showed a resurging tumor that had escaped five months of Coley's Toxins—we'd immediately scheduled a surgery with Dr. Kaplan. But as we awaited the procedure, we vacillated again, afraid that the fear-driven impulse to cut out the tumor was a mistake.

Immunotherapy was not part of the "flowchart" for treating sarcoma. There were zero guidelines on how to incorporate it, let alone in the urgent context of a fast-rebounding tumor. This is still the case in 2016.

Would surgery prolong my life more than if I were to double-down on immunotherapy? Or would surgery instead accelerate existing micro-tumors in my head, sealing my death? And how would I know whether the cryoablation would lead to abscopal effects?

"I feel strongly that this is a significantly poor decision. The tissue is deep such that cryo access is a problem. Are you sure you don't want to rethink your decision?" wrote Dr. Kaplan. "Both MD Anderson and Stanford have, with unanimity, recommended this be removed surgically, and that opinion is evidence-based. Cryo is not recommended and may make surgery more difficult later. I strongly recommend you reconsider."

Dr. Kaplan, my fiercely caring surgeon who'd saved me from the burgeoning original tumor in 2008, sent this email urging us to reconsider our decision. He'd called earlier, sacrificing his precious surgeon's time. He had our best interest at heart. He'd supported me in my journey over the years, ordering scans even after Dr. Ganjoo dropped me. He'd always been open-minded, never heavy-handed, always wanting to make sure we had the right information for balanced decisions. This time, he spent three hours on the phone to convince us we were diving into a mistake. When someone you trust goes out of the way to warn you, you can't help but seriously reconsider.

All the experts recommended surgery: Dr. Kaplan, Dr. Benjamin, Dr. Hanna—even Dr. Old. Earlier in May, when we'd struggled over Coley's Toxins versus surgery, Dr. Old had supported our decision to do Coley's Toxins. But now, he felt that surgery offered the advantage of analyzing tumor tissue. Finding T cells in my tumor would tell us the vaccine-induced T cells had reached their target—but that maybe something else was preventing them from destroying the tumor. That insight could prove useful in charting the next step.

Despite the views of our trusted experts, we couldn't discount cryo. Our physicians had the ethical and legal duty to recommend "proven" surgery—but it was proven only to eliminate the detectable tumor. We couldn't ignore the low likelihood that surgery would "get it all"—as my doctors and the medical literature had corroborated.

Also, none of my doctors could speak to the recent advances in cryoablation technology. Like immunotherapy, researchers had tried cryoablation in the 1970s and 1980s and found it inferior to surgery. Older, crude cryoprobes had caused too much collateral damage to surrounding healthy tissue, leading to unacceptable complications that stemmed from permanently damaged organs, such as bowels, bile ducts and urethras.[7] Like immunotherapy, only a small group of researchers tracked the latest advances in cryoablation technology. But modern cryoablation was yielding dramatically improved results. Newer machines were forming consistent ice balls that could reliably kill tumors. Finer and stronger needles, able to penetrate deep into most parts of the body, could sculpt precise ice balls that encompassed tumors, while minimizing damage to surrounding tissues.

Lesson learned: Patients who use fast-evolving medicines and techniques (such as immunotherapy and cryoablation) often have to consult leading specialists. They then have to carefully assess whether these procedures are advantageous over conventional treatment. They may also face opposition from their conventional doctors, who may deem these techniques experimental.

For a meaningful opinion on cryoablation, we had to consult Dr. Littrup. We'd learned about him from the mother of a sarcoma patient. The patient,

John, a young man in his twenties, was still alive *seven years* after being diagnosed with metastatic sarcoma in both lungs. Every few months, new lung tumors would appear. Instead of debilitating lung surgeries that required weeks of hospitalization, John opted for simple outpatient cryoablation. He'd cryoablate the lung tumors, then go right back to running ten-kilometer races.

Dr. Littrup had performed over 1000 cryoablations in all parts of the body. He explained that cryoablation caused much milder side effects than surgery. He also explained that, unlike radiation, tumors cannot become resistant to freezing. If a first cryoablation fails, it can be repeated in the same spot.

Dr. Littrup also explained that the success rate for treating small tumors (less than 3 cm) approximated that of surgery. Even larger tumors could be treated effectively. In other words, very few tumors cryoablated by an experienced physician would regrow, making it an attractive alternative to surgery.

Since surgery alone had a low chance of curing me, my best bet was to try again to harness my immune system against my cancer. Cryoablation offered the possibility of generating the abscopal effect by leaving dead tumor cells in my head as a vaccine. At the same time, it would destroy the main tumor and therefore buy me some time. These advantages made cryoablation a strong candidate as one part of a complex strategy (soon to be discussed).

In addition, we would pursue surgery after taking advantage of the dead tumor cells in my head—just in case our efforts at immunotherapy would fail to cure me.

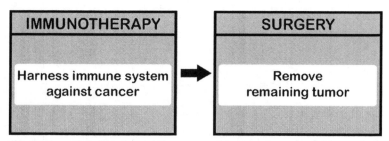

Figure 33: Our overall strategy to beat the recurrent sarcoma in my head (September 2011).

Delayed in Detroit

At the Detroit Medical Center, I recuperated for three days in the ICU, connected to the mechanical ventilator. It forced air through my breathing tube. At one point, Eddy observed that my torso movements seemed grossly exaggerated, like a blow-up toy being mercilessly inflated and deflated over and over.

Finally, it was time to be unhooked. The doctors said I hadn't needed it anyway. Even without steroids, the swelling in my throat wasn't as bad as they'd feared.

A rather huge man—maybe twice my 100 pounds—came by to wheel me downstairs for the tube to be removed. While transporting me, he operated a hand-pump to ventilate my lungs in place of the machine. I felt a sudden sharp pain in my lungs. Alarmed, I gestured to him, then wrote a note asking he not pump so hard.

"Your blood work looks good. I'll sign the discharge papers," said the ENT (ear, nose and throat) resident, leaving the room.

Cryoablation was supposed to have been minimally invasive—maybe even an outpatient procedure—but because I required the breathing tube to protect my airway, I'd been hospitalized for four days already.

We'd planned to fly to Germany right after the cryoablation to receive an immunotherapy called a dendritic vaccine. And it was important that we get there as soon as possible after the cryoablation.

Antsy to leave, I awaited the nurse.

Two hours later, she entered with discharge papers and instructions for home care. Eddy had already packed my belongings. As I got up to change out of my hospital gown, I felt weak and unsteady.

"I feel kind of weak," I said to the nurse. "Maybe I should take a walk around the ward … see if I'm able to do that before you discharge me?"

"You're probably just weak from lying in bed for so many days. But go ahead," she said.

Mom steadied me as I walked down the corridor. She'd flown in from California two days earlier. As we turned the corner, I began to wheeze and lost my breath. Mom rushed me back to my room.

I sat on the bed, out of breath. Seconds later, the doctor who had authorized my discharge came rushing in a panic.

"You can't go!" he said. Apparently, he hadn't checked my chest X-ray (taken hours earlier) before discharging me.

Catching his breath, he said, "Your left lung has collapsed."

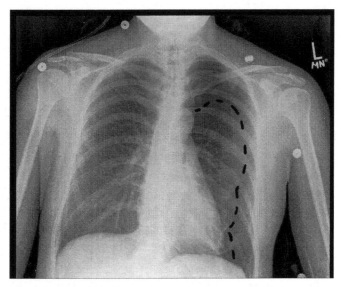

Figure 34: X-ray showing my left lung had collapsed—a 40 percent pneumothorax (boundary of left lung outlined in dashed line for easier viewing). A normal lung occupies the entire rib cage, as with my right lung. (September 17, 2011)

Devising a Combination Strategy

In the days leading up to the cryoablation procedure, we'd devised a two-pronged strategy to harness an immune response against my cancer. We spent every minute of the day (outside the continuing Coley infusions) obsessing over this strategy.

Dr. Old had taught us that training the immune system to attack cancer (with T cells) was only the first step. Stripping away tumor defenses was crucial to improve the odds of success.

Eddy and I were drawn to this "combination approach." We'd already used it when combining my NY-ESO-1 vaccine with Coley's Toxins. Our plan was to continue with more of this strategy.

By now, Dr. Old's cancer had advanced further, and our communication with him had lessened. It was time for us to chart our own course, with what we'd learned about the immune system.

The first part of our plan was to ensure that T cells were created against a broad array of tumor antigens. While we hoped for the abscopal effect, we didn't think that cryoablation was a foolproof method of creating T cells. After all, the abscopal effect is not always observed in patients receiving cryoablation. Seeking to increase our chances of creating T cells, we planned to add another immunotherapy—dendritic vaccination.

Dendritic vaccines were an established method of creating T cells against cancer. Over a year earlier in April 2010, the FDA had approved a dendritic vaccine (Provenge) for treating prostate cancer in the U.S.[8] From the cancer journalist Ralph Moss, Ph.D., we'd learned that the German FDA allowed physicians to create their own dendritic vaccines for *any* cancer, not just prostate cancer.[9]

One German physician, Thomas Nesselhut, M.D., Ph.D., had been offering the procedure for years. Since 2003, he'd presented the results of his vaccines at the annual conferences of the American Society of Clinical Oncology (ASCO), thus boosting his credibility.[10]

After contacting Dr. Nesselhut, he'd agreed to remove dendritic cells (DCs) from my body, stimulate them with certain compounds, then re-inject them near the dead tumor in my jaw. Dr. Nesselhut's own experience had shown that these stimulated DCs were better able to "capture" dead tumor antigen and activate T cells against cancer.

We also surveyed other methods of creating T cells besides cryoablation and dendritic vaccination. Adoptive T cell procedures were the premier approach, but I didn't qualify for clinical trials. Radiation was another method—amazingly, this conventional therapy that's normally thought to harm the immune system can act as an immunotherapy. However, I'd already received the maximum dose of radiation possible to my head. Scientists even believed that chemotherapy could create T cells by killing tumors in the body.[11] All of these methods are being tested in clinical trials today. But in 2011, the safest tools we knew of were cryoablation and dendritic vaccines. Like Coley's Toxins, they had few side effects beyond temporary fevers or inflammation.

For the second part of our strategy—the stripping away of tumor defenses—we hoped the months of Coley's Toxins, including up to two days before cryo, would have depleted Tregs from my tumors. Tregs are those fearsome bodyguards that protect tumors by killing T cells. Aside from Coley's Toxins, another inexpensive method for reducing Tregs was a low-dose course of the chemo drug, cyclophosphamide (which you might recall from chapter 7). For five days leading up to the cryoablation procedure, I took cyclophosphamide pills under the supervision of my doctor.

The most powerful ways to remove tumor defenses were checkpoint inhibitors. The FDA had already approved Yervoy (the CTLA-4 inhibitor) for melanoma, so I could get it off-label—perhaps travel to a foreign country where I could buy it at the cost price of $30,000 per infusion (instead of the marked-up $150,000). Besides the exorbitant cost, we were concerned about the potential autoimmune side effects Yervoy might trigger, such as inflammation of the lungs, inflammation of the gut or even intestinal perforations.

Opdivo (a PD-1 inhibitor) was safer, but it was years from approval. Our plan was for me to stay alive long enough for it to be approved. Once approved, we could incorporate it into our combination strategy.

In summary, the two-pronged strategy we devised was to generate T cells (with cryoablation and dendritic vaccination), while stripping tumor defenses (with low-dose cyclophosphamide and Coley's Toxins). We'd then follow this strategy with surgery as an "insurance policy"—just in case these efforts at immunotherapy were to fail.

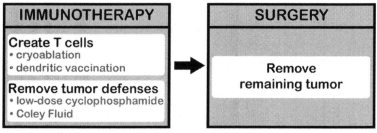

Figure 35: Overall strategy expanded to show details of complex immunotherapy plan (September 2011)

Combination immunotherapy was still a young concept in 2011, still being tested in mice. But MD Anderson experts had confirmed that my immunotherapy efforts had halted my sarcoma for three months. The partial success inspired us to double-down on combination immunotherapy. It gave us the courage to cancel surgery with Dr. Kaplan and proceed with cryoablation. Instead of settling for the temporary delaying of my cancer by surgery, we were determined to achieve the cure that Dr. Coley had proved possible.

Unleashing Cryoablation's Abscopal Effect on Mice and Men

Although few physicians were paying attention to the immune effects of cryoablation, there were some who, in 2011, had recognized its potential. One such person was Dr. James Allison, the discoverer of CTLA-4.

Dr. Allison and his colleagues performed a study of mice injected with prostate cancer cells.[12] In each of the mice, the cells grew into a tumor.

In one group of mice, the tumor was cryoablated when it reached a certain size. A second group of mice received only CTLA-4 blocking antibodies. The third group received a *combination* of cryoablation and CTLA-4 antibodies.

All mice were then *re-challenged*, meaning they were injected again with cancer cells—on the opposite side of the body—to create a second tumor.

The researchers found that in 44 percent of the mice treated with the combination, the second tumors never grew. Their immune systems had become capable of rejecting prostate cancer. The remaining combination-treated mice experienced slower growth of their second tumor. In contrast, all other mice that received either cryoablation or CTLA-4 antibodies alone experienced no benefit. The results suggested that the combination therapy could somehow mobilize the immune system against cancer.

Following this mouse experiment, a human trial of cryoablation with Yervoy commenced at Memorial Sloan Kettering (where Dr. Allison was based at the time).[13] That trial would employ a similar strategy to what we'd devised: cryoablate the tumor; harness dead tumor in the breast to activate the immune system; strip tumor defenses (with Yervoy); then surgically remove the breast "just in case" the immunotherapy alone couldn't destroy the main tumor. The researchers hoped that the combination of cryoablation and Yervoy would activate the patients' immune systems, thereby preventing recurrence or spread of breast cancer beyond the main tumor.

The synergy observed in Dr. Allison's mouse study could be explained by the reduction of Tregs by CTLA-4 inhibitors. Tregs are those fearsome bodyguards of tumors described in chapter 7. By reducing Tregs, CTLA-4 inhibitors allow the T cells created by cryoablation to attack tumors. Similarly, Dr. Old believed that Coley's Toxins could also deplete Tregs, allowing my vaccine-induced T cells to attack my tumor.

Inspired by Dr. Allison's mouse study, we planned to follow my cryoablation with more Coley's Toxins after we returned from Germany.

Another way to deplete Tregs was to use low doses of cyclophosphamide.[14] In another mouse study performed at Johns Hopkins, cryoablation combined with cyclophosphamide cured 45 percent of mice implanted with tumors, making them immune to further re-challenge.[15] The results were similar to Dr. Allison's study.

Also inspired by the Johns Hopkins mouse study, we decided to incorporate low-dose cyclophosphamide into my combination strategy.

Doubling-up on Checkpoint Inhibitors

Combination approaches do not merely seek to marry the creation of T cells with the removal of tumor defenses. Combination approaches can also strengthen the chances of achieving each of these goals.

One strategy Dr. Old had mentioned was to combine CTLA-4 and PD-1 inhibitors. As CTLA-4 and PD-1 are two separate pathways by which tumors evade the immune system, it made sense that combining them would yield better results.

In the summer of 2013, this powerful combination would be tested in a large 945-patient trial of melanoma patients.[16] The trial showed that more patients experienced tumor shrinkage, and their tumors stayed away for longer than if either checkpoint inhibitor was used alone. (At the same time, the combination also led to a higher incidence of autoimmune side effects.)

Galvanized by the early success, scientists and companies today are testing all sorts of combinations in clinical trials, hoping to unleash the immune system against cancer.

Radiation: An Immunotherapy Accessible to All

As mentioned, one approach we considered for creating T cells was radiation. Because it's a conventional therapy and so widely available, it's an essential tool that anyone seeking immunotherapy should be aware of.

Radiation has earned a reputation as one of the feared triumvirate of "slash, burn, poison" (surgery, radiation, chemo). Large doses to certain parts of the body can damage the immune system. But surprisingly, radiation can also help awaken the immune system to tumors.

We were in touch with a researcher at Harvard Medical School, Vikas Sukhatme, M.D., Sc.D. Professor Sukhatme was interested in Coley's Toxins, and we'd been in communication ever since our adventure in Tijuana. Professor Sukhatme was the first to point us to the evidence that even small doses of radiation can act like a vaccine.

Like cryoablation, radiation is thought to achieve this vaccine effect by killing some tumor cells, which are also left in the body. Like cryoablation, radiation also causes acute inflammation, attracting immune cells to the site of cell death and activating T cells against tumor antigens.

The radiation-induced vaccine effect is likely what had caused my Graves' Disease. The radiation treatment I received in 2008 probably killed some cells of my thyroid gland, thus "vaccinating" me against my own thyroid. This led to the unrelenting attack of my thyroid by T cells.

American physicians have observed the abscopal effect since 1956. Two surgeons at the University of Illinois—Tilden Everson, M.D., and Warren Cole, M.D.—published an analysis of 47 spontaneous regressions across many cancers.[17] Intriguingly, some of these patients had received small amounts of radiation—not enough to kill cancer, yet their cancers mysteriously vanished. Eddy and I believed that radiation had sensitized these patients' immune systems to their cancers, leading to the regressions.

This powerful abscopal effect was also observed by Dr. Jedd Wolchok and his colleagues at Memorial Sloan Kettering; their findings would soon be published in the New England Journal of Medicine. A patient in a Yervoy clinical trial had progressive disease despite receiving the CTLA-4 inhibitor since August 2009. She had new tumors growing in her spleen and one next to her spine, causing back pain. To ease the pain, her doctors administered radiation in December 2010. One month after radiation, her tumors were still enlarging.

In February 2011, her doctors gave her another dose of Yervoy. The next scan in April 2011 showed the tumor next to her spine had shrunk significantly. Amazingly, the other tumors in her body that *weren't* irradiated had also shrunk. Six months later, they remained regressed. Based on the timing of shrinkage, Dr. Wolchok and his colleagues believed that radiation had led to the abscopal effect, enabling her immune system to eradicate her tumors (assisted by Yervoy).[18]

News of the abscopal effect spread throughout the medical community such that when former President Jimmy Carter was diagnosed with metastatic melanoma to the brain, his informed oncologists didn't just prescribe Keytruda (a PD-1 inhibitor), but gave him a combination of radiation with Keytruda.[19] These informed oncologists likely knew that radiation would help sensitize his immune system to his cancer, creating T cells that recognize various cancer antigens. And Keytruda would strip the tumor's defenses, allowing the T cells to attack his brain tumors.

A final example of the power of radiation can be seen in this case study of a 53-year-old man.[20] He had far advanced melanoma that no longer responded to CTLA-4 or PD-1 inhibitors. A huge 18-cm-long tumor was annexing the back of his neck. Only after receiving radiation to his neck along with PD-1 inhibitors did the enormous tumor begin to shrink. The dose of radiation alone could not generate the dramatic and rapid shrinkage. So, his doctors believed that radiation had sensitized his immune system to his cancer, enabling his immune system to finally eliminate the large tumor (helped by PD-1).

The "salvaging" of failed checkpoint inhibitor therapy by radiation exemplifies why one should not give up too soon with immunotherapy. Unlike Jimmy Carter's doctors, not all oncologists may be aware of these synergies. Therefore, informed patients should talk to their doctors about adding radiation if PD-1 or CTLA-4 inhibitors fail.

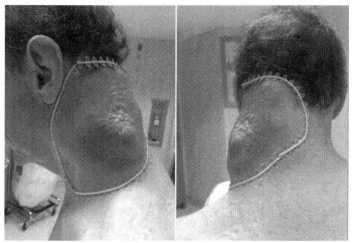

Figure 36: 53-year-old melanoma patient with huge 18x15x8 cm tumor, resistant to PD-1 and CTLA-4 inhibitors.[H]

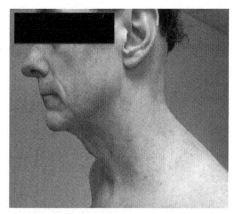

Figure 37: Tumor gone five months later after radiation, while continuing PD-1 inhibitors.[H]

The Chest Tube

We were on a timeline. I'd taken low-dose cyclophosphamide, and then had my tumor cryoablated. The next step of our combination strategy was to fly to Germany, where I'd receive dendritic vaccines to capture dead tumor antigens in my head.

After a four-day delay from the breathing tube nightmare, I'd learned that my left lung had collapsed. I knew then that it would be weeks before I would be allowed to board a plane. With each day that passed, dead tumor antigens were dissipating, cleared out by immune cells.

The resident came to discuss my collapsed lung. Suave, sporting a neat mustache and exuding confidence, he explained what had transpired.

"A lung is like a balloon. When there's a leak, it collapses and can't transport oxygen into the blood. This is called a *pneumothorax*. Air leaks out into the chest cavity, accumulating outside the lung. The trapped air prevents the lung from re-inflating. The only way to fix it—create a path for that air to escape. Only then can your lung find room to re-inflate."

"We'll need to put a small tube into the side of your chest to extract the air. The surgeon will come up soon."

"OK. Small is good ..."

The resident left the room. An hour later, he returned.

"The surgeon's busy. I'll be doing the procedure instead."

"Um, I would really like the surgeon to do it."

"Your pneumothorax is *pretty* major. The surgeon's busy. We need to do this now."

"Err ... OK ... I guess ..."

"I'll need your mother and husband to clear out of the room."

"That's the tube?" I asked. "Looks more like a garden hose!"

"Don't worry, it'll be over soon."

For the next few minutes, I experienced the most excruciating pain I'd ever felt as the resident pushed the garden hose through the incision in the side of my chest, parting muscles between my ribs.

Amid the searing pain, I screamed, gripping the hand of the closest nurse.

Finally, he'd inserted enough—over one foot of tubing.

Without comment, he sutured the tube in place, then cleared out of the room. That was the last I'd see of him.

The Skewer

The chest tube drained into a special container through a few feet of transparent tubing. The container had markings to track the amount of fluid and blood oozing from my chest. It connected to a mild vacuum pump, which sucked out trapped air to help my lung expand.

Now came the wait. The tube would allow my lung to re-inflate. But somewhere in my lung, a small tear needed to heal naturally. If it didn't, I'd need lung repair surgery.

Days passed. Air bubbles kept emanating from my lungs—the leak wasn't healing. The resident never checked on his handiwork. Instead, three other residents took turns.

After one week of daily X-rays, there wasn't improvement. Dejected, stuck with a hose in my side, tethered to the suction device, with no hope of getting on a plane, our window of opportunity to capture dead tumor antigens in my head was closing.

"It's been one week," said the surgeon. "I think we need surgery."

I didn't want to believe what I was hearing. The simple outpatient cryoablation had transmogrified into ten days of medical mishaps. First the horrible retching caused by the breathing tube, then the nurse jamming another tube down my nose, then almost being allowed to board a plane with a collapsed lung, followed by the most painful experience of my life from the chest tube insertion, and now, lung surgery. No wonder they say medical errors are the third leading cause of death in the U.S.[21,22]

After some discussion, Eddy and I agreed to surgery. We had to get moving. If I needed surgery to get to Germany, so be it.

"Before we do the surgery, I'd like a CT scan," I said. Recall that I had three suspicious hollow lung lesions growing very slowly since early 2010. Lately, they'd doubled to 5 mm. We wanted to know where these lesions were located in relation to the chest tube—and how they might be affected by surgery.

"Sure, I'll order a CT," said the surgeon.

The scan complete, the thoracic surgery fellow came in to discuss the results. He asked the nurse to roll in a portable workstation.

Loading up the images, he scrolled to the relevant slice.

Eddy and I stared at the screen, incredulous at what we saw.

The thoracic surgery fellow pulled up the report on the screen. It read: "... portion of tube appears to be traversing through the upper pulmonary lobe with associated hematoma or edema about the tube." In short, the "garden hose" appeared to have skewered my lung.

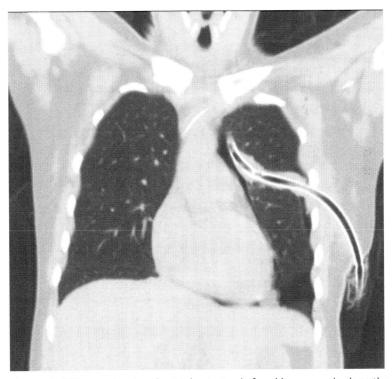

Figure 38: CT image showing chest tube. Instead of snaking upwards along the edge of my chest, the tube traversed my lung (in black), inches away from my heart (gray pear-shape structure in the middle). (September 21, 2011)

CHAPTER 12

Immunotherapy in Germany

"I MAY HAVE TO REMOVE THE ENTIRE LOBE," said the surgeon.

"The entire lobe? Isn't there any way to salvage it?" I asked. Our lungs comprise of five independent lobes: three on the right, two on the left. I stood to lose my upper left lobe—the one apparently skewered by the chest tube.

"I'll try to repair the lobe, but if the damage is too extensive, you need to be prepared to lose it," said the surgeon. "And to prevent further collapse of your lung, I'm going to fuse it to your chest wall. I'll introduce a slurry of talc—the same ingredient found in talcum powder—into your chest cavity. The talc will spark a chemical reaction that'll scar and inflame your lung. In the process it'll fuse the surfaces of the lung and chest wall."

Inflame? Did he say he was going to purposely cause inflammation in my lung? Inflammation that could fuel lurking cancer? Cancer that those three slow-growing lesions in my lung might represent?

"Give us a couple of days to think about it," I said.

Incredulous at how far the situation was spiraling, Eddy and I furiously researched lung surgery and *pleurodesis* (the procedure that fuses the lung to the chest wall). I'd never heard of pleurodesis until now. Nor had I anticipated the need for lung surgery so soon. We had two days to study their ramifications on my future cancer treatment.

The string of complications had stemmed from the precautionary measure of protecting my airway—and were unrelated to cryoablation.

The collapsing of lungs by overzealous ventilation is well-documented.[1,2] Like a balloon popping when over-inflated, my lung may have been over-stretched by air forced in by the mechanical ventilator or hand-pump.

And then, the chest tube—inserted to re-inflate my lung—had made things worse. We would later learn that chest tubes often cause complications. These range from infections to skewered lungs to punctured arteries, or even punctured hearts (that can kill).[3] A study at the Albany Medical

Center in New York found a 25 percent rate of complications.[4] Another study in New Zealand found an up to 40 percent complication rate when inserted by residents.[5] Had I known about these complications, I wouldn't have agreed so quickly to getting a chest tube without exploring less invasive alternatives (such as the thinner *pigtail catheter).*[6,7]

"I don't see any way out of surgery," said Eddy.

"Neither do I," I agreed reluctantly. "Thank God it didn't puncture my heart. I could have died right then." From the CT images, the tip of the tube looked to have gotten within a centimeter or two away from my heart before it angled upwards and away.

"Did you know that talc has been suspected of causing lung and ovarian cancer since the '80s?" said Eddy.[8,9]

"Seriously? And they want to pump it into my chest cavity?!" I said, shocked.

"We should insist on *mechanical pleurodesis* instead," said Eddy.

He'd found an alternative to talc. One that caused less inflammation. One that wasn't embroiled in controversy (for causing cancer). And one that wasn't as permanent.

The surgeon would deflate my lung, then "scratch up" the surface of my chest wall with a rough gauze. The bleeding and scarring would form fibrous bands between the chest wall and re-inflated lung. Like clothespins holding up a shirt hung out to dry, those fibrous bands would keep my lung tethered to my chest wall, preventing further collapse.

Although the procedure wasn't as reliable or permanent, it offered a critical advantage—*the fibrous bands could later be removed, allowing the lung to be deflated, and hence, enabling future surgery.* Think about trying to use scissors to cut out a small piece of balloon, then "sewing" the hole close. You can't do this to an inflated balloon. First, you have to deflate the balloon, then stretch the spot away from the rest of the balloon, and then snip across the stretched portion while sealing the cut. Likewise, a surgeon can't operate until the lung is deflated. And the lung can't be deflated until those fibrous bands are removed. The permanency of talc pleurodesis would render such surgery impossible.

Eddy and I realized just how close I'd come to being excluded from future lung surgery. As the lung is the most common site of spread for sarcomas and many other cancers, preserving the ability to remove lung tumors could mean the difference between life and death. More disturbing was the thought of sealing a potentially cancer-promoting substance in my chest—in direct contact with yet-to-be-recognized malignancy possibly lurking in my lung!

This close call had arisen because we were in a large medical center where doctors didn't know my full history. Their surgeons didn't just treat cancer patients, but also victims of car accidents, stab wounds and gunshot wounds. The Karmanos Cancer Center (where Dr. Littrup practiced) depended on the Detroit Medical Center (DMC) for certain services such as the Intensive Care Unit. Since the cryoablation a week earlier, I'd been transferred from one ward of the DMC to another. The DMC doctors' abbreviated awareness of my greater cancer struggle put me at risk for medical decisions that could compromise my cancer treatment.

Lesson learned: Cancer patients receiving treatment for problems unrelated to cancer have to take care not to let these treatments affect the management of their cancer. This is especially important when receiving care outside of their cancer clinic.

Despair

I found myself again in the basement of the DMC being prepped for lung-repair surgery with mechanical pleurodesis. The surgeon would soon make three one-inch "stab wounds" into my chest (that's how the report would later describe the incisions). Through the wounds, he'd insert three arms of a robot. At the tip of those arms would be precision tools that he'd control from a side monitor, giving him the ability to "zoom in" on the operating field. He would remove the skewered tube, repair any tears (or if unsalvageable, cut out the entire lung lobe), then perform the pleurodesis, where he'd scratch up the surface of my chest wall to create those fibrotic bands.

It was once again time for the anesthesiologist to insert a breathing tube. He would have to put me under and stop my breathing. My left lung would be deflated so that the surgeon could operate. To supply oxygen to my body, my right lung would be inflated with a mechanical ventilator, which is why the breathing tube was needed.

This time, no ICU staff would refuse me sedative after the procedure.

This time, we had met with the anesthesiologist the day before. Dr. Haddad had promised to stay by my side—and to supply me with sedative for as long as the breathing tube was in place.

As I lay in the hospital bed, about to be wheeled into surgery, I began to sob. For over three-and-a-half years, my spirit had remained unbroken. The hopeless survival curves. The debilitating radiation. The chemo that permanently damaged my bone marrow. "Red Death" speeding into my body. Pursuing a century-old immunotherapy in Tijuana. The close call with sepsis. Being dropped by my Stanford oncologist. Graves' disease. Losing my thyroid. Five months of fevers. The stress of charting my own survival plan, while going against doctors' recommendations—I'd endured them all. But this spiraling string of events in Detroit was about to break me.

Feeling helpless and stuck, unable to proceed with immunotherapy in Germany—and literally stuck with a hose in my chest—I broke down and sobbed. An irrational fear overcame me. I was sure I was going to die during surgery—and would soon join the up to 440,000 Americans that perish annually from medical mishaps.[10]

"We're ready to take your wife into the OR," said the nurse to Eddy. "I'll show you to the waiting room."

I handed the iPod to Eddy as they wheeled me away. It contained a tearful video message I'd just recorded for mom, thanking her for always being there for me. A final farewell.

In the distance, I saw Eddy being led away.

The nurse had her arm around his shoulder.

I couldn't see it, but he was weeping.

Destination Duderstadt

The three stab wounds were healing nicely. We were at Detroit Metropolitan Airport, poised to board a nonstop to Frankfurt. Two weeks had passed since surgery.

Surgery had gone well. In a positive twist, the surgeon discovered that the chest tube hadn't skewered my lung. Instead of snaking upward along the side of my chest cavity, the misplaced tube had angled inward, pushing aside the lung lobe. The lung then wrapped itself around the tube, making it look like a skewering. Strangely, he couldn't find the small tear that had collapsed my lung in the first place. Suspecting some blister-like tissue at the uppermost tip of the lung, he snipped off a wedge and sutured it close.

My recovery proceeded without further drama. Ironically, the surgeon had to insert a fresh chest tube to allow the lung to re-inflate and the fluids to drain. But this time, no air leaked from my lungs; within days, the chest tube had been removed.

As the plane soared above Detroit, we left behind the recent trauma. We weren't bitter. Mistakes happen in all hospitals, and one complication had led to another. My doctors had meant well. We were just glad to be liberated. We could now focus on our original goal: to capitalize on the dead tumor in my head and use it to boost immunotherapy.

But how long would the dead tumor cells remain in my head? Would any be left by the time I received immunotherapy in Germany? It was difficult to find concrete information on the subject. But scientific studies showed the increased immune activity after cryoablation significantly abates by week eight.[11] It was now already three weeks post cryo. Dr. Nesselhut would need another two weeks to prepare my first dendritic vaccine. We were cutting it close, but assuming there would be no further delays, we stood a chance of capturing the dead tumor antigen in my head.

Thump. Thump. Thump. The immigration officer inked his rubber stamp, then granted me access into his country.

We collected our luggage, heavy with supplies needed to keep my PICC line sterile. We were now on foreign turf; it was imperative I avoid a repeat of sepsis. With the Detroit mishaps fresh in our minds, we were determined to stay out of hospitals, especially in a foreign land where language could further confound.

Navigating Frankfurt airport was easy. We'd done our homework, mapping out every detail and gleaning tips from an American patient of Dr. Nesselhut, who'd blogged about traveling to Duderstadt. Stopping for a quick snack at McDonalds, we entered our orders on a touchscreen— something we'd never seen before. We maneuvered an ingeniously designed baggage cart up an escalator (the same one we were on). We crossed an enclosed walkway to the *Fernbahnhof,* or long-distance train station, then descended a multistory escalator to the platform, where we unloaded our bags and reclaimed the two-euro deposit for the cart.

Frankfurt airport was intimately connected to the train networks. Long-distance intercity trains reached towns across the country. We soon boarded the Inter-City-Express (ICE) to Göttingen. As German trains are famous for, it arrived on the dot, pausing briefly for us to scramble aboard.

Inside, a clean and serene cabin beckoned. Passengers spoke in reserved tones. Even the noise from the tracks was unobtrusive, given that the ICE reached speeds of 200 mph. Sinking into comfortable reclining seats, we absorbed the scenery, first of the city, then of clean, red trains docked downtown, and then of rolling green countryside hills and quaint little towns with steepled churches and farm houses. Exhausted from jet lag, I drifted off to sleep, Eddy promising he'd rouse me in time to disembark.

Duderstadt is a little north of the center of Germany, located along the former Cold War border that separated East and West. It's a small town, with a population of about 21,000. Trains didn't stop there, so we'd have to disembark at Göttingen, a vibrant university town with a rich academic history.

We reached Göttingen in two hours. There, we caught a taxi to Duderstadt. It took us along miles of single lane roads through rolling farmland, passing fields of yellow rapeseed and a giant modern windmill. As we approached the old town center, it felt as if we were entering a fairytale town—but one where real people lived and worked.

Unlike larger German cities that had been decimated during World War II, Duderstadt had been spared. Two towering, ancient-but-well-preserved stone edifices straddled either end of the town center—one, a majestic 13th-century Catholic cathedral, the other, a stately 14th-century Protestant church. Their bell towers chiming on the hour, they were bridged by a thousand feet of cobblestone thoroughfare known as *Marktstrasse* (or Market Street).

It was about 3 p.m. Townsfolk milled about, sharing ten-foot-wide sidewalks with bicyclists. Our taxi was one of few cars trundling noisily over the uneven cobblestone on Market Street. In small towns such as Duderstadt, not many locals speak English, nor did our taxi driver. But we had no problem conveying our destination, the lone hotel on Market Street—the Zum Löwen ("The Lion"). Checking in, we relished hot showers then ventured out to explore the town center.

Market Street was lined on both sides with cafes, restaurants, a pub, an ice-creamery, a cell-phone store, clothing stores, a trinket shop and pharmacies—occupying the ground floors of three-story linked units. The impressive structure of the Old *Rathaus* (city council building) flanked the eastern end; a mechanized town mascot popped out of its corner steeple tower every half-hour to a repetitive bell tune. For a small town center, there was a curious abundance of pharmacies, five in all.

The linked units were painted in attractive pastel colors. Also peppered around town were picturesque buildings constructed in *half-timber* style with intricate exposed framing, many of them over 500 years old. Some had walls that leaned outward toward the top, and upper-level floors that slanted oddly. (We'd later learn these peculiarities were due to the settling of building materials.)

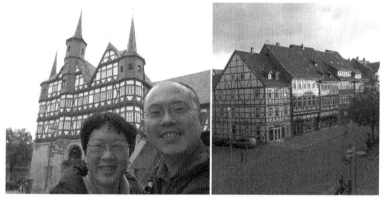

Figure 39: In front of the 700-year-old Rathaus also constructed in half-timber style (left). The main street of Duderstadt (right).

An absence of music shrouded the shops in a tranquil hush. Children behaved respectfully as their families browsed stores and enjoyed local eateries.

"Who needs Disneyland when you have this!" I said.

"It's beautiful … and peaceful," said Eddy.

This idyllic setting was where I'd soon receive more immunotherapy. A surge of fresh optimism welled up, bringing healing to the recent trauma. It made me believe again that a cure was possible.

As the sun set, we walked back to the hotel, grabbed a bite at the café across the street, then turned in early.

Exhausted from the transatlantic journey, we sank into a deep slumber on a blustery October evening in 2011.

The Dendritic Cell Vaccine

Dr. Nesselhut's clinic was a five-minute walk from the hotel. A small plaque affixed to the outer wall identified it. We entered through heavy ornate wooden doors.

On time for our appointment, we checked in at the front desk, manned by four English-speaking nurses. Dressed in smart white uniforms, they busily answered phones, processed paperwork and shuttled between rooms. A nurse showed us to the waiting room where we sat among five German couples, presumably there for fertility treatment (the other therapy Dr. Nesselhut's clinic specialized in).

Silence permeated the room. An hour passed. Apparently, waiting for the doctor was a universal experience, even in punctual Germany. But I wasn't complaining—I'd once waited seven hours to see my surgeon in the U.S. Finally, a nurse called, pronouncing my name as Germans do: "*Mrs. Shee?*"

Dr. Nesselhut greeted us warmly. Soft-spoken and patient, he listened intently to my medical history. We described our previous attempts at immunotherapy—the NY-ESO-1 vaccine, the Coley's Toxins, the recent cryoablation, the low-dose cyclophosphamide. He seemed familiar with them all, perhaps less so the immune effects of cryoablation.

We were here for two things: dendritic vaccination and a newly added component to our already complex strategy—infusions of Natural Killer (NK) cells.

After explaining the therapies and their safety aspects, he went straight to logistics. The first thing he did was schedule me for a *leukapheresis* for the very next day.

Leukapheresis collects white blood cells from which dendritic cells can be extracted. Warning that I'd be bed-bound for a few hours, the nurse encouraged me to use the restroom. She brought me upstairs into a modest, airy room with natural light. She had me lie down in bed, then covered me with warm blankets. She proceeded to prepare the leukapheresis machine, a task that involved threading and connecting sterile tubing into channels and grooves. A sterile collection bag was connected to the tubing; it would accumulate my white cells.

With the machine prepared, she had me stretch out both arms. Placing pillows under them for support, she inserted an IV into each. The IVs were, in turn, connected to the ends of the aforementioned tubing, forming a sterile, closed loop.

The machine came alive. Blood streamed out of my right arm, snaking through the tubing, moved along by the machine. The nurse then injected anti-coagulant into the closed loop to prevent my blood from clotting and clogging up the tubing.

The machine contained a centrifuge, which separated out my white blood cells from my blood. They only needed my white cells; the other components—the plasma, the platelets, the red cells—were returned into my body through my left arm. Over the course of three hours my entire blood volume cycled through the machine more than once, as it hoarded my white cells.

Finally, enough white cells had been collected. The nurse initiated the shutdown. My arms were tired and stiff from being held in position. She unhooked me, gave me orange juice and had me linger a while in bed.

Dr. Nesselhut was also there, making sure I was all right. As we engaged in conversation with him, the nurse finished shutting down the machine, then whisked away the bag of my precious cells to the laboratory down the street.

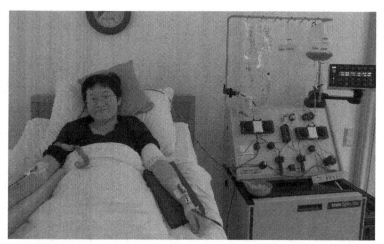

Figure 40: Undergoing my first leukapheresis to extract dendritic cells. Blood exited from my left arm, and returned through my right arm after passing through the centrifuge machine.

The laboratory was a brand new, two-story, government-certified facility for processing human cells. Dr. Nesselhut and his practice partners had built this multi-million-dollar facility to provide cell-based immunotherapy to their patients—therapy that involved extracting, modifying, and reintroducing a patient's own cells. The achievement was impressive for a small group of private physicians. As far as we know, similar facilities in the U.S. are limited to large research centers or biotech companies.

The science and technology behind dendritic vaccines had long been available in the U.S. But the unholy combination of strict FDA laws and the exorbitant cost of running clinical trials meant that dendritic vaccines couldn't be administered as treatment in the U.S. until someone was willing to invest hundreds of millions to validate them in clinical trials. A single product, Provenge, had recently been approved, but only for prostate cancer. Trials were being run for other cancers, but it could be years before approval.

In contrast, Germany—known for its strict regulations—allows this safe, science-based therapy to be accessed by patients with any cancer. Doctors are allowed to treat patients with life-threatening diseases (such as advanced cancer) with experimental therapies, as long as there are no effective standard solutions, and the experimental therapy has reasonable odds of benefit.[12,13]

Despite having to travel to Germany, we were thankful that each dendritic vaccine cost less than $6,000 per injection. In contrast, Provenge ran $93,000 per course of three infusions—a price apparently justified by the expense of running U.S. clinical trials.[14]

Dr. Nesselhut explained that he'd funded the construction of his laboratory with a large subsidy from the German government. He encouraged us to visit the lab, where a biologist gave us a tour. We observed clean rooms where my immune cells were being processed, replete with equipment such as centrifuges and tissue-culture hoods, much of which I was familiar with from years working in biology labs. The elaborate facilities and professionalism of the staff impressed us. Remembering how I had almost been injected with a contaminated syringe in Tijuana, it was reassuring that the processing of my cells was governed by strict German laws and overseen by staff with Ph.Ds.

At the lab, my white blood cells were filtered to extract the dendritic cells (DCs). Most of the DCs were frozen and stored for future vaccines; only a fraction was needed for the first. The DCs were placed in a tightly controlled culture, where they were grown over the course of ten days. At the right time, they would be stimulated with special proteins (cytokines), making them highly active, better able to engulf tumor cells and activate T cells.

Two weeks later, we were back at the clinic for my first vaccine. The nurse brought in the stimulated DCs in a small vial. Dr. Nesselhut drew half of the contents into a syringe, then deftly injected it into my right cheek, near the cryoablated tumor. We hoped the DCs would encounter tumor cells—dead or alive—then migrate to lymph nodes where they'd activate T cells against my cancer.

Dr. Nesselhut then injected the other half into my right upper arm, near where I had received the NY-ESO-1 peptide vaccine in early 2010. The DCs might engulf any lingering peptide, acting as a "booster" shot to the NY-ESO-1 vaccine.

The injections stung a little. The sites grew red and slightly swollen. I was told to expect fever or fatigue. But I experienced neither and enjoyed dinner at a local café. Like Dr. Old's NY-ESO-1 vaccine, the injection had virtually zero side effects—a stark contrast to chemoradiation.

Receiving my first dendritic vaccine gave us a sense of achievement. Even if there weren't assurances that it would improve my survival, it felt empowering to take rational action that might alter my prognosis.

Variations of DC Vaccines

Some DC vaccines are made by priming (feeding) DCs with whole-tumor samples. As I had no tumor sample to prime my DCs with, my first vaccine contained unprimed DCs.

Other DC vaccines are made by priming with a specific antigen found in the patient's cancer. For example, the FDA-approved Provenge is primed with prostatic acid phosphatase (PAP), an antigen expressed in prostate cancer. The priming causes DCs to activate tumor-killing T cells that recognize that antigen.

My later vaccines would be primed with a harmless virus: Newcastle disease virus (NDV). I'd be injected with NDV a day before my DC injection. The NDV would preferentially infect cancer cells in my body. My DCs would also be primed with NDV. Once injected, the DCs would activate T cells that hunt for NDV-infected cancer cells.

In 2011, Dr. Nesselhut presented data at a major cancer conference (ASCO), showing that NDV-primed DC vaccines led to longer survival of patients with brain cancer.[15]

Natural Killer Cell Therapy

During the two weeks that I had been healing from lung surgery in Detroit,

Eddy corresponded with a doctor in New York, an out-of-the-box thinker by the name of Raymond Chang, M.D.

We'd first learned of Dr. Chang while researching alternative medicines in 2009. His clinic treated patients using acupuncture and Chinese medicine. But he also employed common prescription drugs in creative, off-label ways to help cancer patients survive longer. Examples of drugs he used were common antibiotics (like tetracycline), cholesterol-lowering drugs (statins) and medicines for weaning addicts off narcotics (naltrexone). These generally safe drugs have anticancer properties that are supported by studies.[16] Like us, Dr. Chang believed in combining treatments to attack cancer, especially if there was evidence of synergy between them.

One of the core components of Dr. Chang's multi-layered strategy was dendritic vaccination. For years, he'd been sending patients to Dr. Nesselhut. He supported the idea of dendritic vaccination, but also suggested adding another therapy—infusions of NK cells.

Recall from chapter 4 that NK cells can attack cancer cells that lack a certain protein found in healthy cells. But one problem is there are too few NK cells in the body to destroy large tumors. Even so, the known tumor in my jaw had been cryoablated. It seemed logical that NK cells might eradicate small amounts of remaining cancer (such as the microscopic tentacles that may have survived cryoablation).

Also, NK cells can complement T cells, as they can destroy certain cancer cells that are invisible to T cells. This meant the NK cell infusions might complement the other immunotherapy strategies we'd devised.

Finally, the procedure had zero side effects.

Given the dismal prognosis I faced, we decided to layer-on this safe and complementary immunotherapy to my already-complex plan. So, during the two weeks that I recovered from lung surgery in Detroit, Eddy was busy arranging for the NK cell infusions.

The Pros and Cons of NK Cell therapy

Research to harness NK cells against cancer accelerated in the 1980s. But scientists hit roadblocks. One roadblock was the low number of NK cells in the body.

There are an estimated 500 million NK cells circulating the average human body. Each NK cell can kill between two to four cancer cells before it dies.[17] But not all circulating NK cells will reach a tumor or get past its defenses. A small tumor measuring 1 cm wide may already contain a billion cancer cells. It's no surprise then that NK cells were found to be generally ineffective for shrinking large tumors. Despite their limited value against large tumors, Dr. Nesselhut had observed greater benefit in patients with microscopic disease.

Another benefit of NK cells was their ability to attack certain cancer cells that lack a common protein found on normal cells (known as MHC Class 1). Interestingly, these cancer cells cannot be attacked by T cells, as T cells need to latch onto that same protein in order to recognize cancer. In this way, NK cells can complement T cells, helping to attack cancer cells invisible to T cells.

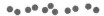

Dr. Chang and Dr. Nesselhut believed that NK cells from other healthy donors would better attack my cancer. This was based on the notion that my own NK cells were probably ineffective against my cancer.[18]

Dr. Chang suggested I enlist multiple donors. They had to be willing to travel to Duderstadt and undergo a leukapheresis to extract their NK cells. Their cells would be cultured, expanded in number and stimulated with special compounds, then re-infused into me. Dealing with live cells is always tricky. Not all cells survive manipulation. And not all that survive become active and able to kill cancer. For these reasons, I needed enough donors.

In discussing with Dr. Chang, we decided to aim for 3 billion NK cells. The cultivation process yielded an average 500 million active NK cells per donor, meaning we needed six donors.

We emailed friends and family. Overwhelmed by an outpouring of willing responses, we had 12 volunteers consult with Dr. Chang by phone. (Not all would qualify, which is why Dr. Chang suggested we screen 12.) Dr. Chang interviewed them and arranged for the requisite blood tests to satisfy German law.

Coordinating the effort was difficult. Our volunteers were spread out across the U.S. in different states. They were busy with jobs, and some had young children. Tricky logistics required meticulous attention. For example, to check that our volunteers' NK cells were functioning well—blood samples needed to be shipped to a specialized laboratory. The samples had to be drawn on certain days of the week, by a specific cutoff time. Coordinating all this required constant communication. But it all came together. The lab results returned in time to certify my donors, enabling them to book flights for a month later.

While all this was going on, Eddy became my first NK cell donor. We'd been in Duderstadt for two weeks when Dr. Nesselhut, seeing an opportunity, suggested Eddy donate his NK cells. Eddy was at the tail end of a flu, having caught it shortly after arriving in Germany. Dr. Nesselhut explained that Eddy's cells were likely "supercharged"—activated by the large number of viruses circulating his body. These naturally activated NK cells could be more effective against cancer.[19]

The next morning, while it was still dark, we walked hand-in-hand past a local bakery, the smell of fresh Brötchen (German rolls) wafting through the crisp morning air. We passed by the stone cathedral on the east end of Market Street, its twin gray steeples indiscernible, as they towered beyond the illumination of the street lamps. At the lab, the nurse was already preparing the leukapheresis machine.

"Guten morgen," she said, as she swiftly hooked Eddy up, placing an IV in each arm and draping a thick blanket to keep him warm.

As dawn began to break, the machine greedily accumulated Eddy's flu-incensed NK cells.

Advancements in NK cell therapies

Ever since the 1980s, scientists have experimented with ways to increase the killing capability or the number of NK cells in the body (for example, by injecting cytokines such as IL2, IL-12 or IL-15). However, the benefits were limited and the results, short-lived.[20] Research interest in NK cells tempered. But in recent years, breakthroughs in immunotherapy have reignited interest. Advances in genetic engineering have enabled scientists to modify NK cells (similar to Dr. Rosenberg's modified T cells).[21] An example is making NK cells home in on specific antigens (just like T cells). Patients in the U.S. now have the option of enrolling in these modified NK cell clinical trials.[22]

Angry Cells from Loving Friends

We had to wait ten days for Eddy's NK cells to multiply. Looking to save money, we asked around about short-term rentals. A nurse at the clinic gave us a lead. A local store owner was renting an apartment directly above her store. Located in the town center, the apartment was clean, comfortable and well kept. We checked out of The Lion hotel, dropped our luggage off at the apartment, and sneaked off to Paris—a six-hour train ride from Göttingen—for a week-long jaunt.

"Make sure you have a working cell phone," Dr. Nesselhut had said. In the event that the finicky NK cells matured faster than expected, I'd have to return instantly to receive them the moment they were most *lytic* (capable of killing cancer cells, or "angry" as I would call them).

The cell culture went as planned. We reveled in what Paris had to offer, forgetting for a week Dr. Benjamin's 80 percent odds that my cancer would return, and the MD Anderson survival curve's 100 percent odds that the cancer will ultimately kill me.[23] Pretending that we'd planned a romantic vacation all along, we celebrated almost five years of marriage, four of which had been consumed by a fight for survival.

It was time to receive Eddy's NK cells. A nurse situated me in a small room, then brought in a very large syringe, filled with a murky white fluid. Dr. Nesselhut appeared, asking questions to ensure I was generally well. He was enthusiastic about Eddy's cells—the lab analysis had revealed them to be extremely lytic, almost certainly activated by the flu.

The nurse secured the syringe to a machine I'd never seen before. It had a mechanized telescoping arm that would slowly depress the syringe plunger, infusing the NK cells at a controlled rate over the next 15 minutes. And so, I received Eddy's "angry" NK cells. I felt no pain, no swelling, no fever, nothing. But it warmed my heart to receive potentially life-giving cells from my husband.

Three weeks later, our NK donors, including Monica (who'd helped us think through the cryoablation-versus-surgery decision) and one of my younger brothers, began to arrive. It was the third week of November in 2011—the week before Thanksgiving. We'd intentionally staggered their arrival as Dr. Nesselhut had only two leukapheresis machines, which we shared with other patients.

One by one, my donors appeared at the apartment doorstep. They had requested time off work, parted with loved ones and young children, and traveled across the Atlantic for the three-hour procedure. Because travel took so long, most would only stay a day or two before having to rush back. Eddy and I were overcome with emotion. After two months of communicating by phone and email, we could finally hug and thank them.

It was cold this time of the year—almost freezing. But the little apartment was filled with warmth and cheer as we shared meals with our donors, some of whom stayed with us. We enjoyed the charm of Duderstadt, checking out bakeries, admiring the unique local architecture and visiting the museum on the west side of Market Street.

We were already amazed that so many friends and family had volunteered their NK cells. But we were floored by the kindness of two strangers.

Dave, a police officer, and Scott, a homebuilder, had heard about my need from close friends of ours, Steve and Grace. They knew it wasn't going to be a simple blood drive donation. They knew it involved screening, blood tests, taking supplements for a month (to activate their NK cells) and almost a full day of travel each way. Both had demanding jobs and young children. Yet, they volunteered. Both ended up being selected by Dr. Chang as donors.

Receiving just shy of three billion NK cells from these six loving human beings was a healing experience in more ways than one. I won't lie—we'd experienced our share of hurt and betrayal. It's not uncommon for cancer patients to feel abandoned by friends, family, employers, even doctors.[24] Seen as "damaged goods" with "expiration dates," friends go silent. Husbands leave. (A study showed husbands are six times more likely to leave their sick spouses.[25]) But this experience had shown us the opposite. Even though there was no guarantee the NK cells would cure my cancer, the sacrifice of these individuals permanently excised the cancerous cynicism that had crept in, preventing it from metastasizing into a full-blown disease of the soul.

Dr. Old's Call

It was the Sunday before Thanksgiving 2011. Four of our NK cell donors had already donated their cells and left. The fifth was resting in our apartment from the transatlantic flight from Virginia.

It was a crisp November evening. Sunday nights were serene in Duderstadt, the only distinct sounds were the hourly chimes from the nearby cathedral and the repetitive bell tune that accompanied the Rathaus mascot. We were finishing dinner when the cell phone rang. It was Dr. Old, calling from New York.

Our communication with Dr. Old had waned ever since cryoablation in Detroit. His cancer had advanced, causing debilitating pain. Not wanting to trouble him with my own struggles, we kept the trauma of Detroit to ourselves, only sending him a letter and photos of us before and after cryoablation.

As mentioned earlier, Dr. Old had favored surgery, preferring to have tumor tissue to analyze. In contrast, we had opted for cryoablation, as we wanted every chance to generate T cells against all tumor antigens. The choice was a subjective one; neither path could guarantee benefit. It was a matter of philosophy.

The letter we'd sent showed pictures of us gallivanting around Duderstadt, my face already well-healed, the pinprick scars from cryoablation barely discernible. He was surprised at how well I looked, and particularly struck by how minimally invasive the cryoablation had been.

We'll always remember and treasure that last conversation. With soaring words of encouragement, which seemed to arise from the depths of a commiserative struggle for survival, Dr. Old asserted how crucial it was that we had developed a philosophy and stuck with it.

"You were right to have done the cryoablation," he said, repeating himself, as if to make certain that we'd heard him.

Probably more than anyone else, Dr. Old understood the complexities of the human immune system—how there wasn't yet a concrete formula for an immune-based cure. Mine was a high-stakes experiment, with tantalizing clues grounded on solid science and hundred-year-old anecdotes—but no guarantees.

We cried that night, partly because he'd touched us with kindness—reaching out despite his pain—and partly because we were helpless to alleviate his discomfort.

Dr. Old extended an invitation for us to visit him. We'd yearned for the opportunity since learning of his cancer, and we counted it an honor. We told him of our plans to consult a surgeon in New York in two weeks' time, and that we would come see him then. We considered flying to New York sooner, but our travel was constrained by the ongoing NK cell donations and the need to remain in Duderstadt to receive the fickle NK cells.

Dr. Old seemed a little quiet. Looking back, perhaps he sensed he didn't have that long to live.

One week after that phone conversation, Dr. Old passed away from his cancer.

CHAPTER 13

Taking No Chances: Consolidative Surgery

In the middle of a packed schedule in Germany, we eked out a short trip to New York City. It was December 7, 2011. We disembarked at JFK international airport. Less than 24 hours earlier, I'd received my fourth infusion of NK cells in Duderstadt. In three days, I'd have to rush back to Germany for the fifth.

Manhattan glittered with Christmas lights. Decorations adorned the city. The Rockefeller Christmas Tree had just been lit. Holiday cheer filled the air. But we were despondent, our hearts in mourning. A week earlier, Dr. Old, our mentor, advocate and co-adventurer for over two and a half years, had passed away, losing his life to cancer.[1]

We arrived too late to bid him farewell. But we were there to consult with someone he'd recommended, a head and neck surgeon at Memorial Sloan Kettering (MSK), Dr. Jatin Shah.

Recall from chapter 11 that, upon learning of my recurrence, we'd eschewed surgery, instead doubling down on immunotherapy. We believed that immunotherapy was our best shot—maybe our only chance—at eliminating diffuse micro-tumors in my head.

But what if I didn't have diffuse cancer? What if that single bright spot on the MRI had been the only focus? The apprehension persisted. Even though the odds of a contained recurrence were low, I could've been squandering my only chance of a surgical cure. For this reason, we had planned on following immunotherapy with surgery.

Dr. Littrup was confident that cryoablation had eliminated the tumor. We trusted his experience and skill, but four years of obsessive research and care had primed us not to underestimate the insidious nature of sarcoma.

Cancer doesn't care what you think. How hopeful you are. Or how well you believe your latest treatment will work. We'd seen too many patients die. One moment things seemed under control. Within the blink of an eye, cancer had killed them.

A family friend had recently suffered the sorrow of losing his sister to lung cancer. It had spread to her brain. Her oncologist told her, "You're going to live a long life."[2] One month later, she was comatose. Her family was told, "There's nothing more we can do but to keep her comfortable."[3] She passed away soon after.

Recall from chapter 4 that Eddy had befriended three sarcoma warriors in 2009—Martha, Charlie and Joe. Each had battled advanced sarcoma in their own way. They had experienced success with alternative approaches. Sarcomas that were supposedly invincible had disappeared. One of them, Joe, had a tumor perceptibly vanish, leaving his doctor to claim he'd been misdiagnosed. But their tumors returned with a vengeance. The last email from Martha was in May 2010. Joe went silent two months later. Charlie— the valiant warrior who woke up every two hours to intermittently take supplements and drugs—succumbed in August that year. Within a short span, Eddy had lost three of his valiant friends.

These stories and others from the sarcoma online forum instilled a great respect for the disease. Not unforgotten was the humbling experience of seeing my tumor regrow in August, after initially shrinking from Coley's Toxins. So, despite Dr. Littrup's skill, we both felt consolidative surgery was prudent.

But we still needed to figure out how much to cut around the cryoablated mass. My Stanford surgeon, Dr. Kaplan, continued to recommend a more conservative approach: cut around the tumor, taking a wide margin of flesh, but leave the jaw bone intact. He didn't think the tumor had invaded the bone. Dr. Hanna at MD Anderson recommended a more extensive surgery. He would take all surrounding muscles and the adjacent jawbone. Which approach made more sense?

Again, we debated. If immunotherapy were to fail, and if diffuse cancer persisted in my head, then no surgery would cure me, meaning I was going to die anyway. In that case, surgery would only buy time, and I should focus on quality of life—perhaps leave the jaw bone intact so I could at least enjoy steaks and Korean barbecue.

On the other hand, if the cancer concentrated in one spot, then surgery might just "get it all." In that case, one could justify aggressive surgery to ensure a cure (sacrificing my jaw joint and my ability to chew).

The choice hinged on the extent of dissemination. For this reason, we'd come to New York to see Jatin Shah, M.D., the Chairman of Head and Neck Oncology at MSK. Dr. Shah was an experienced surgeon who had written six books on head and neck cancer surgery and had published nearly 400 scientific articles.[4] Months earlier, Dr. Old had suggested we consult him. Given the rarity of my disease and the differing recommendations from Stanford and MD Anderson, it seemed fitting to seek a third opinion from a surgeon with decades of experience operating on sarcomas of the head.

Thousands of Tumors

Dr. Shah entered with an entourage of three understudies. He'd read the cover letter we provided upon checking in.

Polite and soft-spoken, he asked incisive questions to understand my history and present situation. To probe the extent of trismus (scarring of jaw muscles), he asked to see how wide I could open my mouth. Brushing a finger lightly over different areas of my face, he checked for damage to facial nerves.

Dr. Shah then wanted to view my MRI images. Although we'd supplied CDs to the administrative staff a day earlier, they hadn't been uploaded. Having anticipated this, Eddy had the images ready on his laptop. Dr. Shah asked to see the MRI of the original tumor from 2008—before surgery, radiation and chemo.

"Which sequence would you like? The T2 images?" asked Eddy.

"Yes, T2. And all three views—axial, coronal, sagittal," replied Dr. Shah. These were sequences of my head from the bottom-up, front and side. He wanted all three to gauge how far the tumor had invaded critical structures.

He scrutinized the images, deep in concentration.

"Your original tumor was *truly* well-circumscribed," he said. "Notice the scalloped edges next to the mandible—they imply the tumor had been there for quite a while, and had eroded the jaw bone.

"OK. This gives me my baseline."

Dr. Shah then launched into a lengthy discourse, building a detailed case for how wide a margin to cut around the recurrent tumor.

"So, let's go back to 2008. That will put things in perspective … Here's the basic principle, starting with an example of sarcoma in the leg," he said.

Decades ago, Dr. Shah explained, a sarcoma in a limb (for example, the thigh) would've required amputation of the entire limb, as sarcomas often sprout long tentacles along muscle planes. Later, as the biology of sarcoma became better understood, surgeons developed a limb-sparing technique. They performed a *muscle group resection*—where the tumor, the muscle of origin, and all surrounding muscles were removed—followed by radiation.[5]

"Now, when you transpose that to sarcomas of the head and neck, all bets are off. There are *no* margins one can pursue—unless you want to do *this* operation," he said, gesturing a slicing motion across his neck with his hand, miming a beheading.

As we absorbed the implications of his words, Dr. Shah reinforced his point. "Talking about margins for a sarcoma in the location where you had your tumor is a *myth—it is not a reality*."

Until now, no other doctor had conveyed my prognosis in such unequivocal terms. This time, there was no 10-or-20 percent chance that surgery might cure me. This time, my odds of a cure were zero.

Dr. Shah explained that the first operation in 2008 had been my best chance of a cure. The cutting of tissue from prior surgery and the dense scarring from radiation made subsequent surgery complicated. It also made it easier for recurrent tumors to invade other areas of my head. In simple terms, there were more grooves and channels for it to squeeze into and spread its tentacles.

"Add to that the complexity of surrounding vital structures: the carotid artery, lower cranial nerves—which are indispensable … and even if you could hypothetically take those structures—everything from skin to spine—you still won't have clear margins," said Dr. Shah, explaining that the proximity to my spine, throat and sinuses implied micro-tumors had spread beyond the reach of surgery.

Dr. Shah's proclamations evoked a sense of finality, obliterating any vestige of hope that we could fall back on surgery in case immunotherapy were to fail.

The forceful assertions of incurability demoralized us. But on the other hand, we needed the undiluted perspective from a surgeon who had decades of experience cutting out sarcomas and witnessing their inexorable regrowth.

Having established that no surgery would cure me, Dr. Shah then described the operation he'd offer.

As the tumor had eroded the adjacent jaw bone, he would remove it along with the jaw joint and all surrounding tissue and attached muscles. To kill off microscopic remnant, he'd apply a high dose of radiation during surgery. For aesthetic purposes, he'd pad the gaping hole in my face with soft tissue from another part of the body. He'd also reconstruct the jaw bone—for which, he'd need to extend the incision along the neck crease to include a four-inch cut from my neck upwards to the middle of my lower lip. The procedure would take ten hours. Three for the actual resection; the rest for reconstruction. This surgery was even more extensive than what MD Anderson had recommended.

I was stunned. I could see it in Eddy's eyes too. The moment Dr. Shah had declared I was incurable, I assumed he'd recommend a *conservative* resection, like what Dr. Kaplan at Stanford had suggested. Why go through all that trouble if I was going to die anyway?

Before I could say anything, Eddy raised the issue. "If she's going to die regardless, what's the point of such an extensive surgery?"

"It's difficult to say. Does it mean you'll live months, years, tens of years? Hard to say."

Half an hour had passed. Sensing we weren't convinced, he asked an assistant to bring in a model skull. Flipping the skull upside down, he pointed to the location of my tumor.

"Here's your tumor. Here's the bone that will be resected. And here's the carotid artery. Now, tell me how much distance is there between your tumor and the carotid?"

"Not much at all," I whispered in defeat. It was barely over a centimeter.

"Thank you. Now here's the top part of your tumor, and here's the *foramen ovale* (a hole in the base of the skull, leading into the brain). How much distance is there between them?"

"I see your point," I said.

This object lesson showed us how close the recurrent tumor had been to these critical structures—and that it had almost certainly spread beyond the reach of the knife.

"But there's only one small locus of tumor. Plus, the cryoablation would have killed any cancer in her jaw bone. Do we really need to take the bone?" asked Eddy.

Then came the emphatic rebuttal: "What you see is one locus on the scan. Biologically, there are *thousands of microscopic tumors.*"

We'd been visualizing in terms of microscopic tentacles, spreading from a mother tumor. Dr. Shah's imagery of cancer everywhere seemed more ominous.

"There's no operation that can get it all.

"I'm not giving you what you'd like to hear—but I'm giving you the truth."

Grateful for the Clarity

We were grateful for Dr. Shah's frankness. For the object lesson. For the forceful statements. They began to erase all traces of wishful thinking that might cloud future decisions.

Deep down, we'd already suspected that surgery wouldn't cure me; the survival curves had declared it. But human beings are optimistic by nature; we were no different. The rarity of my disease, and paucity of data gave an excuse to play angel's advocate and pray that my prognosis of death wasn't so categorical. It didn't matter if the glass was mostly empty; we'd clung on to the drop at the bottom.

Still wrestling with Dr. Shah's declarations, Eddy asked what the odds were that my cancer would return, despite extensive surgery and intraoperative radiation.

"Let's put it this way. First, this is your only chance. Second, if it remains under control, the odds of it coming back end up being zero; on the other hand, if it recurs, the odds become 100 percent. Any statistical percentage in between has no meaning to any one individual. So, if I throw out a number, say—65 percent disease control—what does that mean?"

And there it was again—the oft-repeated argument we'd heard from various physicians along our journey, that statistics don't matter to the individual.

We beg to differ. Statistics do matter. They offer an objective sense of an outcome when a certain path is taken. That information allows patients to make informed decisions: whether a treatment is worth the side effects, whether to try something else (such as immunotherapy), or perhaps not do anything at all.

The ability to make informed decisions had been important to Dr. Old. He often recounted a story about a friend of his—someone prominent in the medical community. Facing terminal cancer, his friend declined chemo, favoring quality of life in his last days. Dr. Old always spoke admiringly of his friend's courage to decline the recommendations of well-meaning physicians, instead trusting his own informed analysis of the medical literature.

Grateful for the time he'd spent educating us, we thanked Dr. Shah and said we'd think it over.

We left MSK with a strange mix of sentiments. On the one hand, there was a pit in our stomachs from being assured I was going to die from cancer in my head. On the other hand, we felt an indirect affirmation of what we'd believed all along—that immunotherapy was my only *realistic* hope for survival.

Finally, a Decision

On December 10, we returned to Duderstadt to receive the last two batches of NK cells, along with a third dendritic vaccine. Five days later, we were back in California.

We celebrated a quiet Christmas with family. The sky was overcast in the San Francisco Bay Area, just as it had been in Germany. We were glad to step away from the battleground and pretend for a moment that life was normal. Despite my dismal prognosis, I was still alive—almost four years after diagnosis. Fellow warriors we'd met along the way had succumbed much earlier. There was a lot to be thankful for despite the dangerous situation in my jaw.

The cryoablation had bought us time to get immunotherapy in Germany and to consult Dr. Shah. His frankness was the best thing that could've happened.

It clarified our thoughts.

"Since surgery can't cure you, the choice is clear—we should go all-in with immunotherapy," said Eddy.

"I agree," I said. "Dr. Shah said no surgery can get those thousands of tumors. So, why do surgery at all?"

"There's one good reason—an established tumor might be harder to kill with immunotherapy," said Eddy. "Remember how Dr. Old had described how established tumors may have stronger defenses than microscopic disease? There's a chance that cryo and immunotherapy may not have gotten all of the recurrent tumor."

"You don't think the cryo would've gotten it all?"

"It may have—but given the high stakes, we need surgery ... as an insurance policy."

"How about the bone? Both Dr. Hanna and Dr. Shah think it needs to go," I said.

"The risky spots for cryo are at the edges of the ice ball—where it isn't as cold. But the bone was engulfed deep within the ice ball. I'm not worried about it. I'm more concerned about the soft tissue at the edges of the ice ball."

And so, we had our decision. We would go with Dr. Kaplan's limited resection, using surgery as a backup to remove the cryoablated mass.

It was nice that Dr. Kaplan's opinion matched ours. He'd operated on me before, saving my life in 2008. Not having to travel to Houston or New York for surgery had its advantages. We'd have family around for support during recovery.

We scheduled surgery for January 25, 2012, allowing time to return to Duderstadt for more immunotherapy the week before the operation. We wanted to pre-shrink as many of the micro-tumors before cutting out the main cryoablated lesion—just as Dr. Coley had done.

Two days before surgery, we went to Stanford Hospital to speak with the anesthesiologist and for a preoperative MRI. Checking in at the radiology front desk, I discovered that the MRI wasn't a full diagnostic scan. It was a simpler one that would reveal less detail, mainly for establishing reference points for a 3D coordinate system so that Dr. Kaplan would know exactly where to cut.

I called Dr. Kaplan's physician assistant and asked for a full scan, waiting two hours for him to change the orders. The last full MRI had been taken over two months earlier during a quick trip back to Stanford, just before our donors had arrived in Duderstadt.

Given how fast sarcomas can grow, I needed to know if new tumors had appeared. They could completely alter our strategy.

After the MRI, we rushed to the imaging library and waited for a CD. In the lobby of Stanford Hospital, we pulled up the images on Eddy's laptop, comparing them with the two-month-old scan.

"The cryoablated tumor looks dimmer and smaller!" I said, elated. Dimmer and smaller were very good things. It suggested the mass was continuing to shrivel as it turned into scar tissue.

I turned to Eddy; he had a serious expression on his face.

"There's a new tumor!" he said, flitting back and forth through the images.

"What? Are you sure? I don't see any—"

And then I saw it.

Almost a centimeter wide, the teardrop-shaped lesion clung to the rear of my jawbone, a centimeter below the jaw joint.

It had recurred just outside and above the cryoablated area.

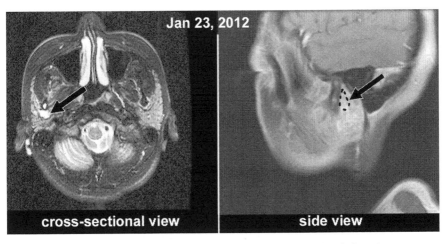

Figure 41: Head MRI, January 23, 2012. LEFT: Cross-sectional view shows re-recurrent tumor right behind the jaw bone. RIGHT: Side view reveals teardrop-shaped tumor (dotted black line).

Thrown for a Loop

Back at home, we sat at the dining table, staring at the MRI images. Deep in thought, we had two days to revise a plan that had taken months to conceive.

Trying hard to suppress a mounting panic, I grasped at alternative explanations for this second recurrence: "Is there a corresponding spot on the other side of the head? Maybe one of those many round circles that appear on both sides of the MRI—representing blood vessels or something like that?"

"No. it's unilateral—only on one side," said Eddy.

"How about the previous scan—was it already there?"

"No."

"Could it be inflammation from cryo?"

"Unlikely, it's next to the cryoablated tumor. Why would inflammation appear suddenly after four months, and only in that spot?"

"Or maybe it's tumor flare caused by immune cells?"

"Possible. But even if it is, we have to assume there's cancer not fully controlled by the immune system," said Eddy, mercilessly shooting down each attempt to rationalize away the tumor.

We'd spent incredible amounts of time, effort and money on the dendritic vaccines and the NK cell infusions. We'd dipped heavily into life savings that would've gone into a down payment for a home or to start a family (assuming I'd even survive). The NK infusions alone had cost around $120,000 in all. Although we had not asked for it, friends and relatives had donated huge sums of money. My NK donors had sacrificed so much to travel to Germany. And yet, my tumor had recurred. Guilt and sadness overcame us. Had we frittered away the goodwill of friends and family for nothing? Perhaps the dendritic vaccines would have been enough? Or maybe we should have just gone back to Coley's Toxins?

"We can't afford to think about that now. We need to focus on one thing," said Eddy. "Surgery is in two days. Dr. Kaplan is planning on a limited resection. We need to figure out if that's still the best way."

●₀ ●● ₀●₀ ₀● ●₀

Gathering Courage

It was the night before surgery. For two days, we'd debated intensely, going back and forth over the pros and cons of limited versus extensive surgery.

We had seen Dr. Kaplan earlier in the day. The Stanford radiologist confirmed that the new bright spot was a re-recurrent tumor, abutting the jaw bone, a centimeter below the jaw joint. Dr. Kaplan again helped us think through the pros and cons. But after an hour, he had to tend to other patients.

"We can continue this discussion later this evening over phone or email," he said, gracious as always, bearing with our vacillation.

That night, I stood in my bedroom, gazing at the mirror, thinking to myself.

If we decide to remove my right jaw, I'm going to look forever different. Maybe I should take pictures to remember how I look.

On second thought, maybe I won't.

No matter how I end up looking, I will accept it. I will adjust to my new reality.

Duderstadt was headquarters to Ottobock, a worldwide prosthetics company. Many amputees traveled there to be fitted with custom limbs. Once when walking along Market Street, I saw a young man without a leg, talking and laughing with his friends at a café. Even though it must've devastated him to lose his leg and mobility, he seemed to be making the best of the situation, living life with joy.

In the recent weeks, I'd read about Roger Ebert, the famous movie critic—how he'd lost his entire jaw to complications from surgery for cancer. He couldn't speak, eat or drink. Having forfeited vital parts of himself, he still found ways to compensate and continue living. As a movie critic, speaking had been essential to his livelihood and persona. Now that he couldn't, he turned to writing and used technology to communicate with a computer voice. No longer able to savor food, he obtained nutrition through a feeding tube.[6]

These amazing human beings inspired me. Their indomitable spirits and ability to adapt to new realities gave me strength. If I had to lose my right jaw, and if it would forever affect two things I loved—eating and talking—I would adjust, just as they had.

Down to The Wire

The alarm jolted us awake at 4 a.m. Only five hours had passed since we'd hung up the phone with Dr. Kaplan. That evening, we'd continued discussing surgery with him, yet hadn't been able to arrive at a conclusion. By around 11 p.m. or so, we had to let him go. It's not a good idea to keep your surgeon up late the night before surgery!

"Tell me what you decide on when I come by to see you before the operation," said Dr. Kaplan, hanging up.

In the cold of the morning, my parents drove us to Stanford Hospital along the winding 280 freeway. Few cars were present. The sky and highway were pitch black. Sitting in the rear, we were mesmerized by the snaking lane markings, their raised markers glittering in the headlights.

Forcing ourselves out of our sleep-deprived stupors, we turned and faced each other, concentrating hard. We had about half an hour to make our final decision on the extent of surgery.

Dr. Shah had convinced us that no operation could cure me. To us, it confirmed immunotherapy as my only real hope, and despite his recommendation of extensive surgery, we felt it argued for a limited resection. My ability to chew would be less compromised. I would be better able to maintain weight, continue dendritic vaccinations in Germany and resume Coley's Toxins.

But there was a problem. The twice-recurrent tumor looked as if it may have bloomed from a tentacle that had originated from the cryoablated tumor, crawling upwards toward the jaw joint, hugging the bone. The only way to cut out the tumor with surrounding margin was to take the jaw bone and jaw joint.

Circumstances now forced us to go for the bigger surgery.

"Please tell Dr. Kaplan we want an en-bloc resection—tell him to cut wide around the tumor. Tell him to take the jaw bone, take the jaw joint, and take all surrounding muscles," I said to the surgical fellow.

As the anesthesia dripped in, I again entrusted my life into the hands that had removed my original tumor almost four years earlier. I had peace about the decision. We had contemplated the pros and cons for months. Whatever the outcome, I wouldn't regret it.

The Mysterious Invisible Tumor

The anesthesia had worn off. It felt like I'd just finished a nap. Only, I no longer possessed a right jaw.

I looked in the mirror expecting to see a gaping hole—I'd declined reconstructive surgery. (Eddy and I had felt that reconstruction would involve more healing. And more healing could lead to more growth factors—proteins that might accelerate the remaining 999 micro-tumors.)

Hmm. Doesn't look too bad. Just a slight depression.

The swelling from surgery had masked the indentation, making my face look almost normal.

The incision along my neck crease line—the one Dr. Kaplan had elegantly sliced in 2008—now extended all the way up and behind my right ear. I didn't remember him saying he'd cut all the way up there! But whatever he'd needed to do was fine by me.

Hours passed. My strength began to return. Then, they let Eddy visit. I was so glad to see him. He'd been my faithful companion all these years, staying by me, fighting for me, thinking through every difficult problem.

"Hey there," he said.

"Hey," I whispered, my throat still raw from the breathing tube that had just been removed.

We kissed and hugged, happy to be together again in the land of the living.

At the end of surgery, while I was still under, Dr. Kaplan had gone out to update Eddy and Dr. Agah, my primary care physician. (Dr. Agah had taken time out of his day to wait with Eddy.) Dr. Kaplan conveyed the news about the margins, and also described the rest of his findings to Eddy.

"Good news. All margins were negative!" said Eddy, holding my hands in his.

Relieved, I smiled. It was the best possible outcome—no microscopic cancer at the surgical boundaries.

"What about the lesion? Was it cancer?" I asked.

"Yes. It's confirmed. Recurrent synovial sarcoma," said Eddy. "But there was something strange."

"What?"

"Dr. Kaplan said he couldn't see any tumor."

"What do you mean?"

"He carved up the resected tissue, looking for the tumor … but still couldn't see it with the naked eye."

"How then did he know it was cancer?"

"Microscopic analysis."

"That's so strange," I said, wondering why the tumor wasn't visible to the eye, but clearly defined on MRI.

"He did say that it felt firm to the touch—it just didn't *look* like a tumor."

"It looked like a tumor on MRI though," I said.

"Yes, I know. And the MRI was taken only two days earlier."

"Wait a minute! Do you think the immune system could have shrunk the tumor in the past two days?" I asked, excited at the prospect.

"Hmm. Why suddenly though? Seems like too big a coincidence," said Eddy. "Although … We did receive the last NK cell infusion and a DC vaccine just last week."

As we continued to wonder about the mysterious invisible tumor, a thought crossed our minds.

Perhaps the lesion represented tumor flare—the influx of immune cells. That might explain the well-defined lesion on MRI. We knew that scans couldn't differentiate between tumor flare and an actual tumor. Perhaps the MRI had captured a mass of immune cells mixed with microscopic cancer.

"We'll just have to see what pathology says," said Eddy.

Excited at the possibility of an immune response against my cancer, we asked Dr. Kaplan if there was any way the resected tumor could be analyzed for immune cells. Immunotherapy was still highly experimental in 2012, and analyzing tumors for an immune response wasn't part of standard pathology practice, so Dr. Kaplan connected us with a professor of pathology at Stanford. The pathologist analyzed my tumor and confirmed our suspicion.

Just as Dr. Kaplan had observed, the pathologist also couldn't see tumor with his naked eye. Absent from my tumor was the distinct fibrous outer layer common to synovial sarcomas, known as the "pseudo-capsule." He could only see cancer cells when he looked at the sample under a microscope.

Secondly, about 40 to 50 percent of the lesion comprised inflammatory cells—meaning various cells of the immune system had swarmed my tumor.

Thirdly, some of the cancer cells appeared to be necrotic—meaning they were dead. The dead cells were all over—not congregated in any one spot.

As the interpretation of immune cells within tumors was still nascent science, the pathologist couldn't offer any conclusions. But taken together, these tantalizing clues convinced us that my immune system had attacked my tumor.

Large tumors can sometimes spontaneously necrose when they outrun their blood supply. But these fledgling clumps of cancer were microscopic—unlikely to have outgrown the capacity of supporting blood vessels. The microscopic necrosis along with the inflammatory cells suggested that immune cells had attacked and killed some of the tumor. It warranted further investigation.

Evidence of T Cells in My Tumor

It was March 18, 2012. We were in New York City for Dr. Old's memorial service. Two months had passed. My surgical wounds had healed nicely. I'd already resumed Coley's Toxins. We were intent on following Dr. Coley's practice of sandwiching surgery with the toxins.

"Where should we eat?" asked Eddy.

"I really miss New York bagels … but they're going to be difficult to chew," I said.

Now that my right jaw had been removed, I had only half the biting power of a normal person. As most of the surrounding muscles had been removed, my lower jaw pulled hard to the right. My upper and lower jaws were misaligned. Upper teeth no longer contacted lower, with the exception of a few mismatched ones. This made chewing difficult.

"I think I'll go for something soft … maybe Korean tofu soup."

"Make sure you eat enough," said Eddy. "If we're going to fit in a Coley infusion today, we'll have to start soon and skip lunch."

After walking off breakfast, we returned to the cramped hotel room on West 32nd Street, in the middle of Koreatown. Eddy turned on the TV to drown out noise from the traffic and thronging pedestrians. A rerun of *Twilight* played as we prepared for the Coley infusion.

As Eddy connected my PICC line to the saline bag hanging from the portable IV pole, I turned to him and asked, "How does my smile look?"

We were to meet people we knew at the memorial service the next day. I wanted to figure out the best way to smile—so I'd look as normal as possible when taking pictures. Missing a jaw joint made it tricky.

"Try opening your mouth a tad as you smile," said Eddy.

"That's too much. Close it a little … there we go. That looks pretty normal."

The next day, we took a cab to the MSK Rockefeller Research Laboratories auditorium. Luminaries in the field of cancer immunology had come from all over the world to honor Dr. Old. The world-famous Shanghai Quartet played pieces by Beethoven and Mozart. (Before he became a scientist, Dr. Old had trained to become a violinist.[7])

Dr. James Allison, the discoverer of CTLA-4, to whom Dr. Old had once introduced us when we visited his research laboratory in the summer of 2010, took the podium. He honored Dr. Old as his mentor and friend.

For the first time in person, we met Ronny, a tall, cheerful, intelligent young man in his 20s. Ronny was one of the many other patients Dr. Old had helped get into immunotherapy clinical trials. We instantly bonded. Not just because he, too, had synovial sarcoma—but because he exuded hope and inspired us with his can-do fighting spirit. His loving fiancée and parents were by his side. Like Eddy had done for me, they'd cared for Ronny, traveling with him for years in search of a cure.

Also there were members of Dr. Old's team who'd freely given their time to put together my NY-ESO-1 vaccine protocol: Linda Pan, Pharm.D., the clinical trial coordinator who'd helped organized the entire effort; Sacha Gjnatic, Ph.D., the immunologist who'd analyzed my blood to confirm presence of NY-ESO-1 T cells; and Achim Jungbluth, M.D., Ph.D., the pathologist who'd examined my original tumor for presence of NY-ESO-1.

After the service, Dr. Jungbluth invited us over to his lab where he showed us slides of my most recent tumor. We had sent him a sample weeks earlier. Peering through the lenses of a four-headed microscope (where up to four people can view the same sample simultaneously), Dr. Jungbluth took us on a journey into the microscopic world of my tumor.

First, he showed us a lymph node. He then showed us areas of fibrosis, scar tissue probably caused by prior radiation or cryoablation. Next came the cancer cells. Still expressing NY-ESO-1, they were stained brown and easily distinguishable.

And then came the exciting part—the necrosis.

"Here's an area of necrotic tumor ... and another one here ... and here," said Dr. Jungbluth.

Dr. Jungbluth pointed out that the "islands" of necrotic tumor were surrounded by rings of T cells, along with other immune cells.

We already knew that immune cells had swarmed my tumor. But to see this vivid picture of my actual T cells—those soldiers of the adaptive immune system—surrounding dead tumor, strongly suggested the T cells had killed some cancer. Although the science of interpreting immune cells within tumors is nascent, Dr. Jungbluth's findings implied that our back-breaking efforts at creating T cells may have succeeded after all.

Dr. Shah had said it was a matter of time before the cancer would kill me. That was predicated on the idea that no therapy could eliminate the "thousands of microscopic tumors." But evidence of T cells changed that assumption, making a cure plausible.

Lesson learned: Would my T cells have eventually eliminated all of the tumor had I waited longer (as in Mr. Telford's case)? I'll never know. But I didn't regret cutting out my jaw.

Immunotherapy can produce mixed responses: some tumors may shrink, while others continue to grow. What good would it do if my T cells killed the 999 micro-tumors—but the single visible lesion kept growing and eventually killed me? The precarious location meant I couldn't afford to take the chance.

A Renewed Faith

Two months earlier, the second recurrence had demoralized us, filling us with guilt for wasting a fortune on seemingly fruitless efforts. Had we not tried to find out if my tumor contained immune cells, we might've assumed that the entire tumor contained unchecked malignancy and abandoned immunotherapy altogether. But the image of T cells besieging dead tumor buttressed our faith in immunotherapy.

By now, I had completed a year's worth of Coley Fluid infusions—117 fevers in all. These infusions were different from how Dr. Coley had administered his toxins. Intravenous infusion of medicines were not widely available until the 1950s.[8] Instead, Dr. Coley injected his toxins directly into tumors, or sometimes, into large muscles.

A year earlier, we'd wanted to inject Coley Fluid directly into my tumor—but there wasn't a safe and practical way to inject through the jaw bone. With my right jaw gone, a carefully placed syringe could easily reach into the surgical bed—right where the tumor once resided. (This was another reason I'd declined reconstruction, as the transplanted bone or tissue would impede injections.)

Dr. Coley advocated injecting the tumor bed within days after surgery, a practice we labored to reproduce. Two weeks after my surgery in February 2012—even before receiving evidence of necrosis from Stanford, and later from Dr. Jungbluth, we began injecting Coley Fluid into the post-surgical bed.

Dr. Shah had affirmed what the survival curves showed: I was going to die.

But I was not ready to.

The tumor-killing T cells renewed our hope.

We were going to unleash the full fury of Coley's Toxins at the site of my tumor.

CHAPTER 14

Injecting Tumors

I tensed up as Eddy positioned the small syringe containing the Coley Fluid at the edge of my cheek. His hands trembled as he checked and re-checked the needle position.

I lay in bed on my left side. A disposable blue, translucent bouffant cap—worn by doctors to prevent hair from contaminating sterile fields during surgery—covered my head. Eddy taped up the small tuft of exposed sideburn. Using a disposable razor, he shaved off all hair from the crater in front of my right ear.

Donning disposable gloves and a face mask, he tore open a pack of disinfectant swab sticks—sterile Q-tips soaked with povidone iodine. Starting at the injection point, he painted my skin brown, working a swab stick outward in concentric circles. The outward motion would sweep bacteria away from the injection point, helping to disinfect it. He waited three minutes for the iodine to dry (a necessary step to sterilize the skin).[1] Paranoid about sepsis, he repeated the process—five more times—each time using a fresh swab stick.

This was to be the first injection into my jaw. It was two weeks after Dr. Kaplan had removed my right jaw bone. Unlike the previous infusions—where we diluted Coley Fluid into a bag of saline and slowly infused it into my bloodstream, this would be a concentrated injection into the side of my face. With my jaw bone gone, we could now inject Coley Fluid right where my tumor once sat.

We had studied my head MRIs to find the safest injection site. Using a tape measure, Eddy had measured and re-measured distances from various points of my right ear to confirm the spot he was about to pierce.

Earlier, we'd asked Dr. Kaplan to show us the location of the carotid artery on MRI. We needed to understand the risks of injecting within the now-transformed landscape of my jaw—the greatest being accidental puncture of critical blood vessels such as the carotid artery.

We identified a safe spot far enough from the carotid but still within the surgical bed. A needle entering about one centimeter in front of the ear at nose-level would reach it. As long as the needle angled forward and downward, there'd be no risk of hitting the carotid. To reduce the risk of damage, we'd use a fine 28-gauge insulin syringe, its needle only 1.3 centimeters long.

Dr. Coley had injected his first patient (Mr. Zola) with live erysipelas. The bulky tumor was just underneath his right ear, perhaps even closer to the carotid. The injections were safe for Mr. Zola. We believed they'd be safe for me.

We'd hoped to find a doctor willing to administer the injections. But it became clear that none would be willing to inject Coley Fluid. They didn't have experience with it. And in the U.S., the fear of lawsuits made it even riskier.

We concluded we had to do it ourselves. I couldn't safely inject the side of my face so Eddy took up the responsibility.

"What choice do we have," said Eddy. "Dr. Shah confirmed there's no way of getting all the cancer in your head. We have to do everything possible to make immunotherapy work. Otherwise the sarcoma's going to kill you. The MDA curves agree."

"I know," I said. "But aren't you afraid?"

"Terrified. But we've done our homework ... We'll start with the tiniest dose. And ramp up *real* slow."

"Gosh. This is scary!" said Eddy, still hesitating to proceed.

"Don't worry," I said. "I'll keep giving you feedback."

The needle pierced my skin. He gently advanced the needle, while asking if I felt anything. Satisfied he'd reached deep enough into the surgical bed, he began to inject the Coley Fluid.

"I'm feeling resistance. I'm afraid to push too hard on the syringe," said Eddy, his hands still trembling. Sweat streamed from his forehead, drenching the surgical mask over his mouth.

"I can't afford to drip sweat on you. It'll contaminate the area," he said. Making sure the syringe could stand by itself, he left it embedded in my jaw, told me not to move, then ran to dry himself and change his surgical mask.

He ripped off the disposable gloves. Sweat had pooled in the finger sheaths. Drying his drenched palms, he donned a new pair, then resumed his position bedside.

"OK, I've injected 0.1 ccs. Keep telling me how you feel," he said.

I stared at the wall to my left, mumbling feedback, afraid to move my jaw in case it would shift the needle.

"No pain."

"Good. 0.2 ccs have entered. Another 0.3 left. It's getting even harder to press."

Suddenly, I winced. A bolt of sensation shot from my cheek to my temple.

"Might be hitting a nerve. I'm going to back up and try a different spot," said Eddy.

Gingerly, he retracted the needle. Making sure not to contaminate it by touching unsterilized skin or hair, he repositioned it about half a centimeter closer to my nose. The remaining fluid went in easily.

The rest of the afternoon was anti-climactic. We had used such a low dose of Coley Fluid that I experienced nothing. No fever. No redness on my face.

Two days later, we injected a higher dose. This time, my cheek grew hot, inflamed and swollen. It was painful to chew my dinner. The increased dosage had elicited a reaction in my jaw. Still—no fever.

By the next day, the pain mostly subsided. But the swelling persisted for days, filling out the depression in my jaw.

Why Inject Tumors?

Dr. Coley and his colleagues had injected tumors directly with the toxins. They injected tumors to shrink them before surgery. They also injected the post-surgical bed (after tumors had been removed) to destroy remaining micro-tumors. They performed these injections not based on scientific theory. Experience and observation guided their practice; injected tumors shrank more readily and stayed away longer.

But weren't intravenous infusions good enough? How did injections into tumors differ from intravenous infusions?

When Coley's Toxins is injected into a tumor, dead bacterial fragments are concentrated in a small area, acting as a homing beacon for immune cells. Innate immune cells (such as neutrophils and macrophages) are awakened, alarmed by the bacterial signatures. Thinking that foreign bacteria have invaded the body, they swarm the location, secreting inflammatory proteins to call for reinforcements.

Dr. Old had mentioned that this acute inflammation may convert the environment within the tumor to one that enables immune cells to attack cancer. Attracted into the tumor, the swarming immune cells may kill some cancer. Dying cancer cells are then engulfed by dendritic cells drawn to the site of danger. The dendritic cells may activate T cells against cancer antigens, triggering a full-fledged adaptive response against cancer throughout the body.

In contrast, when Coley's Toxins is infused into the vein, the bacterial toxins are quickly diluted in the blood and circulate the entire body. Some toxins may still reach the tumor, but at a much lower concentration. The dispersed toxins still attract immune cells, causing systemic inflammation and fever. But the inflammation isn't concentrated at the tumor. It quickly disperses; the fever subsides within hours. In contrast, the inflammation and swelling from injections into tumors can last for days, as it takes longer for the trapped bacterial fragments to clear out from tissues.

Scientists still don't fully understand how tumors respond to Coley injections. But it is clear that the benefits of injecting tumors aren't confined to Coley's Toxins. Immunologists are actively studying the effect of *intratumoral immunotherapy* (where various immune substances are injected into tumors). One of those researchers is Ronald Levy, M.D., a renowned immunologist at Stanford University.

Dr. Levy has researched intratumoral immunotherapy for many years.[2] In 2008, the year I was diagnosed, Dr. Levy published fascinating results of a study.[3] Dr. Levy's team treated fifteen patients with refractory low-grade B cell lymphoma (a cancer of the white blood cells). They treated a single tumor from each patient with a low dose of radiation. The radiation killed some tumor cells, creating a vaccine within the patient's body. In addition to radiation, the team injected the tumor with CpG, a substance that resembles bacterial DNA. Like Coley's Toxins, CpG tricks the immune system into thinking that bacteria have invaded the body.

The results were astonishing. The low doses of radiation and repeated injections of CpG in a single tumor induced systemic responses in a majority of the patients. Cancer throughout the body shrunk or stopped growing. One 38-year-old patient experienced complete disappearance of disease. It was as if these patients had received powerful systemic chemotherapy—but without toxic side effects.

Eddy and I were intrigued by Dr. Levy's research. His philosophy of using low doses of focal immunotherapy to awaken the immune system to cancer reminded us of Dr. Coley's injections into tumors.

In addition to CpG, Dr. Levy is attempting to improve on his results by injecting checkpoint-inhibiting antibodies (like PD-1 and CTLA-4) or immune-activating antibodies (like OX40) into tumors.[4] The antibody that seems to work best is OX40. Dr. Levy thinks that OX40 may work by eliminating Tregs (those fearsome bodyguards of tumors that Dr. Old had suspected could be depleted with Coley's Toxins).[5,6]

Perhaps that's how intratumoral injections of Coley's Toxins can cure some patients. First, it may kill some cancer at the site of a tumor, thereby "vaccinating" the patient. Second, if Dr. Old's hunch was right, it may deplete Tregs or other tumor defenses, thus fully activating the immune system, unleashing it against cancer around the body.

Laudable Pus

Intent on unleashing the full effects of Coley's Toxins, we continued with the jaw injections every two or three days. On the off-days, I continued with the intravenous infusions. We watched for side effects and for signs of infection. None came. Satisfied we'd figured out a safe system to inject Coley Fluid, we ramped up the dosage.

The higher dosage caused a painful tightness in my right upper cheek. Patches of red appeared, just under the skin. The pain and swelling would subside after a few hours. But the swelling would resurge when I received intravenous infusions, sometimes causing a pricking sensation on my right ear lobe or just inside the ear canal. All of these were consistent with symptoms of acute swelling, caused by the influx of immune cells.

Mostly, the side effects of the injections were minor and transient, even mundane. But on three occasions, the swelling and pain were intense.

I whimpered and cried, tossing and turning in bed for half an hour before the pain subsided.

The first time it happened, Eddy freaked out. He wanted to give me Tylenol to kill the reaction. But I knew the pain would pass once the toxins cleared out of my system. So, in the midst of my whimpering, I tried to reassure him I'd be OK.

In time, we became acquainted with the symptoms. And Eddy became adept at administering the injections. Over the next four months, I'd receive 30 injections, alternating them with intravenous infusions—sometimes doing both on the same day. We'd continue these wherever our adventures took us—California, New York, Texas, Germany and Singapore.

On May 17, 2012, we were in a hotel, about seven miles south of Frankfurt Airport. We were to fly home to San Francisco the next morning. I'd received a dendritic vaccine in Duderstadt two days earlier and had immediately followed it with an intravenous infusion of Coley Fluid.

Wanting to draw Dr. Nesselhut's dendritic cells to my jaw and provoke them into action, we contemplated injecting a large dose of Coley Fluid.

Our hotel room was on the third floor. Eddy opened the wide window, letting in crisp spring air. A view of a lake ringed by lush, green vegetation greeted us. It was a clear spring day, the temperature in the 60s.

"It's so pretty! Let's take a walk before we start the injection," I said.

We approached the narrow paved path that circled the lake. A man rode past on a bicycle. A picnic basket sat on the rear rack. A corner of red and white plaid cloth peeked out from under its lid, flapping in the wind. I imagined the delicacies it held that would soon be relished. Another man walked past with his fishing pole. Everywhere, the chirping of crickets could be heard, emanating from dense, long grass. Twenty feet ahead of us, a rabbit froze on the path.

"Let's sit here a minute," said Eddy, as we came upon a wooden bench.

"We've come a long way, haven't we?" He gazed contemplatively at the lake.

"Four years and three months since diagnosis," I said.

"Do you feel down about it?" Eddy flung a little pebble, trying to skip it across the water. It sank.

"No. I think we're doing quite well. Bessie Dashiell's olive-sized tumor killed her in three months. It's been 15 months since my jaw tumor recurred, and I'm still alive …"

"If you had to guess, which immunotherapies have helped the most?" asked Eddy.

"Well, the T cell necrosis came sometime after the cryo, the DC vaccines and the NK infusions. I don't think there's any way to figure out which contributed the most," I said.

"I really wonder which one did it," said Eddy. "The blood analysis shows that your T cells can attack other segments of the NY-ESO-1 protein. Not just the ones you were vaccinated against."

He was referring to a recent blood test Dr. Gnjatic had performed. (Dr. Gnjatic was the colleague of Dr. Old who'd been analyzing my blood since the NY-ESO-1 vaccine.)

"That my T cells can target more than what they'd been trained to do suggests a broader awakening of my immune system. If I had to guess, I'd say it was the cryo," I said. "The freezing destroyed billions of tumor cells and unleashed a wide assortment of tumor antigens, acting like a broad vaccine."

"Do you think there's any point in keeping up these Coley injections then?" Eddy asked.

"I do. It's been our philosophy to layer multiple strategies," I said. "Remember what Dr. Old said about sticking to a philosophy?"

"Right … I keep thinking how Mrs. Gruver's son injected her abdominal tumors for almost three years. What perseverance," said Eddy. Injections of her twin tumors with the toxins had cured Mrs. Gruver of terminal metastatic cervical cancer.

"Even if it doesn't cure me, I'll be glad if it kills the micro-tumors in my head."

"I agree. Let's try to get a strong immune reaction going in your jaw." Eddy grasped my hand and began to get up.

It was about 4 p.m. We finished our stroll around the lake, went back to the room and prepared for the injection.

The first half of the needle didn't go in easily. Perhaps the skin had scarred from prior injections. But the second half went in without problem. I felt no pain or sensation.

A short while later, my jaw felt sore. By 7 p.m., Eddy noticed a slight swelling in my cheek. My right upper eyelid seemed pinkish. But there wasn't obvious redness.

"Seems like this one's going to be mild. Should we add an intravenous infusion to boost it?" asked Eddy.

"Let's try for a strong reaction in the jaw. Let's inject more in the same spot," I said.

Again, the first half of the needle met with resistance. And again, I felt no pain or sensation. Eddy injected the second dose.

As he retracted the needle, he noticed some thick, whitish pus on the metal. A small amount oozed from the injection site.

"I see pus. Probably just dead immune cells from the first injection," said Eddy.

Pus comprises white blood cells that have died from fighting an infection. But in this case, the pus signified white cells fighting harmless dead bacterial fragments from Coley Fluid.

Tired, I closed my eyes. It was 9 p.m. As the sun set, I fell into a deep sleep.

The next morning, the skin around my right cheek bone and temple displayed a slight reddish hue. At Frankfurt Airport, my right teeth ached when I chewed on a pork chop and sautéed onion sandwich. I sulked as I surrendered the sandwich to Eddy, settling for a yogurt drink.

We boarded the plane to San Francisco. Fatigued from the ongoing immune reaction in my head, I slept through the flight, missing my meals—something that never happens, as I loved the simple thrill of savoring in-flight meals.

By the time we landed, the entire right side of my face—including my cheek and eyelids—had become swollen and bright red. It looked as if I had erysipelas—that disease with which Dr. Coley had infected his first patient. Passengers and flight attendants stared, then looked away when I caught their eye. Thankfully, the Customs and Immigration officer didn't stop me from re-entering the country.

Back home, the swelling and redness lasted a good three days. The skin at the injection site—about the width of a pea—became soft and blister-like, then turned dark purple. A two-millimeter hole broke. Thick sterile pus oozed out. We weren't concerned. A century earlier, Dr. Coley and his colleagues had documented this benign side-effect of intratumoral injections.

Before antibiotics were discovered, surgeons paid careful attention to pus in surgical wounds. They identified different types of pus to predict how patients would fare. There was the "bad" kind of pus—watery, tinged with blood and foul smelling, portending infection and death. And there was the "good" kind—thicker, cream-colored and odorless, described as "laudable pus." Surgeons considered this beneficial pus as a sign that the wound would heal because, "nature [the immune system] ha[d] put up a bold fight against the invader."[7]

Antiquated notions of pus notwithstanding, we lauded the odorless pus oozing out of that little hole in the side of my face. We hoped it meant we'd succeeded in bringing the fight to the micro-tumors in my head. The hole healed within days. But subsequent injections would cause it to open up more easily, prompting us to decrease the frequency of injections.

Turning Attention to My Lungs

While the battle against the legion of micro-tumors in my jaw raged, another battle was brewing—in my lungs.

Recall that shortly after the NY-ESO-1 vaccine in early 2010, CT scans had revealed three small lung lesions, one of which had grown. As they were only two to three mm wide and growing slowly, Dr. Benjamin at MD Anderson wasn't certain they were cancerous, but advocated close monitoring.

Eddy and I had tracked the growth of these hollow lesions over the past two years. By now, they'd grown to eight mm wide. Oddly, the one in my left upper lung had begun to "fill in." It was located in the same lobe that had almost been skewered in Detroit. We were concerned that the changes represented advancing cancer.

Having been steeped in years of driving my own care and charting my own treatment, we had developed a proactive proclivity toward intercepting problems early on. We'd seen too many patients struggle with advancing lung tumors that caused disruptive symptoms like bleeding, coughing and difficulty breathing. These symptoms made travel difficult, if not impossible. Now was the time to consult lung surgeons.

Through the online sarcoma forum, we'd befriended Agnes, the mother of John (the young man mentioned in chapter 10). Eight years earlier, John had 130 sarcoma tumors in both lungs and should have died within months. But Agnes refused to accept her son's demise, scouring for alternatives and finally finding an "experimental" surgical technique in Germany. That technique gave her son what conventional surgery or che-motherapy couldn't: the ability, not just to stay alive, but to run 10K races.

Axel Rolle, M.D., Ph.D., Director of the Center of Pulmonology and Thoracic Surgery at a specialist hospital in Coswig, Germany, had been honing this experimental technique since 1995. Instead of using mechani-cal tools to cut out cancerous pieces of lung, Dr. Rolle used a laser to burn away lung tissue.

Conventional mechanical tools make it difficult, if not impossible, to operate on numerous tumors dispersed throughout the lung. Think of a balloon with a hundred defects spread across its surface. You'd first have to deflate the balloon. Then, you'd have to isolate each defect, stretching it away from the rest of the balloon. Then you'd cut across the stretch, sealing (or suturing) the cut. You'd have to repeat this a hundred times. By the time you're done, you'd have cut away all of the healthy surface of the balloon— there'd be no balloon left. In such hopeless cases, surgeons would remove the entire lobe. If the tumors are spread across all five lobes, the patient is deemed inoperable.

In contrast, using his laser, Dr. Rolle could burn away small tumors without needing to cut away healthy lung tissue. Larger tumors could be circumscribed by the laser, sparing as much healthy tissue as possible, while "sterilizing" the cut edges with heat to reduce recurrences. Patients no longer had to lose entire lobes. These advantages made it possible to dramatically extend the life of patients who'd otherwise die.

More on Laser Lung Surgery

Laser lung surgery was first proposed by an American surgeon at Northwestern Univer-sity in 1985.[8] Medical centers in the U.S., Japan and Europe began experimenting with lasers. But technical limitations led to their abandonment. Even so, Dr. Rolle had con-tinued research in this field and developed a solution that overcame the limitations. For example, by using a different wavelength, the cutting laser would better coagulate blood, thereby "sealing" lung tissue simultaneously.[9]

Many cancers spread to the lungs, where tumor cells get trapped in small veins and capillaries finer than the width of a human hair.[10] Dr. Rolle's tissue-sparing tech-nique made surgery possible for patients deemed inoperable with conventional tech-niques. In 2006, Dr. Rolle published a study showing that patients with various cancers could be successfully operated on with his laser—even patients with numerous tumors spread throughout their lungs.[11]

The Journey to Coswig

It was the end of June in 2012. I'd just received my eighth dendritic vaccine in Germany. Seeking to get ahead of the possibility of advancing cancer in my lungs, we decided to consult Dr. Rolle. We took a four-hour train ride from Göttingen to Dresden, a magnificent city near the Eastern border alongside the Czech Republic and Poland.

The city has since been meticulously rebuilt after being leveled by Allied forces in 1945. In between infusions and injections of Coley Fluid, we toured the city by bus, reveling in the view of magnificent edifices. Cruising down the Elbe river in a tourist boat, we waved to locals sunbathing on the banks.

On July 3, we took a taxi to Coswig, a small town of 12,000, twenty minutes outside Dresden. We checked in at the nondescript specialist lung hospital. A nurse showed us to Dr. Rolle's office.

Dr. Rolle was gentle and kind. He scrutinized the CT images of my lung, examining the growth of the three lesions from 2009. He believed they were sarcoma metastases, as they had once been round and solid, but had become hollow. He suspected the NY-ESO-1 vaccine had created T cells against cancer in my lungs. But he surmised that if all of the cancer had died, the lesions should have eventually shrunk and become scar tissue. Since the hollow cysts were still expanding, there was likely cancer at their edges, eating away at surrounding lung tissue.

Dr. Rolle said the tumor in my right lower lobe would be tricky to locate during surgery. Unlike the other two that were closer to the surface, it was deep, closer to the bronchi (the main airways of the lung). Unlike surface tumors, he wouldn't be able to see this embedded tumor and would have to rely on the ability to feel it. A solid tumor can normally be palpated, as it feels like a hard lump. But since this lesion was hollow, he could end up crushing it and never finding it.

Dr. Rolle also described how it was important to wait for other lung tumors to reveal themselves before operating. Open-chest lung surgery is one of the most painful surgical procedures.[12] It requires weeks of recovery. Furthermore, these lesions had arisen before my head recurrences. The head recurrences could have seeded new lung tumors. These later seeds could still be invisible. For these reasons, Dr. Rolle recommended we wait a little longer before operating.

We were grateful for the hour-long meeting with this world-class surgeon and astonished at how inexpensive the consultation had been—it cost 50 Euro (about 65 U.S. dollars). But as the taxi took us back to Dresden, we left with mixed feelings.

On the one hand, finding an alternative to conventional surgery encouraged us. Metastatic sarcoma is a death sentence for most. Chemo may extend life by weeks, maybe months, but not years. But for a subset of patients, whose only site of disease is in the lungs, surgery can buy years of life.[13] In short, lung tumors can be continually "weeded" with surgery, keeping the patient alive, until there's no more lung tissue left to sacrifice. And Dr. Rolle's tissue-sparing technique could extend my life longer than conventional surgery would.

On the other hand, Dr. Rolle had corroborated what we had feared all along—that my cancer had already gone metastatic—that is, it had spread beyond the original site. Frankly, the majority of patients with metastatic sarcoma soon die. Unless I fell into that lucky subset of patients for which "weeding" worked, I would too.

The Beginning of the End?

Sobered by the reality of metastatic disease, we pivoted our attention toward my lungs. Having learned the value of expert opinion, we pursued more perspectives on lung surgery.

Two weeks later, we consulted the Chief of General Thoracic Surgery at the University of California, San Francisco (UCSF), David Jablons, M.D. Affable and energetic, Dr. Jablons also suspected my lesions had hollowed out in response to the NY-ESO-1 vaccine. He confirmed that the hollow cysts would be difficult to find and might be inadvertently crushed. We recounted the lung collapse in Detroit and the subsequent mechanical pleurodesis—the repair procedure that had fused my left lung to the chest wall. Dr. Jablons warned that the pleurodesis would complicate surgery. Like Dr. Rolle, he said to keep watching for more tumors to declare themselves.

As the reality of having metastatic sarcoma sank in, we realized that our still-intensifying battle—now having dragged on for over four and a half years—was likely in the early innings of a dangerous new phase. After two years of indolent growth, the signs of accelerating lung tumors could portend the soon-to-come exponential spread that sarcomas are notorious for—like what had happened to Bessie Dashiell.

We planned a trip to see Eddy's parents in Singapore. Because of my protracted battle, he had not seen his parents for over five years already. The last time they'd met had been at our wedding, one year before my diagnosis. My mother-in-law's birthday was coming soon, and I wanted us to see her before my treatment intensified further.

In early August, 2012, I received my ninth dendritic vaccine in Duderstadt. Three days later, we were back in the Bay Area. The day after, we boarded a plane to Singapore. We surprised Eddy's mom, glad to celebrate her birthday with her. In the heat and humidity, I continued my Coley infusions and injections. A month later, we were back in Duderstadt for my tenth dendritic vaccine. The zigzagging across the globe was wearing us out and rapidly depleting our savings. But the back-to-back tumor recurrences in my head, and now, the advancing lung lesions, had launched us into an all-out frenzy to ward off full-blown sarcoma.

Validation

In late September, we were back in Houston for another lung CT. (By now, I was getting all scans at MD Anderson, no longer at Stanford.) The scan showed the once-hollow lesion in my left lung had become almost fully solid. With this latest change, Dr. Benjamin concurred the lesion represented metastatic sarcoma. He suggested surgery.

We reminded him that my left lung was fused to the chest wall, and recounted Dr. Jablons' concern that surgery would be complicated. To circumvent that problem, Dr. Benjamin suggested we consider ablation techniques. MD Anderson offered radiofrequency ablation, a technique similar to cryoablation, but one that generated heat instead of cold. He was also open to cryoablation with Dr. Littrup in Detroit.

During that same trip, we saw Dr. Patrick Hwu, M.D., Chairman of Sarcoma and Melanoma Oncology (now Head of Cancer Medicine at MD Anderson). Dr. Benjamin had suggested we seek counsel with Dr. Hwu, an internationally respected physician-scientist with over 25 years of experience in cancer immunotherapy.

Meeting Dr. Hwu was a turning point. For the first time, I was speaking with an oncologist at a conventional cancer center who understood every aspect of our immunotherapy effort. In 2008, my original sarcoma oncologist at Stanford had told me that sarcomas do not respond to Coley's Toxins. When she retired, the younger oncologist who took over dropped me after I went to Mexico for Coley Fluid. In contrast, Dr. Hwu agreed with us that sarcomas are immunogenic. He agreed with my efforts at getting Coley's Toxins. He agreed that cryoablation can sometimes act as a vaccine to create T cells. And he said to keep up with these immunotherapies.

Déjà vu: Debating Cryo Versus Surgery

It was time to get serious about getting rid of the growing tumor in my left upper lobe. We already had two surgical opinions. Both surgeons had said that prior mechanical pleurodesis would complicate surgery. We thought of Agnes and John. After Dr. Rolle had lasered away John's initial 130 lung tumors, John began going to Dr. Littrup in Detroit to cryoablate a tumor or two every few months. Instead of painful surgeries, many of his procedures were outpatient. He had employed this strategy for years, enjoying a high quality of life, taking part in active sports. John was a living inspiration and a medical marvel. Could cryo be a suitable alternative to surgery for me?

We were already familiar with Dr. Littrup's skill from my jaw cryo, done a year earlier. We had studied the medical literature and concluded that lung cryo was safe and effective, especially for small tumors. Even if it failed to destroy a tumor, it could be repeated in the same spot, without cumulative side effects. Unlike radiation, tumors cannot develop resistance to the freezing cold. Side effects were low, as evidenced by the outpatient nature. As it relied on CT imaging to locate tumors, it was ideal for hollow lesions that could not be palpated.

But most attractive was cryo's ability to act as a vaccine, sensitizing my immune system to antigens within my lung tumors. Tumors in different parts of the body may not necessarily harbor the same antigens.[14] For example, the recurrent tumor in my head could have expressed different antigens from the tumors in my lungs. If so, T cells created by the head cryo would fail to target my lung tumors, which could account for their continued growth. Perhaps it was prudent that we cryo at least one lung lesion?

To confirm our understanding of lung cryo, we flew to Detroit to consult Dr. Littrup. Dr. Littrup said the success rate for destroying small tumors was over 90 percent.[15] He confirmed what Agnes had told us—that side effects were low, and the pain afterwards was minimal. He also described how cryo is often used to ease debilitating pain from lung surgery or cancer that has spread to the bone.[16,17] As my lung had been fused to the chest wall, the risk of further lung collapse was low. Dr. Littrup also said he would bracket the tumor between two cryoprobes, instead of inserting a single needle into the tumor. This strategy would increase the odds of complete kill while reducing the risk of seeding tumor along the needle track. Leaving Detroit, we were heartened that cryoablation seemed to be a strong candidate for my lung tumors.

As if our research had not been thorough enough, in the two weeks after seeing Dr. Littrup, we saw another lung surgeon back at UCSF (whom Dr. Jablons had recommended), and then a lung surgeon at MD Anderson that Dr. Benjamin had referred us to. Both surgeons felt that the lesions in my lung were cancerous, affirming Dr. Rolle and Dr. Benjamin's opinions. In two weeks, we had seen three doctors in three different states, all the while continuing Coley infusions and injections in hotel rooms. Despite the overkill, we were grateful to glean insights from these experienced physicians. It would help us to once again weigh conventional surgery against "experimental" cryo.

In the end, we decided on cryoablation. Aside from the low side effects that would allow me to resume immunotherapy faster, it offered three irresistible advantages.

First, it could act as a vaccine against my lung tumors.

Second, the prior pleurodesis (that would complicate surgery) would instead help cryo, making it safer by preventing lung collapse.

Third, the tumor was at the edge of the lung and may have invaded the adjacent chest wall; the cryo ice ball could kill the tumor while sterilizing the adjacent chest wall at the same time.

Satisfied we had done our homework and having Dr. Benjamin's approval, we forged ahead with plans to cryoablate the left lung tumor.

Bringing The Fight to My Lungs

On December 8, 2012, we flew to Detroit for the lung cryo. Ten days and one year earlier, our beloved mentor, Dr. Old, had passed away. We remembered his lifelong efforts to defend immunotherapy—even when some considered it quackery. It gave us strength to hold fast to our conviction that immunotherapy was my only realistic hope for survival.

We were battle-hardened and ready for the next skirmish.

We'd been faithful with the Coley infusions. Three days before landing in Detroit, I'd completed my 202nd intravenous infusion into my blood. A few days earlier, I'd received my 38th injection into my jaw. We'd continued Coley's Toxins all over the world, lugging bulky supplies to keep my PICC line sterile for over two years to avoid sepsis.

"Come February, you'd have been alive five years since diagnosis," said Eddy, holding my hand as we waited in the surgical staging area.

The cryo was supposed to have started late morning. It was now past 5 p.m. But we weren't antsy. We knew how hard Dr. Littrup and his small team labored, working to extend the lives of patients who had flown from as far as Finland for his cryoablation.

Finally, they came to wheel me in.

"Thanks for fighting so hard for me all these years," I said, letting go of Eddy's hand. "I love you."

"I love you, too. I'll see you in a bit," he said.

Two hours later, I was back in the post-surgery recovery area.

The short-acting anesthetics had worn off. I'd been given conscious sedation, not general anesthesia. I had been awake as Dr. Littrup and his colleague, Dr. Aoun, inserted two cryoprobes straight through my chest wall into my lungs, freezing the tumor to death.

Despite the intentional skewering, I felt no pain.

I was fatigued. It had been a long day and I'd had my last meal almost 24 hours earlier.

Behind the curtains to my left, a nurse tended to a patient coughing violently. Voices murmured from a TV.

A while later, Eddy came by.

"Hey there. How do you feel?" he asked.

"Just really fatigued. But no pain at all," I said.

"Did you cough that out?" asked Eddy, pointing to the plastic cup in my hand that contained a smattering of blood.

"Yes. Don't worry. It looks scarier than it is."

Despite the unnerving image, coughing up a little blood after lung cryo is a normal and benign side effect. Unless a patient has clotting problems, the internal bleeding quickly stabilizes, aided by the freezing.

"It looks like the procedure was a success," said Eddy. "Dr. Littrup said the nodule had become fully solid, suggesting a cancerous nature. He ablated a bit of the chest wall—just in case the tumor had invaded it."

As it was late, Dr. Littrup ordered that I be kept overnight for observation. In the ward, I wolfed down a meal of baked sole and mashed potatoes, chicken soup and cling peaches. Eddy slept by my side in an arm chair.

Out of an abundance of caution, we stayed in Detroit for another two weeks, in case of late side effects such as a collapsed lung. But this time, there were zero complications. We visited the beautiful Somerset Collection mall in Troy, a half-hour drive from Detroit, marveling at giant, intricate Christmas decorations—angels and fairies—dangling from the ceiling. We joined thousands at the Holiday Nights festival at the Henry Ford Greenfield Village in Dearborn—a historic recreation of Christmas past, spanning 200 years of American history—where we savored the smell of roasting chestnuts, the sounds of carolers, and the sights of horse-drawn wagons and Model T Fords.

Adapt or Die

The first lung cryoablation had been a success. In the coming months, we continued immunotherapy, shuttling between Germany, San Francisco, Houston and New York.

In January 2013, I had another round of scans. We remembered how my head recurrence in February 2011 hadn't been reported—until it doubled in size three months later. We sat side by side, poring over every MRI and CT slice, scouring for evidence of new tumors in my head and lungs, checking for growth of existing lesions. We found no new tumors, but we would adopt this practice for all future scans.

In April of 2013, I was back at MD Anderson for more scans. The radiology report noted "no evidence of progression or metastatic disease." But our own scrutiny of the images told us otherwise. The lesion in my right lower lobe had "filled in," just as the previously cryoablated lesion had. A hazy ring surrounded it, perhaps indicating a bleeding tumor. We believed these changes represented tumor growth. Dr. Benjamin—one of the few oncologists we know who goes out of his way to scrutinize patients' CT scans—had analyzed my chest CT. He concurred with our findings.

On April 23, I had my second lung cryo in Detroit. As I had done with the jaw cryo, I took a short course of low-dose cyclophosphamide to deplete Tregs, hoping to unleash the immune effects of cryoablation. This time, cryoablation turned out to be an outpatient procedure with zero complications—not even an overnight stay for observation. The next day, we toured the Detroit Art Institute, admiring the works of Goya, Rembrandt and van Gogh, as there was talk that the city might soon have to auction off paintings because of bankruptcy woes.[18]

The messy growth of this second tumor alarmed us. Despite our continuing efforts at immunotherapy, our fears seemed to be unfolding. We were already struggling to prevent death by a thousand micro-tumors from materializing in my head. Now, like weeds sprouted by first rains after a multi-year drought, the disease in my lungs seemed to be entering a sinister, aggressive phase.

Maybe my cancer was adapting to our efforts. Maybe it had found ways to evade my immune system. But we weren't about to give up. We would adapt as well.

We reviewed Dr. Coley's cases and the early results of PD-1 inhibitors. We noticed that some patients experienced *mixed responses*—some tumors shrank, while others kept growing.

We believed mixed responses happen because each tumor within the body may have a different makeup. A tumor's ability to evade the immune system depends on its makeup—for example, the immune cells it recruits as bodyguards, or the "scaffolding" that it surrounds itself with.[19]

The Tumor Microenvironment

The tumor microenvironment refers to the other cells and structures surrounding tumors. This includes "bad" immune cells, blood vessels and structural scaffolding (known as the *extracellular matrix*). Scientists are learning that the tumor microenvironment plays a pivotal role in repelling "good" immune cells and allowing tumors to evade the immune system.[20,21]

The prospect of a mixed response compelled us to supplement immuno-therapy with cryoablation.

We'd rely on my immune system to wipe out micro-tumors in my head and lungs. These micro-tumors might have underdeveloped defenses, and therefore be more easily attacked by immune cells.

Simultaneously, we'd leverage the low side effects of cryoablation to physically destroy intransigent tumors before they became intractable. We'd known patients on immunotherapy who had died when one or two tumors had grown too large (even as other tumors vanished).

Finally, each cryoablation would act as a custom vaccine to generate T cells against my cancer. Tumors can evolve; antigens they express can change. Each cryo would generate T cells to attack the new antigens in the ablated tumor, thereby keeping my immune system "up to date."

Having adjusted our strategy around cryoablation, we waited for the next scan.

An Omen

On June 30, 2013, I had my next CT scan in Houston. Again, the radiology report didn't note any new tumors. But again, our own analysis of the images showed otherwise (later independently confirmed by Dr. Benjamin's own scrutiny).

Since 2010, only three slow-growing lesions had besieged my lung. But this time, sitting near the bottom of my left lung, we found a new solid lesion, half a centimeter wide.

Analyzing previous scans, we traced it back to January 2013.

Plotting its growth against the other tumors, the difference was plain to see.

The others had grown over three years; this one was doubling every three months.

This new, fast growing tumor was an omen.

My disease was accelerating.

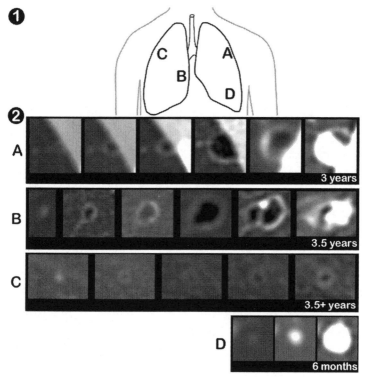

Figure 42: Location of four lung lesions (1) and appearance over time (2).

The Importance of Catching Tumors Early

For patients with metastatic disease, intercepting tumors early may be viewed as worthless. What's the point of treating one small tumor when ten—or a hundred—are soon to come? Seen as a futile endeavor, some surgeons may decline to operate.[22] Furthermore, debilitating procedures like lung surgery cannot be performed too frequently; it makes sense to "wait for more tumors" before operating.

In contrast, we adopted a different philosophy. We relied on immunotherapy to destroy disseminated invisible tumors. Simultaneously, we used cryoablation to destroy larger tumors not responsive to immunotherapy. With cryoablation, there is no advantage in waiting for tumors to grow—you can't ablate multiple tumors with a single needle. Also, the tumor kill rate with cryo is higher when tumors are smaller.

Finally, the more tumors a patient has, the less likely immunotherapy may work.[23,24] For example, tumors can secrete proteins that suppress the overall immune system. Because we were relying on immunotherapy to destroy invisible tumors, we viewed the early "weeding" of tumors as an advantage. For these reasons, we sought to detect tumors as early as possible, scrutinizing my scans instead of relying on radiology reports.

CHAPTER 15

Diet-Based Immunotherapy

"Do you think this fourth lesion appeared because we stopped Coley's Toxins and the dendritic vaccines?" asked Eddy, in between mouthfuls of a burger.

Three months earlier, just before cryoablating the second lung lesion in April 2013, I'd received my final Coley infusion. I hadn't been feeling well. I became fatigued. I lost weight. My appetite vanished. I experienced two attacks of shingles—the reactivation of dormant chickenpox virus often suffered by the elderly; it signaled a weakening of my immune system. In early May, I received my fourteenth (and final) dendritic vaccine. For the next few weeks leading up to the June 30 scan, I felt unwell and did no further immunotherapy. Now, this fourth, fast-growing lesion had appeared. Was it because we'd stopped our frantic efforts?

"Maybe this fast growing lesion isn't necessarily a bad thing? Maybe it's tumor flare—just like my last jaw tumor?" I picked up a mouthful of fried noodles—a favorite of mine—with chopsticks, but my appetite languished; nothing was appealing.

"Could be," said Eddy. "Maybe it became visible after you cryoablated the other two. Maybe the cryo taught your T cells to attack cancer in your lungs. And maybe the T cells swarmed that fourth lesion, making it visible on the scan."

"But tumor flare would still mean there was cancer to start with," I sighed, toying with a piece of fried eggplant. "This means I have cancer in four corners of my lungs."

"Had ... two of them are dead. We'll get the other two as well. A handful of tumors we can handle. It's the thousands of invisible ones that will kill you. Let's just hope the cryoablations you did in December and April managed to create T cells," said Eddy, finishing the last of his burger and getting up. "We have to get to the gate."

We rushed from the food court to the boarding gate for the United Airlines flight from Houston to San Francisco and joined the line for United's Premier Gold members.

"Nice to have this early boarding privilege from all that air travel. I can't believe how many flights we've taken these two years," said Eddy.

"At the cost of depleting our life savings," I said, reflecting on the inordinate amount of money we'd spent to keep me alive.

"Cheer up. Think of it this way—we're doing what others do when they retire ... seeing the world." Eddy handed his ticket to the gate attendant. "We'll worry about the future later ... If we beat this cancer, we'll just have to work until we're 80."

"That'll be a good problem to have," I said, thinking about Mrs. Gruver—how, cured of metastatic cervical cancer with Coley's Toxins, she lived almost 80 years.

It's nice that she'd had kids before her cancer struck. I wonder if there'll still be time for us to start a family, assuming I somehow survive the cancer.

As the plane soared above Houston International Airport, we turned our thoughts to our overall strategy. What did the faster growth of this new lesion mean? Was my cancer accelerating? Was it related to my fatigue and loss of appetite? Had we done something wrong?

Cachexia: A Wasting Syndrome

Back home at my parents' dinner table, we continued to discuss my symptoms. Mom had cooked a delicious pan-fried tofu with chicken dish. A steaming bowl of chicken broth warmed our stomachs after the flight.

"Do you think this fourth lung lesion means my cancer is about to go exponential?" I asked. "The fatigue and weight loss remind me of the original tumor. I had these symptoms when the tumor was in my head, remember?"

"Fatigue. Weight loss. Lack of appetite ... they're all symptoms of *cachexia*," said Eddy.

Also known as "wasting syndrome," cachexia is characteristic of cancer and many other serious diseases. It's often seen in end-stage cancer. Patients waste away, unable to maintain or gain weight. Fat stores rapidly deplete. Muscles atrophy as the body cannibalizes its own tissue to sustain itself. The complete causes behind cachexia are not yet understood. But research implicates inflammation as a prime suspect.[1,2,3,4]

"I thought cancer-related cachexia is usually seen in patients with larger tumors?" I asked.

"I think you're right ... Plus, you began experiencing these symptoms in ... what ... March? That was months before this fourth lesion appeared. There were no new tumors—only the filling-in of the second cyst. That small bit of tumor inside the cyst was probably too tiny to cause cachexia," said Eddy. "I doubt your symptoms are caused by cancer. I suspect they're related to too much immunotherapy."

In two years, I'd completed 223 Coley infusions—that's 223 high fevers, most reaching 103°F to 104°F—and 40 injections into my jaw. I received 14 dendritic vaccines in Germany. A jaw cryo. Two more to my lungs. Three billion NK cells. Had all of this been too much for my body? Had excess immunotherapy weakened my immune system? Could this explain the recent fatigue, weight loss and shingles?

"Maybe all that immunotherapy tipped me into a state of *chronic inflammation*?" I said.

"That would be my guess," said Eddy.

Inflammation, the Fuel of Tumors

Inflammation has become a buzzword in health circles. Books abound that describe it. All kinds of supplements are sold that claim to conquer it. But what is inflammation? How did it relate to my immunotherapy? And what does *chronic* inflammation mean?

When we speak of inflammation, we're most often speaking about *acute* inflammation. Acute inflammation is the body's healing response to finger cuts, ankle sprains, sore throats and so on. It is characterized by well-known signs: pain, swelling, redness and warmth. When a wound opens and foreign bacteria invade, immune cells rush in. These cells secrete cytokines (inflammatory proteins). These cytokines help immune cells kill pathogens, repair wounds and clear away dead tissue. Acute inflammation is temporary and purposeful. When the problem is solved, immune cells stand down, and the inflammation and symptoms subside. So then, inflammation is fundamentally an immune response.

When Coley Fluid was infused into my blood, immune cells rushed in to attack and clear away the dead bacteria. When Coley Fluid was injected into my jaw, immune cells swarmed there, causing temporary swelling, redness, warmth and pain. When my jaw and lung tumors were cryoablated, the sudden "frost-bite" triggered an intense inflammation deep within my body, drawing immune cells to repair and clear-away dead tumor cells. For my dendritic and NK cell treatments, Dr. Nesselhut inflamed those cells in the laboratory (with cytokines) before re-injecting them into me. But in all these cases, the acute inflammation subsided quickly, within hours to days.

When the immune system is overstimulated, the acute inflammation may tip into a state of *chronic* inflammation.[5] Instead of finishing their job and standing down, immune cells stay stuck in a heightened state. They begin secreting different cytokines. The cytokines recruit other immune cells not typically involved in acute inflammation. Instead of healing and repairing, these immune cells may harm the body. The beneficial acute inflammation morphs into a damaging, chronic form that can last for months or years.

In contrast to acute inflammation, chronic inflammation is insidious, usually showing no symptoms. It often arises in the presence of triggers that provoke a chronic immune response. Examples are unresolved infections (caused by bacteria, viruses or parasites), asbestos trapped in the lungs, constant exposure to ultraviolet light from tanning beds, autoimmune diseases and repeat physical trauma.

In recent years, science has revealed the pervasive role of chronic inflammation in many major diseases, one of which is type 2 diabetes. Almost one in ten Americans have type 2 diabetes.[6] Often thought to be caused by a mix of factors, including lack of exercise, "eating too much sugar" or "bad genes," studies increasingly implicate chronic inflammation as the root cause.[7,8] Exercise has powerful anti-inflammatory effects on the body.[9] And sugary foods promote inflammation.[10] So, lack of exercise and consumption of sugary foods may be contributing to a common root cause—chronic inflammation.

Likewise, coronary artery disease (clogged arteries) that can lead to heart attacks were once thought to be caused by eating cholesterol-rich foods, or even "old age." Like diabetes, it's linked to lack of exercise and unhealthy diets. But research implicates chronic inflammation as the root cause.[11]

Chronic inflammation continues to be implicated in an expanding array of diseases: osteoporosis, hypertension, Alzheimer's, depression, asthma, allergies and cancer. Even if inflammation has yet to be established as the cause of these diseases, it is becoming clear that inflammation fuels them. These "diseases of affluence"—seen in developed nations—are strongly associated with lifestyles that promote chronic inflammation. As chronic inflammation is, in essence, an unbalanced immune response, these diseases—once attributed to other factors—may essentially be diseases of the immune system.

But what role does chronic inflammation play in cancer?

First of all, chronic inflammation can actually spark cancer. Rampaging immune cells stuck in a state of inflammation may damage the DNA of normal cells, causing mutations that spawn tumors.[12]

Once spawned, chronic inflammation helps tumors recruit immune cells into their fold. Tumors subvert these immune cells, using their capabilities to grow and invade the body.

For example, tumors use the ability of immune cells to form new blood vessels.[13] Originally meant for repairing damaged tissue, these blood vessels now supply nutrients to fuel tumor expansion.

Tumors also use immune cells to invade surrounding tissues. These cells secrete enzymes, allowing tumors to digest their way as they infiltrate and annex neighboring tissues.[14]

Tumors even use immune cells to speed up their growth. Immune cells secrete *growth factors* to help damaged tissues regenerate. But tumors use these to propel their own hyper-growth.[15]

Finally, tumors subvert certain immune cells to repel T cells and other immune cells that would otherwise attack them. For example, they recruit allies such as Tregs—those fearsome bodyguards of tumors. The Tregs kill and maim other immune cells that attempt to attack the tumor.

All these subversive actions of tumors are fueled by chronic inflammation. Perhaps too much immunotherapy had tipped my body into a chronically inflamed state? Perhaps chronic inflammation was empowering my tumors to grow faster and act with aggression?

> **Examples of Cancers Caused by Chronic Inflammation**
>
> Chronic inflammation caused by infectious agents drives more than 15 percent of cancers worldwide.[16] The following agents, when they cause chronic inflammation, result in various cancers: *H. pylori* bacteria, which leads to stomach cancer; Hepatitis C virus, which leads to liver cancer; Human Papillomavirus (HPV), which leads to ovarian, cervical and anal cancer; and Epstein-Barr virus (EBV), which leads to lymphoma.
>
> Chronic inflammation can also arise after trauma.[17] Ronny—the other synovial sarcoma patient that Dr. Old had helped—was an avid soccer player; his primary tumor grew on his foot, right where he'd kicked the ball for years. A young mechanic had Ewing's sarcoma grow on a repeatedly injured thumb.[18] Bessie Dashiell's sarcoma grew on her injured hand. In each of these cases, the trauma-induced inflammation could have fueled cancer.

Quenching the Fire with Fish Oil

As we delved into the study of inflammation, our suspicion grew. In our zeal to harness my immune system against terminal cancer, we may have inadvertently sabotaged our efforts.

What was the sense of creating T cells to attack my cancer if chronic inflammation was helping tumors defend against them? To make matters worse, we learned that chronic inflammation directly impairs T cells, "exhausting" them, rendering them unable to attack tumors.[19]

"It's time we switch strategies. We should try to quell inflammation in your body," said Eddy.

"Should we try curcumin?" I said. Back in 2009, when first experimenting with alternative medicines, I'd taken curcumin supplements. Curcumin is the active ingredient of turmeric, the main yellow spice used in curry. It's famed for its anti-inflammatory properties. Unable to swallow pills, I opened the capsules, pouring the yellow powder into a cup of hot chocolate. The fat in the hot chocolate would help my body absorb the curcumin better.

"The problem with curcumin is the absorption. I know there was a curcumin clinical trial at MD Anderson ... for pancreatic cancer," said Eddy. "But from what I've read, not enough gets absorbed. And even if it does, it gets eliminated rapidly from the body. I think we need something more powerful."[20]

"How about anti-inflammatory drugs like Celebrex or aspirin?" asked Eddy.

"There've been studies showing that anti-inflammatories can lower cancer risk,"[21] I said. "But these drugs are so widely used that if they could actually reverse large tumors, doctors would have noticed by now … Plus, they can have dangerous side effects like bleeding and stomach ulcers."

"Hey, how about that fish oil case study?" said Eddy. "Remember the patient with the huge sarcoma tumors in his lungs that disappeared after taking megadoses of fish oil?"

"You mean the Pardini paper?" I said.[22]

"Yes, that one. The results were unbelievable. His tumors shrunk slowly and almost vanished over four years. The only thing he did was high doses of fish oil," said Eddy.

The paper was a single case report written up by Ron Pardini, Ph.D., Professor at the Department of Biochemistry and Molecular Biology at the University of Nevada, Reno. It documented the case of a 78-year-old man who had metastatic sarcoma in his lungs, patient DH.

DH's doctor told him he had only a few months left to live. He could try chemo, but all it would do is temporarily shrink his tumors while causing devastating side effects. Given his age, DH declined. Instead, he embarked on an unconventional approach suggested by his neighbor, Dr. Pardini.[23]

Dr. Pardini's own experiments had shown that dietary fish oil could dramatically retard the growth of tumors implanted in mice.[24] Tumors of all cancer types such as breast, ovarian, colon, prostate and pancreatic were suppressed by as much as 90 percent. In contrast, mice that were fed corn oil exhibited accelerated cancer growth.

With nothing to lose, DH consumed large amounts of fish oil, which comprised omega-3 fats, known for their anti-inflammatory properties. At the same time, he strictly limited intake of inflammatory omega-6 fats (such as corn oil). After two months, the huge tumors in his lungs began to shrink, shriveling over the next four years. He experienced no side effects and his quality of life was unaffected.[25]

"It doesn't get any better—regression of metastatic sarcoma *and* zero side effects," said Eddy. "Chemo can't keep tumors away for that long, let alone without side effects."

"No side effects?" I asked.

"None."

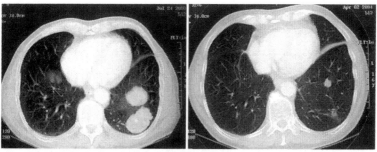

Figure 43: LEFT: Patient DH's largest lung tumors, July 2000. RIGHT: Tumors mostly resolved by April 2004.[j] (His tumors eventually disappeared.[26])

"I think you may be on to something," I said. "Fish oil gets incorporated into every cell in the body ... unlike supplements like curcumin, or drugs like aspirin. Maybe that's why it worked so well for him."

The fats we eat get absorbed into the blood, then become part of the membranes surrounding each cell in our body.[27,28] Tumor cells also have fatty membranes, and the fats we consume enter those membranes.[29]

Omega-3 and omega-6 fats compete against each other to be assimilated into the body. Take too much omega-6, and it will prevent omega-3 from incorporating into cells.[30] DH took megadoses of omega-3 fats in the form of fish oil, while strictly limiting omega-6 fats (like corn oil). By doing this, the fish oil was sure to enter his cells. Once assimilated, the anti-inflammatory properties of fish oil could quell inflammation throughout his body—24 hours a day, every day of the week.

"It looks like, when it comes to fats, you really are what you eat," said Eddy, thrilled at the simple elegance of this promising dietary intervention.

"Right," I said. "Compare that with drugs such as chemo, which have a half-life. The body eventually excretes them, which limits their benefits. Stop chemo and the cancer comes right back."

"This is exciting," said Eddy. "It sounds logical. And the case study is compelling."

"And the treatment seems safe. DH had no side effects."

"Do we have any fish oil capsules?" Eddy got up to look in the cupboard.

"I don't think so."

"Let's spend a day or two to study this more."

And so, we pored over scientific studies of omega-3 fats and their effects on cancer. What we found excited us further.

We learned that fish oil significantly improved the symptoms of cachexia in patients with pancreatic cancer, helping them gain weight and improving their appetite.[31,32] The researchers suggested that fish oil could reverse cachexia by quelling chronic inflammation.

Another study found that high doses of fish oil (18 grams daily) given with the antioxidant, Vitamin E, significantly prolonged the survival of patients with advanced cancer, while reinvigorating their immune systems.[33] Fish oil restored the number of beneficial helper T cells to healthy levels while reducing the number of harmful Tregs. The back-to-back attacks of shingles I'd experienced suggested that my immune system was weakened; this study gave us hope that fish oil could restore it.

Once incorporated into the membranes of tumor cells, omega-3 displaces omega-6, the fats responsible for promoting inflammation. By so doing, it begins to quell inflammation within the tumor. We know that omega-3's ability to enter tissues and quell inflammation is real and profound, as seen in startling reports where it has healed brain trauma—and even awakened patients from comas.[34,35]

By quelling chronic inflammation, omega-3 robs tumors of their fuel, and may slow the progress of cancer.[36] Omega-3 also retards tumors by quenching growth signals in tumor cells and stopping angiogenesis, the formation of new blood vessels which feeds tumors.[37,38] In addition, the active components of fish oil (EPA and especially DHA) have direct anticancer properties. In other words, fish oil may act like a mild form of chemotherapy, destroying cancer directly.[39]

Although the human studies were small, the science was compelling. So was the notion that I could alter the environment in my tumor with a simple and safe dietary modification.

We also pondered the many diets believed to curtail cancer and prolong life: the Gerson diet, vegetarian and vegan diets, the Mediterranean diet, the Okinawan diet. Common aspects of these diets include lots of vegetables, some fruit, a modest (or no) amount of meat and lower carbohydrates. But on closer look, all of these diets naturally exclude foods or preparation techniques that tend to be rich in omega-6s (e.g. frying with corn oil). Some, like the Okinawan diet—famed for its centenarian adherents—naturally contain omega-3s, while precluding omega-6s. Could it be that these diets conferred benefit by quelling chronic inflammation through the balancing of omega-3s and omega-6s?

Above all, we marveled at DH's success. Having studied sarcomas for five years, we knew their tenacity. They withstood the most toxic chemo that could kill patients or damage bone marrow. Yet, DH's metastatic tumors had crumbled under the onslaught of this inconspicuously powerful fat.

The cryo of my fourth lung lesion would happen in a month. Meanwhile, we sought to leverage this promising weapon against my cancer.

One Cup of Peanuts

"Did you know that the typical American diet contains 14 to 25 times more omega-6 than omega-3?" I asked.[40]

"Yes, I've read that before," said Eddy.

"Maybe that's why some fish oil clinical trials showed no benefit," I said. "The patients could have been eating too much omega-6.

"One tablespoon of corn oil has over seven grams of omega-6 … and just one cup of peanuts has 23 grams!"

"You're right," said Eddy. "Many of the fish oil trials gave patients low amounts of omega-3s—just two or three grams in some cases … That's nothing compared to the omega-6s in the typical Western diet."

"The omega-6s found in those foods would have eclipsed the omega-3s," I said. "I wonder why none of the trials restricted omega-6 fats?"

"Good question," Eddy said. "Maybe it was too difficult to control their diets? Maybe they wouldn't have been able to recruit participants? Anyway, at those ratios, probably little-to-none of the omega-3s would have made it into their cells."

After a while, Eddy asked, "So … What's our strategy going to be?" as he pulled up the Pardini paper on his laptop. "Are you going to try to achieve DH's ratios?"

Unlike other human studies with fish oil, DH's case was unique. Using computer software, Dr. Pardini had taken care to calculate the amount of omega-6 fats in DH's diet. Despite DH's efforts to cut corn oil and other inflammatory oils from his diet, he still ended up consuming an average of 12.6 grams of omega-6 daily. For at least two years before he was diagnosed, DH had already been taking 2.0 grams of fish oil daily (containing 0.6 grams of omega-3s, slightly more than the recommended daily intake[41]). Obviously, this amount of omega-3 didn't prevent his cancer.

To replace the inflammatory omega-6 fats in his body with anti-inflammatory omega-3s, DH ramped up the fish oil to 12.4 grams of omega-3 per day—achieving a one-to-one ratio of omega-3 to omega-6.

This initial dose of omega-3s shrunk all but one of DH's tumors. The single, stubborn tumor was biopsied and confirmed to be sarcoma. Galvanized by the overall success, DH upped his dosage of omega-3s to 17.2 grams. He now consumed more omega-3 fats than omega-6. It worked. The stubborn tumor began to shrink.

"I know what I'm going to do. I'll take more omega-3s than DH took. And I'll limit my omega-6s to less than what he consumed." I said.

"Sounds good. It's going to be really hard to limit omega-6 though," said Eddy. "It's in everything! Anytime you eat out, the food will probably be cooked with corn, soy or vegetable oil. They're all high in omega-6."

"No more fried noodles or fried eggplant, I guess …"

"Yeah, and no more peanuts. The 23 grams in one cup will negate your entire dose of fish oil," said Eddy. "Walnuts are even worse—effectively 29 grams of omega-6s in one cup. But macadamias are fine—only two grams of omega-6s in a cup."

"Also, you might want to cut tofu products. After cooking oils and nuts, condensed soy products like tofu seem to have the highest omega-6s."

"I'm going to miss all those foods," I said.

"Well, you can eat anything you want … so long as you tally the omega-6s."

"At least meats and butter are OK!"

I'd discovered that butter consists mainly of saturated fat and contains very little inflammatory omega-6s. Also, most lean meats—organic or not—contain little omega-6s. A nine-ounce sirloin, trimmed of fat, has less than a gram of natural omega-6 oils.[42] I could eat ten of those steaks and still stay under my daily quota of omega-6s.

"As long as you cook your own meals, you can control the oil. Otherwise, you could easily consume two tablespoons of corn oil for every meal eaten out … especially with Chinese or fried foods. Let's see … seven grams per tablespoon … that's 14 grams of omega-6s—in just one meal," said Eddy.

"Would you mind cooking with butter or coconut oil from now on, mom?" I asked.

"No problem. I'll use whatever oil you want," said mom.

Having determined a strategy, I recorded everything I ate, tallying the omega-6s every night, referring to online resources to figure out the omega-6 content in my food.[43] Eddy reigned in my love for eating out. Meanwhile, I took liquid fish oil supplements by the tablespoon, ramping up to 24 grams of omega-3s daily—the equivalent of 48 fish oil capsules (each containing 500 mg of DHA and EPA). Thankfully, I didn't experience diarrhea or gas as some do. Perhaps taking it on a full stomach helped.

A few days into the diet we were at the grocery store. I grew depressed as I surveyed the foods I used to eat. I felt shackled. Not only had I lost my right jaw, making it hard to eat certain foods, but I also had to avoid the foods I loved. *Why is there so much omega-6 everywhere?*

No more mayo.

No more soy products.

No more nuts—especially peanuts and walnuts.

No more Honey Walnut Shrimp, my favorite dish at Chinese restaurants—it has walnuts, the shrimp is battered in mayo (which is high in omega-6) and it's fried in high-omega-6 oils.

"Hang in there," said Eddy, putting his arm around my shoulder. "We'll get through this. We'll just double your fish oil occasionally so you can eat out."

Combining Fish Oil with a High-Fat, Low-Carbohydrate Diet

We viewed this omega 3-6 regimen (our hereafter shorthand) as a possible form of immunotherapy. EPA and DHA (the omega-3 fatty acids from fish oil) can directly kill cancer cells. But perhaps the omega-3 had also helped DH's immune system attack his cancer.

Sarcomas are immunogenic, and some sarcoma patients' immune systems may spontaneously create T cells against cancer. Perhaps these tumor-killing T cells had been created in DH's body, but the T cells were unable to penetrate his tumors' defenses.

The subsequent omega-3-6 diet would have quelled inflammation throughout DH's body, including within his tumors. Perhaps this made the tumors less aggressive and weakened their ability to subvert immune cells for defense purposes, thus enabling the T cells to attack them?

Whether omega-3-6 worked by direct kill or by indirect immune effects didn't really matter. If we could reproduce DH's results, we'd be ecstatic.

Around the time we began omega-3-6, Eddy suggested a supplemental intervention—the ketogenic diet. The ketogenic diet is a high-fat, very low carbohydrate diet used to control epilepsy in children.[44] It starves the body of carbohydrates and propels it into a fat-burning mode. Like omega-3-6, Eddy had reason to believe it could change the environment around tumors, allowing my immune system to better attack cancer.

You might recall Professor Vikas Sukhatme, the Harvard oncologist and researcher we had been in touch with since going to Tijuana for Coley's Toxins.[45] Eddy had contacted him to let him know we were beginning the omega-3-6 regimen. During the conversation, Professor Sukhatme recommended we study the effects of the ketogenic diet on immune cells. His own research in mice showed that the diet can deplete a certain immune cell that tumors recruit and subvert to their benefit. Known as the myeloid-derived suppressor cell (MDSC), it's a formidable ally of tumors.

Cancer's Fierce Enablers

In the early stages of formation, tumors secrete signaling proteins to recruit MDSCs into their fold. Like Tregs, MDSCs suppress beneficial immune cells such as T cells, dendritic cells and natural killer cells. But beyond protecting tumors from immune cells, MDSCs assist tumors in many other ways.[46]

For example, MDSCs help tumors form new blood vessels. All cells need oxygen and nourishment; they also excrete waste products that must be carried away. A vast network of blood vessels transports nutrients and waste products. Like highways leading to main streets branching to side streets, larger blood vessels taper down to the smallest of capillaries. These capillaries supply life-sustaining blood into cells. Without an increasing supply of blood vessels, a tumor cannot thrive and expand. Unfortunately, the MDSCs around a tumor constantly secrete proteins that accelerate the forming of blood vessels. The mass—comprising cancerous cells, MDSCs and other subverted immune cells—expands, fed by a growing network of new blood vessels.

MDSCs also help tumors invade neighboring tissues. They secrete enzymes to break down surrounding tissues, making it easier for tumors to expand their territory.

But one of the most fearsome traits of MDSCs is that they help tumors metastasize.[47] Like Marines storming a beach to secure the way for other armed forces, MDSCs help cancer cells travel to distant parts of the body and establish new colonies.

First, MDSCs secrete enzymes that make it easier for cancer cells to squeeze through the walls of blood vessels.

Once in the bloodstream, MDSCs coagulate cancer cells into little clumps, ready to be swept away by rushing rivers of blood to distant parts of the body. Solo cancer cells are susceptible to damage and less able to survive the long journey. But clumps of cancer cells mixed with MDSCs are bigger, stronger and more able to withstand physical damage. Furthermore, MDSCs protect these clumps from being killed by roving immune cells.

To form new colonies, these cancerous clumps must first stick to the walls of blood vessels at new sites. MDSCs secrete proteins that make the clumps "stickier." Once stuck, MDSCs secrete enzymes that help cancer cells squeeze back out of the bloodstream, enabling them to invade new tissues and ensconce new colonies. These colonies flourish into new tumors, protected and propelled by these fierce enablers of cancer.

How Very Low Carbohydrate Diets Can Deplete MDSCs

Dr. Old had warned us that certain inflammatory cytokines such as GM-CSF may promote the growth of MDSCs.[48] (GM-CSF is also the active ingredient of a drug given to cancer patients to increase their white blood cells after stem cell transplants.[49]) Perhaps too much immunotherapy had flooded my body with such inflammatory cytokines, thereby increasing the number of MDSCs and spurring the recent growth of my lung tumors.

Depleting Tregs and MDSCs has become an important goal of immunotherapy. Drugs such as low-dose cyclophosphamide are being tested to reduce both of these tumor allies. But Dr. Sukhatme's research hinted that simple dietary modification might achieve the same results.

Spend time researching alternative cancer cures, and you'll quickly come across the "Warburg effect," which describes the deranged metabolism of cancer cells. Normal cells burn glucose in the presence of oxygen to create energy. Cancer cells, however, ferment glucose, using a highly inefficient process that extracts only 1/15th of the energy compared to normal cells. The process creates a large amount of a byproduct known as lactate, which acidifies the environment within tumors. Lactate and the acidic environment have been found to impair immune cells, rendering them less able to attack tumors.[50,51] Furthermore, Dr. Sukhatme's research suggested that lactate increases the number of MDSCs and causes them to accumulate within tumors.

The relationship between lactate and MDSCs raises an important question. Since MDSCs are such feared allies of tumors, could we deplete them by reducing lactate? What if we deprived tumors of glucose? Less glucose, less lactate byproduct. And with less lactate, wouldn't there be fewer MDSCs?

Dr. Sukhatme would soon publish a study showing that a three-week ketogenic diet could indeed deplete MDSCs from tumors in mice.[52] Besides depleting MDSCs, the diet also reduced Tregs and boosted the number of beneficial T cells. In other words, a short course of this simple dietary regimen stripped tumors of two powerful allies, making them more susceptible to immune attack.

We were drawn to Dr. Sukhatme's research despite it being conducted on mice. We had also learned of the anti-inflammatory effects of ketogenic diets.[53] Even if the ketogenic diet failed to deplete MDSCs, perhaps it would synergize with fish oil to quell cancer-promoting inflammation?

❧ ❧ ❧ ❧ ❧

"We have a little over three weeks before your cryo with Dr. Littrup," said Eddy. "Just enough time to try this ketogenic diet."

"Do you think we can find a diet that will satisfy both the omega-3-6 *and* the ketogenic requirements?" I asked.

"Let's see … For ketogenic, you'll need high fats but very low carbs. And for omega-3-6, you'll need to take a large amount of fish oil, while limiting omega-6. You can limit omega-6 if you eat at home and avoid bad oils and nuts and tofu and snack foods," said Eddy.

"And the fish oil plays right into the ketogenic—it's all fat, which is what I need," I said. "All I have to do it cut all carbs, and take gobs of fat—like butter and coconut oil."

"For just three weeks," said Eddy.

"I think I can do that."

And so, we embarked on the ketogenic diet together.

The first five days were crippling. It takes a while for the body to exhaust its stores of glycogen (carbohydrates) and to switch over into fat-burning mode. Until our bodies adjusted, plunging blood sugar debilitated us. We lay in bed, incapacitated, minds foggy, bodies frail from pseudo-starvation despite the copious fats we consumed. Thank God mom was there to help with our meals.

But once our bodies acclimated, we felt great. It was as if a switch flipped. Our bodies now burned fat. No longer prone to sugar spikes from large meals, our minds became sharp. We ate modest amounts of baked meats, letting their natural oils drip off. We ate heaping green salads drenched in olive oil. We whipped butter into decaf coffee. I ate all the cheeses I wanted. And at the day's end, we rewarded ourselves with a square (or two) of 90 percent dark chocolate.

We aimed to continue this diet for three weeks. I took 24 grams of omega-3 daily and limited omega-6s to less than 10 grams. We left nothing to chance, weighing all food items and tallying carbs and omega-6s. I consumed no more than 20 grams of carbs daily—the amount found in two slices of wheat bread.

Was this extreme? Yes. But the circumstances warranted it.

For over three years we'd labored to create T cells against my cancer, starting with Dr. Old's NY-ESO-1 vaccine, then Coley Fluid, then cryo and dendritic vaccines and jaw injections and more cryo. But my accelerating tumors suggested something was confounding the T cells.

All those years, we'd operated on a best-guess effort, with no access to clinical trials. We considered off-label Yervoy to strip my tumors' defenses, but were concerned about autoimmune side-effects. We'd found an oncologist in Singapore who'd administer it at the "bargain" cost price of $30,000 per vial—no 400 percent markup. But Yervoy was the nuclear option. If we could keep "weeding out" tumors a while longer, perhaps the safer PD-1 would soon be approved?

For now, a hunch told us to give diet-based immunotherapy a shot. It was the safest and cheapest option—and the easiest.

As the cryo approached, our anticipation grew.

My Third Lung Cryoablation

On July 30, 2013, we returned to Detroit for my third lung cryo. I lay in the hospital bed in the preoperative staging area. Dr. Haddad, the anesthesiologist who'd taken care of me during previous lung cryos, came to see me. Three hours had gone by while we awaited results of the *thromboelastogram* (TEG), a comprehensive test of my blood's clotting capacity. Standard tests, such as the *prothrombin time,* had shown up as normal. But a *platelet function assay* had come back abnormal, suggesting compromised clotting. The TEG would give a clearer picture.

We had done our homework.

Contrary to copious warnings on the internet, fish oil is generally safe, even when taken before surgery.[54,55] Studies even show that 10 grams given a few days before major abdominal surgery can significantly reduce death and help patients heal faster with fewer infections.[56,57] But isolated reports of compromised clotting cause some to advocate stopping it before surgery.[58] Secondly, the large amounts I'd taken posed an unknown risk.

Also, the ketogenic diet can impair platelets (the blood cells involved in clotting). A study found that one third of children treated for epilepsy with the ketogenic diet experienced excessive bruising. Their blood took longer to clot.[59]

A week before the cryo, I noticed a spontaneous bruise on my knee. I stopped the ketogenic diet and fish oil but continued restricting my intake of omega-6 fats. We emailed Dr. Haddad and Dr. Littrup, intent on working with them to ensure my safety. After all, poking very sharp cryoprobes into my lung could quickly turn treacherous if my clotting was impaired.

The TEG came back fine. Although Dr. Haddad didn't think extra platelets would be needed, he ordered some on standby.

Lesson learned: Patients on blood-thinning medicines or those taking high-dose fish oil (or the ketogenic diet) should consider stopping these at least two weeks before surgical procedures for safety.

It was time for the cryo.

Dr. Littrup had said this lesion would be easy to obliterate. It wasn't near anything—no large blood vessels. No heat source to compromise the freezing temperatures.

The procedure went swiftly. I experienced no bleeding problems. By late afternoon, we were back at the patient apartment. After a shower and food, I felt tired. I lay down in bed. Eddy came by to take my temperature.

"One-o-three degrees!" said Eddy, surprised. This was the first time I'd developed spontaneous fever after cryo. Ecstatic, we hoped that cryo had triggered a strong acute inflammatory response, generating T cells against my cancer.

"Maybe the omega-3-6 and ketogenic diet managed to strip my tumor defenses!" I said, smiling weakly. I closed my eyes, visualizing dendritic cells munching away at dead tumor, migrating to lymph nodes, activating billions of T cells against a plethora of antigens. I drifted off to sleep. When I woke four hours later, the fever was gone.

The next day, we went to the image library to order a CD of the procedure. Loading the images onto Eddy's Macbook, we identified the image showing the tumor before Dr. Littrup had ablated it.

"Look! Do you see that?" said Eddy, barely able to contain his excitement as he measured the width of the lesion.

"It looks a tad smaller than it was a month ago!" he said.

"Are you sure?" I said, scrutinizing his measurements. "You may be right ... Either way, it definitely doesn't look any bigger!"

A month earlier, the tumor had measured 0.6 cm in diameter. It'd been doubling every three months. At that rate, we'd expect to see it approaching 0.8 cm.

Instead, the lesion measured 0.5 cm, maybe even 0.4 cm.[60]

Had the two short weeks of omega-3-6 and the ketogenic diet stopped it from growing? Had we replicated DH's success? Had we quelled inflammation or lactate or depleted MDSCs or Tregs? Was my immune system suddenly attacking my cancer? Did the 103°F fever hint at this?

We'll never know the answers. But it didn't matter. I had survived five and a half years of sarcoma, metastatic to my lungs. Having ablated the lesion, I was "tumor-free." The symptoms of cachexia vanished; my appetite returned. PD-1 inhibitors were marching along in trials. I just needed to keep weeding tumors until they were approved.

And now, I had two more weapons in my arsenal to suppress micro-tumors: fish oil and the ketogenic diet.

The glass was no longer almost empty. Once again, it brimmed with hope.

PART III
Immunotherapy Today

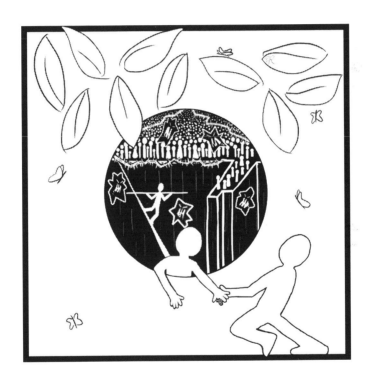

CHAPTER 16

Seizing the Cure

It was October 1, 2013. Three months had passed since I'd cryoablated the fast-growing lung lesion.

Encouraged by the possibility of tumor shrinkage, I had resumed the omega-3-6 diet. (I stopped the ketogenic diet a week before the cryoablation when the spontaneous bruises on my knee suggested heightened bleeding risk.)

We were back in Houston. As usual, we obtained the scan images and radiology report before seeing Dr. Benjamin.

We loaded the images with trepidation. Would this scan show even more tumors? If our plans for cryo, omega-3-6 or the ketogenic diet were mere wishful thinking, we would expect to see new tumors. After all, for the past nine months, each lung CT had revealed tumor progression and warranted a cryoablation: the first in Dec 2012; the second in April 2013; the third in July 2013.

"You take the left. I'll take the right," said Eddy. He aligned three-month-old images of my left lung next to the current ones. Scrutinizing them for new tumors or regrowth at the previously cryoablated sites, we found no changes—at least, none we could detect.

Next, we scanned the right lung. This time, we found one change—but it was a change that allowed cautious optimism.

Recall the three cystic lesions first detected in 2010. They had started as small and solid, then hollowed out. Later, two of them filled in, which prompted the cryoablations. But the third had remained small and hollow, with an enhanced rim. Because of the halo-like appearance, radiologists call it a *Cheerio lesion*—a known manifestation of cancer.[1]

We hadn't cryoablated the Cheerio as it was still small, only 0.3 cm wide. Dr. Littrup had suggested we wait until it reached 0.5 cm. But now, we wouldn't have to.

The Cheerio had vanished.

"The omega-3-6 and ketogenic diet might have gotten it! Or maybe the T cells generated by the last cryo!" I said.

"Let's not get ahead of ourselves," said Eddy. "The Cheerio's pretty small ... slightly bigger than the image slice pitch of 0.25 cm. If the slices were taken at the edges of the lesion, it might not appear on the scan."

"You're right," I said, curbing my enthusiasm. "We'll keep checking future scans. If it's really gone, it'll become apparent. Let's move on to the head MRI."

We finished analyzing the lung CT and head MRI, detecting no changes with our untrained eyes. Turning to the radiology reports, we breathed sighs of relief. They, too, noted nothing worrisome.

Later that afternoon, we saw Dr. Benjamin. This was the first in nine months I didn't have to deal with a growing tumor. Dr. Benjamin said the surveillance clock had been "reset" by the cryoablation of my last lung tumor. It meant I needed to continue the aggressive three-month scans for another three years.

As the plane soared westward above the Houston skies, we allowed ourselves to ease into a tenuous calm. With a strategy in place, we could resume our autopilot strategy: Keep up the omega-3-6 diet and hope for another clean scan come January. And another one three months later. And another.

Time would tell if the micro-tumors in my head or lungs had been tamed.

Silence of the Lesions

Three months passed. No tumors materialized. Only visible were the scars where three of the lung lesions had been cryoablated. And the fourth—the Cheerio—was still nowhere to be found.

Another three months passed. Again, no new tumors. Day after day, I consumed 24 grams of omega-3, limiting omega-6s to less than 10 grams.

Soon, one year had gone by since my last cryo. We breathed easier, relieved that the pattern of accelerating lung tumors had been broken. I lowered the omega-3s to 16 grams, bringing the omega-3-6 ratio closer to what patient DH had taken.

By the end of the second year of clean scans (July 2015), our confidence had grown. The trips to MD Anderson became mundane—not that we were complaining! By that time, cancer immunotherapy had taken the oncology world by storm. PD-1 approvals across different cancers were accelerating.

Breathing even easier, I decreased my omega-3s to 8 grams daily, some days taking nothing. Frequent blood tests showed the diet wasn't causing me problems. But remembering how my body had tipped into a state of chronic inflammation after 223 Coley infusions, we thought it wise to avoid "too much of a good thing." Despite patient DH's success and the many human studies that supported the benefits of fish oil, some mice and cell culture studies suggested it could suppress immunity. Since my cancer hadn't returned for two years, why risk tipping my body too far in "the other" direction?

It is now July 2016. For three years, I've done no further immunotherapy. No more trips to Germany. No more Coley Fluid. Only the omega-3-6 diet.

For three years, my scans have shown no change.

For three years, the Cheerio lesion has remained invisible, perhaps forever destroyed by my immune system or fish oil.

It feels strange. Our experience resembles Mary's—the woman in her 30s with lymphoma, whose tumors had vanished with radiation in combination with Opdivo (the PD-1 inhibitor). She endured debilitating side effects from intensive chemo regimens and a stem-cell transplant. But none of these shrunk the large mass in her chest. So, when she first received Opdivo, she wondered if it was working. It seemed "too easy"—the only side effect of itchy skin, too mild. Likewise, the cessation of my tumors after omega-3-6 seems surreal after years of intense travel, Coley fevers, surgery and cryoablations.

Except for the long-term side effects from that single chemo regimen eight years ago, I feel quite normal. The fatigue and low neutrophil counts persist. I lack the strength for sports but I can handle 20-minute walks with Eddy. Even before my cancer, my main recreation had been hanging out with friends over meals and going grocery shopping. I can still do both. Having only one jaw joint makes chewing difficult, but I've adapted by carrying a pair of mini food scissors everywhere. My misaligned upper and lower jaws cause minor sores in the corners of my mouth. But all these are trifling compared to what I'd be suffering had I followed a conventional route and taken more chemo when my cancer returned.

"It'll be awesome if your scans stay quiet for as long as DH's," said Eddy.

"Yes, quite unbelievable. All of his tumors are gone, and he's alive *16 years* after end-stage sarcoma in his lungs."

We'd gotten in touch with DH and have continued correspondence with him over the years. Now 90 years young and still sharp of mind, he's a medical marvel. Like Mr. Fred Stein who had inspired Dr. Coley's foray into immunotherapy, we believe DH's success with fish oil holds scientific secrets that will one day benefit humanity.

Had we succeeded in mobilizing all aspects of an effective immune response against my incurable cancer? Had our combination immunotherapy generated tumor-specific T cells? Had fish oil and the ketogenic diet quelled inflammation, depleted MDSCs and Tregs and allowed the T cells to attack the cancer? Were *memory* T cells keeping my cancer at bay, just as a flu vaccine inoculates against future infection? We suspect that some of these hold true.

Or perhaps my cancer still lurks, merely made dormant by fish oil, robbed of its fuel (chronic inflammation). We'll never know the answers to these ifs and buts. Still, I'm alive! It's 2016. And I have access to PD-1 inhibitors off-label, should I ever need them.

I remember the first Opdivo TV ad. To the backdrop of soaring music, a father and son, a husband and wife hugged as they gazed up at glowing words projected on a skyscraper: "A CHANCE TO LIVE LONGER." Our eyes grew misty. We'd made it. We'd attained the goal Dr. Old had given us—we'd survived long enough to add PD-1 to our growing arsenal of immunotherapies. Countless immunotherapy clinical trials had become available. The longer I lived, the more tools I'd have, should my cancer ever return.

You Can Benefit from Immunotherapy Today

The American Cancer Society (ACS) estimates 596,000 Americans die every year from cancer.[2] That's over 1,600 lives extinguished daily, most never having the chance to try immunotherapies like PD-1. Many patients we've met had never heard of immunotherapy. Those who had were told "it's still experimental," or, "wait for clinical trials to prove it works for your cancer."

Take Emma, for example. Emma had lung cancer that had advanced despite chemo and targeted therapy. As we'd done with Mary, I shared the basis of PD-1 inhibitors. I showed her the compelling early clinical trial data. I described how she could obtain treatment through clinical trials or off-label therapy. At the time, a phase 3 trial of Opdivo for lung cancer was close to completion. Opdivo had already been approved for melanoma, which meant the FDA deemed it safe for human use. But her oncologist wasn't enthusiastic about PD-1, deeming it "experimental." Ironically, he recommended she enroll in a phase 1 experimental trial of a targeted therapy that *hadn't* been FDA-approved for any cancer. Emma died within weeks—from the side effects of the experimental drug. A month later, the FDA approved Opdivo for lung cancer.

Emma's example shows us that not all "experimental" drugs are created equal. As a *Forbes* article suggests, the spectacular failures of experimental drugs occur mostly with novel agents that have never been used to treat humans.[3] In contrast, drugs already approved for one cancer, and are being tested to expand their use in other cancers—such as PD-1—are far more likely to succeed.

Emma's case captures our heartfelt frustration that many are dying or stand at the brink of death without being given a chance to benefit from immunotherapy. Harry (my uncle's friend with stomach cancer) had unquestioningly accepted the word of two oncologists—that "there was nothing else," despite the strong PD-1 Phase 1 data for his cancer.[4] Mary would've died of her lymphoma had she not pursued off-label PD-1.

These are stories of patients whose oncologists either weren't apprised of PD-1 or didn't fully understand its potential. The FDA later approved PD-1 for Emma's lung cancer and Mary's lymphoma. The FDA is also likely to soon approve PD-1 for Harry's stomach cancer. The after-the-fact approvals justify our view that these patients should have been steered toward PD-1— *because the safety was well-established and the early data was already compelling.*

To understand the plight of patients like Emma and Harry, we must first understand the nature of the clinical trial approvals in the U.S.

The first PD-1 approval came in September 2014 for patients with melanoma. Within two years—a breathtaking pace by traditional measures—the FDA has already approved PD-1 for lung cancer, kidney cancer, bladder cancer and lymphoma. This fast-expanding list will likely soon include gastric cancer. PD-1's rapid validation across a broad spectrum of cancers reflects the nature of immunotherapy—instead of targeting weaknesses in specific cancers, PD-1 mobilizes the immune system, regardless of cancer type.

While the science and unfolding data suggest a wide spectrum of cancers may benefit from immunotherapies like PD-1, the reality we live in precludes a blanket FDA approval across all cancers. This is because, in the U.S., drugs are approved for specific *indications*. For as long as different cancers are viewed as different diseases, PD-1 (and other immunotherapies) will need to be validated one indication at a time.

An indication doesn't just refer to a type of cancer; it may require patients to have tried and failed prior treatments such as chemo. For example, the September 2014 approval of Keytruda for melanoma applied only to those who had tried and failed Yervoy.[5] If their melanoma had the BRAF mutation, they had to have failed the targeted therapy Zelboraf. It didn't matter that these drugs were less effective or had more side effects. Patients still had to try them before their doctors could prescribe Keytruda and have it covered by insurance.

It took another fifteen months before the FDA approved Keytruda for first-line treatment in metastatic melanoma. Only then could patients get it without first having to take other treatments.

Despite the accelerating pace of FDA approvals, it won't be soon enough for patients like Emma and Harry. Curious patients will continue to be told PD-1 is "still experimental." Sixteen hundred will continue to die every day.

While these deaths frustrate us, they also impassion us to share the message of immunotherapy with as many who would hear it. Our view is that dying patients need not wait for PD-1 to be approved for their cancers. Its experimental status shouldn't be used to deter patients from clinical trials or off-label use if the early data suggests strong benefit, as in the cases of Emma and Harry.

A Tail of Survival

Besides being labeled as "still experimental," another common refrain we've heard is, "Immunotherapy only works for a small percentage of patients."

We've described the dramatic differences between immunotherapy responses versus those of chemo and other targeted agents. Foremost is that immunotherapy can create long-term remissions. In contrast, the shrinkage begotten by chemo and other targeted agents is short-lasting for solid tumors (excluding blood cancers like lymphoma and leukemia).

Despite the transient benefit, chemo and targeted agents may elicit high response rates, meaning that many patients experience initial shrinkage. In contrast, the first checkpoint inhibitor, Yervoy, achieved a meager overall response rate of between 10 to 20 percent in early trials. Even so, patients who responded to the drug in 2000 didn't just experience temporary tumor shrinkage—they became part of the "vast majority"[6] still alive *16 years later*, effectively cured.[7] On top of that, PD-1 inhibitors are showing even better response rates: 40 percent of melanoma patients who responded to Keytruda are still alive three years later, many having returned to productive lives.[8]

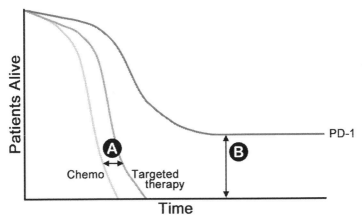

Figure 44: (A) Even though targeted therapy confers longer survival than chemo, the survival curves for both therapies intersect zero: meaning the benefit is short lived. (B) Survival for immunotherapies like PD-1 flatten out, showing a fraction of patients live for many years, perhaps cured.[j]

Besides the long-lived nature of immunotherapy responses, Eddy and I believe that checkpoint inhibitors and other immunotherapies are being underestimated. There are three reasons why we think so.

First, the early trials that validated PD-1 and CTLA-4 were *monotherapy* **trials**—meaning these checkpoint inhibitors were used in isolation. As we've seen, the immune system is complex, and a monotherapy approach is unlikely to mobilize all aspects of an effective immune response.

For example, from chapter 7, we've seen that PD-1 inhibitors are thought to work by blocking the ability of tumors to neutralize T cells. But this implies the T cells existed in the first place, spontaneously created by the immune system against tumors. Perhaps some patients' cancers are more likely to instigate the creation of T cells, which may be why PD-1 inhibitors work better for those patients, but not others.

But what if these trials had first ensured the creation of T cells *before* giving PD-1? In chapter 11, we described the case of a 53-year-old man with the huge 18-cm tumor on his neck. He had failed both CTLA-4 and PD-1 inhibitors. Only after his doctors had irradiated the tumor—thereby creating T cells—and resumed PD-1 did the massive tumor melt away.

Case reports like the above suggest that combination strategies may increase the number of patients who benefit from immunotherapy, possibly garnering success in cancers once thought unresponsive. But we're not the only ones who think so. A quick search on the National Institutes for Health's *ClinicalTrials.gov* website reveals a plethora of combination immunotherapy trials. Leading scientists like Dr. James Allison (discoverer of CTLA-4) are attempting to "elevate the tail end of the curve" with combination approaches that layer chemotherapy, radiation, targeted drugs and other immunotherapies. Already, the FDA has approved the combination of CTLA-4 and PD-1 for melanoma.

A second reason why immunotherapy may be underestimated: many early clinical trials administered it to patients who had already failed chemo and other targeted therapies. Chemo is notorious for weakening the immune system. Logic suggests that immunotherapy may not work as well in such patients, especially if their immune systems haven't had enough time to recover or are permanently impaired. If PD-1 and other immunotherapies are instead given to patients with intact immune systems, we might see better results.

Note, however, that certain chemotherapies and targeted drugs may synergize with immunotherapy. For example, cyclophosphamide may deplete Tregs, allowing T cells to better penetrate tumors. Likewise, drugs like Sutent, Gemzar and Taxotere may also deplete MDSCs.[9] Also, like radiation and cryo, chemo may destroy tumors and generate T cells.[10]

Despite the potential synergies between chemo and immunotherapy, the dosage and timing of the chemo needs to be carefully studied so as not to counteract immunotherapy.

A third reason why immunotherapy may be underappreciated is the negative impact of tumor burden. "Tumor burden" refers to the sheer number of cancer cells in the body, reflected in the number and size of tumors. Tumor burden matters because tumors secrete cytokines that can suppress the overall immune system—the more tumors, the greater the immunosuppression.

Dr. Old believed the best time to attack my cancer with immunotherapy was when I had no visible tumors. Likewise, we believe that patients with heavy tumor burden may benefit by reducing their tumors with surgery or cryoablation, a practice known as *debulking* tumors. Researchers have shown that the debulking of tumors may reduce immunosuppressive cytokines, thereby allowing the immune system to better attack remaining cancer.[11,12] Similarly, Dr. Coley and his colleagues observed better results when the toxins were combined with surgery.

We've outlined three possible reasons why immunotherapies such as PD-1 might be underestimated. We incorporated these optimizations into the treatment choices we made. Perhaps when optimizations such as these are exploited, the long tail of the survival curve will ratchet up, hopefully closer to 100 percent, offering a second chance at life to all patients.

Meanwhile, if you have a cancer for which single-agent PD-1 doesn't seem to work, and you've exhausted all conventional treatments, don't assume the only option is death. You may still benefit from the above optimizations—especially since some of the tools like surgery, radiation and chemo are widely available.

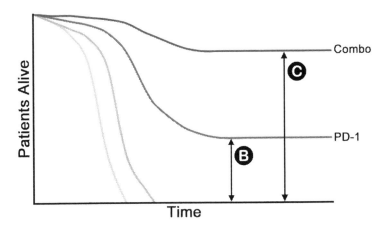

Figure 45: (B) Survival curves for single-agent PD-1 flattens out at 40 percent for melanoma. (C) Researchers aim to ratchet up survival closer to 100 percent with combination strategies.[13,J]

Creating an effective immune response against cancer

In the following table, we summarize various aspects of mobilizing the immune system against cancer discussed in this book. The science is fast evolving and many of these therapies are still being tested in clinical trials. But a key point is that a single-agent approach (such as PD-1 inhibitors) is unlikely to achieve optimal results.

CREATE T CELLS	
Against all tumor antigens	**Against a single tumor antigen**
• Cryoablation	• Peptide vaccines
• Intratumoral injections of CpG, BCG, Coley's Toxins	• Dendritic vaccines
• Radiation	• Adoptive T cells - CAR-T & TCR
• Chemotherapy	
• Dendritic vaccines	
• Adoptive T cells - TIL	
• Whole tumor vaccines	

STRIP TUMOR DEFENSES	
Prevent T cell shutdown	**Deplete Tregs**
• PD-1 inhibitors	• Low-dose cyclophosphamide
Deplete MDSCs	• CTLA-4 inhibitors
• Certain chemotherapies	• Coley's Toxins
• Ketogenic diet	

RELEASE THE BRAKES
• CTLA-4 inhibitors

OTHER OPTIMIZATIONS
Quell chronic inflammation
• Anti-inflammatories
• Omega-3-6
Debulk tumors to reduce immunosuppression
• Surgery
• Cryoablation
Give immunotherapy early
• After surgery before tumors spread
• Before chemo weakens immune system
Inject tumors repeatedly
• Mimic Dr. William Coley's practice
Inject low doses of PD-1, CTLA-4 inhibitors into tumors
• To minimize autoimmune side effects

Table 3: Methods to mobilize various aspects of the immune system against cancer

Like Mary or Like Harry?

Cancer "doesn't care." It doesn't care if the patient is unaware that chemo may only buy temporary tumor shrinkage. It doesn't care if that vaunted new drug extends life by a mere two months (like Votrient for sarcoma[14]). It doesn't care if the patient suffers and dies from debilitating side effects (like Emma). It certainly doesn't care if an oncologist fails to inform the patient about PD-1 and other immunotherapies (like with Harry)—or if profit motivates the prescribing of chemo (like with Mark and my grandmother). Cancer is going to grow and infiltrate and spread. That's what it does. And when side effects of bleeding tumors or chemo debilitate the patient, preventing travel to clinical trial sites, it's not going to care.

So, you have cancer. You've completed first-line chemoradiation. Your cancer has returned. You've done your homework and you realize that chemo will only buy temporary tumor shrinkage. Death is inevitable. You've heard about immunotherapy. You ask your oncologist about it. She says it's "still experimental," and instead offers more chemo. What's your next move?

Will you emulate Mary, who invested time and effort to understand immunotherapy, kept raising the issue with her oncologist, managed to receive off-label Opdivo, avoided hospice, experienced complete remission *one year before FDA approval*, and is now back to normal life?

Or, will you emulate Harry, who accepted the word of two oncologists that there was "nothing else" and died three months later?

Driving Your Own Cure

If you want to emulate Mary and ride the long tail of the immunotherapy survival curve, we have some ideas to offer.

Be prepared to sacrifice. Attempting the miracle of a cure takes time, money, effort and a willingness to travel. But the good news is it's becoming easier by the day.

When we began pursuing immunotherapy, it was inaccessible. We invested years of full-time effort and travel to make it a reality, sacrificing life savings, careers and dreams of children. But today, immunotherapy has become widely available. Immunotherapy clinical trials have mushroomed across the country. You may not even need to travel far. Every major hospital will have oncologists with experience administering checkpoint inhibitors (especially melanoma oncologists). Any outpatient clinic that offers radiation therapy and PD-1 infusions can offer you the combination that Mary and Jimmy Carter received.

Even so, patients seeking to optimize immunotherapy may consider travel to larger academic centers where doctors have deeper experience with immunotherapy for specific cancers. For example, if I was diagnosed with brain cancer (glioblastoma), had completed standard therapies, and was still well enough to travel, I'd immediately enroll at Duke University's clinical trial to receive intratumoral injections of a modified poliovirus.[15] I'd act swiftly, knowing that brain tumors can suddenly incapacitate, preventing travel and disqualifying me from clinical trials.

In the early years, we avoided travel because of cost and effort. We were also attached to our alma mater (Stanford) and assumed there wasn't any benefit to getting a second opinion elsewhere. It took us over two years to realize the value of going to a high-volume sarcoma center like MD Anderson for my rare cancer.

If you have the means, we advocate you not tarry—make the appointment and, if necessary, get on a plane to see that experienced oncologist. If travel is impossible, consider remote consultation services like Partners Online Specialty Consultations which offers expert opinion from Dana-Farber Cancer Institute and other affiliate hospitals (In chapter 10, we described how we used this service to analyze my MRIs for evidence of tumor shrinkage while on Coley's Toxins).[16]

Leverage informational resources. The internet offers instant access to high-quality resources that can aid research. But it is a two-edged sword: the diversity of voices can empower or mislead, wasting precious time.

For a thorough understanding of standard-of-care treatments, we favor *UpToDate.com*—a website written by oncologists for other doctors. Patients can purchase a short term access pass for a reasonable fee.[17] The website offers concise and thorough summaries of how to treat various cancers; you won't have to study complex research papers (unless you need to delve into the nuances). The articles are somewhat technical. But those who persevere will glean a solid grasp of conventional therapies and their benefits (or lack thereof). With this understanding, you'll be empowered to avoid unnecessary or even detrimental therapy (such as the chemo prescribed to Mark and my grandmother, despite their frail statuses).

Besides *UpToDate.com*, other free and reputable resources are WebMD's *Medscape*, the websites of major cancer centers such as MD Anderson, Dana-Farber, Memorial Sloan Kettering and the National Cancer Institute's *cancer.gov*.

For immunotherapy, *cancerresearch.org* contains a wealth of information, listing various immunotherapies and clinical trials by cancer type.[18] This is the website of the Cancer Research Institute (CRI), the organization founded by Helen Coley Nauts (Dr. William Coley's daughter) and nurtured by the late Dr. Lloyd Old. Also, *scholar.google.com* is a powerful tool for culling summaries of the latest published studies.

Finally, we've compiled resources related to this book at *CuringCancerBook.com*, where we also hope to further develop the topics and strategies we've touched upon.

Whatever the resource, we advocate that patients glean a thorough understanding of their prognoses, without which they cannot make informed and rational decisions whether to pursue "experimental" immunotherapy over conventional treatment.

Seek a second (or third) opinion. We hold physicians in the highest regard. They labor daily to save lives and alleviate pain and suffering. But, as our esteemed primary care physician often tells us: don't *just* listen to your doctor. Especially when it comes to difficult diseases like cancer.

Medicine for complex diseases isn't pure science. It involves subjective thinking, skill, experience and intuition. Almost every physician we've encountered has been genuine, caring, respectful and mindful enough to admit that they don't have all the answers. But the nature of their profession requires cancer doctors to project confidence and optimism. In this context, it is sometimes tempting for patients facing the prospect of death to latch onto this confidence—and to entrust our futures without asking hard questions or doing our homework.

The rarer the disease, the more critical it is to seek further opinions. For example, Dr. Benjamin's insistence of scans every three months allowed me to catch my jaw recurrence early. Otherwise, the tumor may have ensnared critical structures and become inoperable.

Even if your cancer isn't rare, a second opinion can be invaluable. Take, for example, our friend Francis. He saw an oncologist at a reputable academic center for his metastatic lung cancer. The oncologist had exceptional bedside manners that garnered Francis' trust. She prescribed chemotherapy, but it didn't seem right to us. Francis' cancer had a specific mutation known as ALK. We looked up his disease on *UpToDate.com* and learned the recommended initial treatment was Xalkori (an ALK inhibitor). Xalkori had far fewer side effects than chemo but comparable-or-better efficacy. We urged Francis to seek a second opinion at another reputable academic center close by. The second oncologist unequivocally recommended Xalkori as the initial treatment—not chemo. Francis ended up taking Xalkori, which kept his disease stable while allowing him to avoid the harsher side effects of chemo. Francis's story shows us why second opinions matter.

Work with a doctor experienced in immunotherapy. The sudden and fast-evolving breakthroughs means the majority of today's medical oncologists were not trained in immunotherapies (unless they've been involved in research or clinical trials). With the recent approvals of PD-1 in skin cancer, lung cancer, kidney cancer and lymphoma, oncologists who treat these would have garnered some experience. Even so, they may not be familiar with other experimental immunotherapies.

In the previous section, we emphasize why a second opinion matters. Here, we emphasize the need to see *the right person*. A case in point: Most of the surgeons we consulted had discouraged me from cryoablation. With the best of intentions, they were trying to keep me on the proven path. But their expertise lay with surgery, and some of the facts they quoted about cryoablation didn't reflect the latest advances. We had to speak with Dr. Peter Littrup (chapter 11) for a state-of-the-art understanding of the pros and cons of cryo.

Likewise, if not for Dr. Old's guidance and affirmation, we would not have persevered so deep into immunotherapy, given the abstruse science and daunting logistical challenges (let alone that none of my other doctors had experience with it).

Recall from chapter 10 that we had befriended a sarcoma patient named Jake. He had consulted a physician in Los Angeles with years of experience administering PD-1. But he enrolled in a trial closer to home in Tulsa, Oklahoma. Nine weeks later, the inexperienced Tulsa doctors, mistaking tumor flare for growth, booted Jake off the trial. Although a scan three weeks later revealed tumor shrinkage, they couldn't readmit him.

More serious is if autoimmune side effects occur from PD-1 inhibitors or other immunotherapies. Although rare, this can lead to major problems like perforated intestines, lung inflammation and even death. Timely administration of steroids is crucial. Experienced doctors will be more adept at identifying warnings signs and managing side effects.

So, due to the fast-evolving nature of immunotherapy, **we feel it is best to consult doctors with experience, not just the one whose clinic is closest to home.** Patients have to decide for themselves how much time and money they're willing to sacrifice. After all, what value does one place on averting wrong treatment decisions, suffering or loss of life?

If you feel intimidated by the science, or if you're overwhelmed by your cancer, don't be discouraged. Get in touch with a *reputable* and experienced doctor—just as the mothers of John and Ronny had. (John was the young man with 130 lung tumors, now alive and well almost 12 years later, and Ronny was the other synovial sarcoma patient whom Dr. Old had helped.) You'll get a more balanced view of the risks and benefits of immunotherapy versus conventional therapies—rather than the cursory proclamation: "it's experimental."

Certain cancer centers have strong histories in immunotherapy research. The National Cancer Institute in Bethesda, Maryland, and the "big three" (MD Anderson, Dana-Farber and Memorial Sloan Kettering) are choice places to look. Centers like the Fred Hutchinson Cancer Center in Seattle and the University of Pennsylvania's Abramson Cancer Center in Philadelphia have strong programs in adoptive T cell therapy (e.g. CAR-T). But now that immunotherapy has captured the imaginations of oncologists worldwide, many other academic centers are ramping up their programs.

Beyond specific academic institutions, it pays to focus on a doctor's experience. Our favorite tool for locating experienced physicians is to search for academic publications on *scholar.google.com*. Look for doctors involved in highly cited studies and find out where they practice.[19] Also, hospital or university websites often list doctors' biographies. Spend time studying these and you'll get an idea of their experience with immunotherapy.

Finally, online discussion forums are useful places to obtain leads. But be sure to ask specific questions about a doctor's experience, not just how friendly, smart or accomplished he or she may be.

Get immunotherapy as early as possible. Most of the patients we've known who tried immunotherapy did so as a last resort. We haven't met anyone else who pursued it aggressively while they had no detectable tumors.

Some of these patients had problematic tumors that caused internal bleeding or incapacitated them (especially those with brain tumors). Some were excluded from clinical trials because of these complications. Others were admitted at first, but shortly after starting immunotherapy, their advancing tumors created complications that disqualified them from the trials. Had they started immunotherapy sooner—when they had fewer, less-problematic tumors—they might have had more time for immunotherapy to work.

Also, clinical trials have strict criteria and favor patients with good functional statuses. For example, most will require patients to have healthy livers and adequate white blood cells. These can be compromised by chemo or targeted therapies. Be sure to consider this when weighing whether to first enroll in immunotherapy clinical trials or embark on conventional therapies.

The choice of when to start immunotherapy is especially critical for patients like Harry, with an advanced disease. As immunotherapy can take time to work—up to three months in the case of PD-1—these patients have no time to lose. Recall that Harry died three months after diagnosis. For him to have experienced the benefits of PD-1, he would've had to begin it immediately, without delay.

The sooner you can start immunotherapy, the more time you'll have to evaluate if it's working, and the better you'll be able to handle side effects and demands of travel. And if immunotherapy were to fail, the generally mild side effects aren't likely to compromise your ability to fall back on conventional therapies.

Study immunotherapy clinical trials. All clinical trials are listed on *ClinicalTrials.gov*.[20] Patients can search for relevant trials by entering keywords such as "PD-1 colon cancer." Trials are constantly being added, so keep checking for suitable ones. Also, we've mentioned the CRI's website as a useful resource that lists trials by cancer type.

In this book, we've discussed the still-evolving principles in cancer immunotherapy: Create T cells to attack tumors. Release the brakes of the immune system with CTLA-4 inhibitors. Strip tumor defenses with PD-1 inhibitors and by depleting Tregs and MDSCs. Bring the fight to tumors with direct injections.

As you survey clinical trials, remembering these principles will help you better understand the rationale behind a trial. Take for example the trial NCT02775292 at the University of California, Los Angeles (UCLA) with the cryptic title *"Gene-Modified T Cells, Vaccine Therapy, and Nivolumab in Treating Patients With Stage IV or Locally Advanced Solid Tumors Expressing NY-ESO-1"*.[21] This trial combines many of the strategies we've discussed:

1) A short course of chemo is first given. It includes the chemo drug fludarabine, which kills off the patient's existing T cells to "make space" for soon-to-be-infused adoptive T cells.[22] Also included is cyclophosphamide, known to deplete Tregs from the tumor microenvironment.

2) Patients are then given adoptive T cells that target the NY-ESO-1 antigen found in many cancers (NY-ESO-1 is the same target in the vaccine Dr. Old gave me).

3) Besides the adoptive T cells, a dendritic vaccine (also pulsed with NY-ESO-1) is co-administered to generate T cells.

4) A low dose of Aldesleukin (the cytokine IL-2) is given to provoke T cells into an inflammatory state so that they attack tumors.

5) A PD-1 inhibitor is given every two weeks to strip tumor defenses, allowing T cells to attack unimpeded.

This UCLA trial exemplifies the multi-pronged combination approach we had adopted in our own efforts. Also, notice that the trial accepts patients with *any* solid tumor that expresses the NY-ESO-1 antigen. As awareness of the broad applicability of immunotherapy spreads, I think we'll see more studies like this that surmount the rigid classifications of cancer types and the notions of drugs that work for specific cancers.

Think out of the box. Clinical trials don't charge patients, but the cost of off-label therapy can be prohibitive. Many large clinics and hospitals charge a 400 percent markup for non-insured drugs. Oncologists at smaller clinics or private practices may have more flexibility to provide PD-1 inhibitors at cost, saving you tens or hundreds of thousands. A four-infusion course of Keytruda obtained at cost may be as "cheap" as $25,000 (compared to $125,000 after markup).

Many clinical trials have been administering PD-1 inhibitors continuously to patients, some for years. Even at cost, long-term off-label PD-1 becomes prohibitively expensive. But the indefinite administration of checkpoint inhibitors may not be necessary. Some patients have experienced continued remission of tumors even after stopping the infusions, their immune systems having learned to suppress the cancer.[23]

It may even be detrimental to receive continuous infusions of checkpoint inhibitors. The longer you receive PD-1, the greater the cumulative risk of autoimmune side effects.[24] Mary, at first, experienced only some itchy skin while receiving PD-1 twice-monthly. All her tumors disappeared by month three, but she continued to take the drug. By month nine, she developed pneumonitis (inflammation in her lungs), causing her difficulty breathing, for which she had to receive steroids. This example reminds us that the human immune system comprises checks and balances. Push it in one direction for too long, and there may be unintended consequences.

Another option is to travel abroad for PD-1. Medicine hasn't become a high-profit industry in all countries. Countries like Germany, Singapore, Australia and Thailand have world-class hospitals and physicians. You can get radiation therapy at a local cancer center to generate T cells, then get PD-1 abroad at cost price, and then return home to have an experienced local oncologist follow you for side effects.

For creating T cells against your cancer, you can enroll in one of many immunotherapy clinical trials (vaccine trials, adoptive T cell trials, cancer-killing viruses). You'd hope that these therapies would help your body develop memory T cells against your cancer, after which you'll have them for life. If the cancer progresses and you're booted off the trial, you can then get PD-1 separately, and hope to unleash those already-created T cells against your tumors.

Finally, patients with tumors amenable to injection can work with experienced doctors to inject compounds similar to Coley's Toxins known as *toll-like receptor (TLR) agonists*.[25,26] This may be done as part of a clinical trial or off-label treatment. You might even explore co-injections of checkpoint antibodies directly into tumors, potentially avoiding autoimmune side effects. This strategy may be worth exploring for patients with known autoimmune diseases that may be exacerbated by systemic infusions of checkpoint inhibitors.[27]

These are just some ideas as to how you might attempt to put all the pieces in place for successful immunotherapy. Ultimately, your immune cells are oblivious to how or where you receive the various therapies, or how much you paid for them. The important thing is to get them into your body without delay.

What I Would Do If My Cancer Returns

I continue to focus on avoiding inflammatory omega-6 fats and sugary foods—my "diet-based" immunotherapy. I hope to extend the three years of clean scans to thirty years. But should my cancer recur, we have a game plan.

We view early intervention as critical.

If a single tumor were to recur, I'd opt for cryoablation whenever possible because, (a) it is minimally invasive, and (b) it can generate an up-to-date repertoire of T cells to keep up with a mutating cancer.

I'd also favor cryo over radiation because tumors can develop resistance to radiation. In contrast, the pure physical effect of freezing destroys all tissue. Also, despite its immune-sensitizing effects, radiation may not be the best immune activator, as it can recruit MDSCs into tumors.[28]

As cryo itself may mobilize my immune system against my cancer, I wouldn't use off-label PD-1 for a single tumor. (Even though the risk of side effects is low, why risk it unless I have to?)

If a handful of tumors recur (say five), I'd cryoablate as many that could be safely treated. The presence of multiple tumors would indicate a cancer that's spreading more aggressively. I'd get a PD-1 inhibitor soon after cryo—perhaps within a week. I'd hope the PD-1 antibodies would neutralize tumor defenses and enable the cryo-induced T cells to eradicate remaining cancer. Even if all five tumors are treatable with cryo, I might intentionally leave a small tumor untreated (perhaps one at a safe distance from critical structures that isn't at the risk of becoming untreatable). I'd do this to *track the efficacy* of PD-1, which could help determine how long I'd need to keep taking it.

I'd work closely with an oncologist who has experience with the side effects of PD-1. And I'd want to pay careful attention to the timing of follow-up scans. I wouldn't scan too soon because tumor flare might give the false impression of tumor growth. But if I were to see clear signs that PD-1 wasn't working, I'd seek more powerful immunotherapy.

A more powerful immunotherapy would be adoptive T cell therapy (TCR, CAR-T or TIL therapy, described in chapter 6). The sheer infusion of billions of T cells can whittle away large numbers of tumors. But the downsides of adoptive therapy—especially with TCR and CAR-T—are the potential serious side effects (such as cytokine storms), the inability to target multiple tumor antigens and the lack of a suitable antigen for solid tumors (antigens that aren't specific enough to cancer can cause collateral damage to healthy organs).[29]

Biotech companies are engineering "off-switches" into T cells to make them safer. With these switches, doctors can force the adoptive T cells to self-destruct in the event of a cytokine storm or attack on healthy organs (by giving the patient a drug that activates the off-switch). So, I'd search for these next-generation adoptive T cell trials. But I wouldn't rely on adoptive therapy alone. I could envision myself using it to eliminate most of my tumors, then following up with cryoablation plus PD-1 for a more holistic approach that creates T cells within the body.

If all else fails, I'd combine PD-1 and CTLA-4 inhibitors with cryo. Although powerful and synergistic, the cumulative risks of autoimmune side effects are not to be taken lightly.

These are some strategies that Eddy and I have conjured over the years of thinking about survival. They are, of course, subject to change as new data arrives.

It's been a long and arduous journey, but we've survived long enough to witness the ongoing revolution in cancer immunotherapy. Sometimes, I have to pinch myself and realize that I'm still alive—and that I now have these powerful tools at my disposal should my synovial sarcoma return.

Real Hope

The study of tumor immunology suggests the need for a multi-faceted, holistic approach to curing cancer. For example, you may kill tumors that express a single antigen like NY-ESO-1, but cancer cells that lack the antigen may escape. You may neutralize PD-1 defenses, but tumors may develop other defenses. And in your attempt to stimulate the immune system against cancer, you may inadvertently promote the bodyguards (Tregs) and enablers (MDSCs) of tumors through feedback mechanisms originally intended to protect against autoimmunity. In short, the immune system is a complex system of checks and balances, and a single-agent approach is unlikely to be enough.

Perhaps one day we'll see a general formula that works for all cancers. Perhaps it will look something like this: First, deplete Tregs and MDSCs with special drugs or antibodies. Next, create T cells against all tumor antigens with cryo, radiation or intratumoral injections of CpG. Then, infuse the patient with a cocktail of checkpoint inhibitors regardless of tumor type. Or, as Dr. Ronald Levy at Stanford has inspired, inject a single tumor with that cocktail to minimize autoimmune side effects.[30]

A century ago, Dr. William Coley aspired to cure his patients. Understanding of the immune system in the 1890s paled in comparison to today's. Dr. Coley had no notion of targeting specific antigens, nor any knowledge of specific mutations. But it didn't stop him from trying. He injected tumors directly, whatever their makeup. His toxins shrunk sarcomas, lymphomas and carcinomas. Some patients like Mrs. Gruver (who had cervical carcinoma) were cured with his "rudimentary" approach.

Dr. Coley's courage and tenacity inspired Eddy and I to strive for a cure and not to settle for the limited benefits of "proven" therapies. At the start of our quest for a cure in 2009, some doctors dissuaded us, deeming immunotherapy as unproven. Back then, it was harder to defend our conviction: the evidence we had was century-old anecdotes of Coley's Toxins and a smattering of encouraging early reports (such as Heather's success with Dr. Rosenberg's adoptive T cells). But even those were enough to stake my life upon. In contrast, patients today have the astonishing successes of PD-1 and other experimental immunotherapies upon which to anchor hope. These are vivid testaments of the immune system's potential to conquer cancer.

We wrote this book partly to honor Dr. Old; we'd promised him we'd do what we could to help others. But first and foremost, this book is for cancer patients and their caregivers. Having gone through years of not knowing if I'd be alive the next few months—let alone the next year—we've grappled with the fear and devastation that cancer brings into lives and families.

We don't claim to know the answer to a cure for every patient. But one thing we know is that the immune system **can** cure cancer.

That I'm alive eight years after diagnosis, with clean scans for the past three years, tells us a cure is plausible.

That Mary, Jimmy Carter and hundreds of other patients are still alive after taking checkpoint inhibitors—some as far back as 2000—tells us a cure is probable.

That many patients of Dr. William Coley had survived *decades* after being diagnosed with terminal cancer tells us a cure is surely attainable. *If he did it a century ago, we can too.*

We hope this book has informed, inspired and empowered you.

Take that step out of the box.

Seize that cure for your cancer.

A Tribute to Dr. Lloyd Old

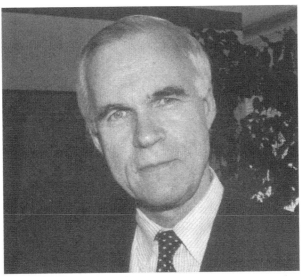

Figure 46: Lloyd Old, M.D. (September 23, 1933 – November 28, 2011).
Picture taken 1995.[K]

Dr. Lloyd Old is internationally recognized as "one of the founders and standard-bearers of the field of tumor immunology."[1] In addition to active scientific research, he captained premier research institutions such as the Ludwig Institute for Cancer Research (LICR) and the Cancer Research Institute (CRI). At these institutions, he served as scientific founder, director and CEO (of LICR). He shaped strategy, vision and policy as an architect of worldwide research efforts.

Even though he didn't treat patients, he touched the lives of individual cancer patients struggling for survival, using his knowledge and influence to help them gain access to cutting-edge immunotherapy.

His compassion was apparent from the first phone call. My boss at Stanford, Lucy Shapiro, had told him about my cancer and our interest in getting Coley's Toxins. We were nobodies, with nothing to offer in return.

He could've sent a terse email, saying, "Call my secretary to set up a time." But despite his myriad responsibilities, he made time to call. We spoke with him for one hour. Instead of objectifying my travails with medical speak, science and statistics, he empathized with the pain I'd endured from the large tumor in my head. But his compassion didn't merely manifest as empathy. It resulted in strong action: he immediately asked me to send a sample of my tumor to his team at LICR, to find out what immunotherapy I might benefit from.

That conversation, and every one that followed for the next two and a half years, would end with deliberate words of encouragement, such as, "You're not alone in this," married with a concrete plan on how to get immunotherapy into my body.

Dr. Old introduced us to other cancer patients he was helping. Like us, they were strangers that somehow found their way to him. Dr. Old walked alongside them, leveraging his network of collaborators and protégés to open doors to immunotherapy clinical trials, transforming theory and talk into tangible chances at life. "It is the responsibility of those who can help to open doors if they can," he once told us.

So embodied was his compassion and chivalry that in his last months of life—while dealing with his own pain and suffering from advancing prostate cancer—he was *still* helping patients, calling them to offer encouragement and strategizing plans of action. One patient's mother conveyed how Dr. Old had told her he'd continue doing everything within his power to help her son until he could no longer do so.

Dr. Old was patient and gracious. He had a towering intellect and had made seminal discoveries. Yet, there was never a hint of condescension or impatience, despite our glaring deficiencies in knowledge. We had no background in immunology and were still struggling to understand key concepts and strategies. He would gently point us the right way, showing us what we needed to study and why it was important.

From Dr. Old, we learned the importance of open-mindedness, grounded on objective science. He would say that every anecdote of miraculous disappearance of cancer held value, should not be dismissed, and should be scrutinized. Many in the medical and scientific community had dismissed

Dr. William Coley's work. But Dr. Old was instead inspired by Dr. Coley's anecdotes. He told us that Dr. Coley's work had motivated his research into Bacillus Calmette–Guérin (BCG), which eventually became a standard therapy for superficial bladder cancer.[2]

Despite his interest in alternative medicines, he would caution us that many alternative therapies lacked basis, saying, "Hopeful thinking is wonderful, but what's the justification?"

His open-mindedness reflected a genuine intellectual humility. Soon after my fourth NY-ESO-1 vaccination, my lung lesions had become visible on scan and lymph nodes had lit up near each axilla. Thinking nothing of it, Eddy asked Dr. Old if the vaccine could have caused my cancer to suddenly grow. I feared Dr. Old would be offended, after the great lengths he'd gone through to set up the single patient protocol. Perhaps some in his position might have grown defensive, even offended at the insinuation that their efforts had caused more harm than good. But not Dr. Old.

"Eddy, when you said to me, 'Could this vaccine make the cancer grow faster?'—that was a profound statement," he said. "It's something I've thought a great deal about. The first thing you learn in med school is "do no harm." But there's no evidence, Eddy. I've gone through all 44 of our trials and found no evidence the vaccines have done harm." Instead of brushing off Eddy's question as a neophyte's ignorance, Dr. Old took the time to ponder the possibilities.

Dr. Old realized the need to translate immunotherapy research into actual treatments. His life's work bears witness to this. He devised a strategy to bring immunotherapy to the masses.

First, to eradicate the stigma of immunotherapy as "fringe science," he mentored a worldwide community of immunologists over many decades, equipping them with training and financial support; together, they advanced the field of cancer immunology. As the CRI website aptly states, "Nearly every major advance, scientist, and research program in the field of tumor immunology can somehow trace its lineage back to him."[3]

Then, realizing that the pharmaceutical industry was beholden to near-term profit goals and lacked the flexibility to invest in the long view, he built up a formidable research institution—the LICR. LICR had the muscle to perform basic research in immunotherapy *and* push those discoveries through the staggering regulatory and financial barriers of early-stage clinical trials.

"It's been very difficult to keep this up," he once said. "To do this, you have to set up so many components. An intellectual property program—otherwise no company would ever take it [into later stage trials]. A production facility [that satisfies stringent safety regulations]. And the staff and resources to manage clinical trials. Many institutions [like universities] have clinical trial programs. But to run Phase Ones of things discovered in the same place—almost *impossible*."

"Our scientific establishment thinks about grants, promotions and appointments. Therapy is left to the drug companies," he said. "Take Coley's Toxins … a classic example. There's no commercial motivation, hence no development. The idea of taking unpatentable dead bacteria and injecting it? In contrast, take the cytokine *interleukin 7*, which might cost $100,000 for three treatments—now, *that* might get done in a clinical trial."

In a later conversation, Dr. Old shared his view that Coley's Toxins hadn't been adequately evaluated. From 2008 to 2012, LICR ran a trial of Coley's Toxins in Frankfurt, Germany. But, as had happened in many Coley's Toxins trials throughout history, limitations prevented an accurate assessment. (In this case, the German authorities didn't allow dose escalation beyond the dosage that elicited first fevers.)

Dr. Old taught us not to give up even when things were difficult. Instead of pursuing the scientific fad of the day, he devoted his life to a field, which, at the time, held no glory. In 1958, he began his career in cancer immunotherapy, at age 25. For the next five decades, he labored to decipher the intricacies of the human immune system, believing immunotherapy would one day yield the most benefit for mankind.

But above all, the plight of cancer patients fueled his perseverance. He once recounted how a journalist had interviewed him about LICR, then portrayed his efforts and the organization in an uncomplimentary slant. She ended her piece by questioning why LICR had invested so much into immunotherapy, with little results to show in the form of approved treatments.

"My point was if we already knew that immunotherapy would pan out, we wouldn't have to do all this [difficult work], would we?" he told us.

With a fire in his voice, he then lamented that patients like myself were forced to turn to unconventional therapies precisely *because* conventional medicine wasn't offering what we needed.

"There's a *tremendous* need for this [immunotherapy research]—a tremendous need."

Dr. Old was a true humanitarian. "You and Eddy are dealing with the forefront of what I'd call 'clinical discovery research.' It's so important that you're recognizing some of the deficiencies [of conventional medicine] and were able to surmount them to a certain extent. But what about the next person? And the next person? And the next?"

He drew inspiration from the philosopher Immanuel Kant's *categorical imperative,* and taught us that, "If you're going to do something good for someone, you'd want it done for everyone else."

•₀ •• •°₀ •• •₀

"Oh, Lloyd, why has it taken so long for people to recognize my father's work?" Mrs. Helen Coley Nauts used to ask him. (Dr. Old shared how Mrs. Nauts—his close colleague and dear friend—had been perplexed at the scientific community's failure to recognize her father's work.)

"Because, Helen, science has taken this long to catch up to your father's work," he'd answer her.

Without Mrs. Nauts' equally passionate determination to preserve and propagate her father's work, immunotherapy would still be in its infancy, or perhaps non-existent. Who knows where we'd be without Dr. Coley's spark that inspired visionaries like Dr. Old.

Dr. Old, you once said to us, "I hope you're right about this pursuit of yours—and when Rene is fine, you can sit back and reflect on all this, then ask yourself what you can do to make the situation better for others."

We can't do much, Dr. Old, for we have little influence. But this book is our tribute to you—our small contribution to mankind. We hope it will help others understand immunotherapy a little better, and in so doing, honor you.

Thank you, Dr. Old. Thank you for devoting your life to science, so that Eddy and I might have the chance of a future together.

Because of your sacrifice, countless patients can now reach for a cure.

Acknowledgments

Eight years ago, we'd never have imagined writing a book. The idea first came from Rene's advisor at Stanford, Professor Lucy Shapiro. With the dire prognosis, survival had been an all-consuming focus. But when Rene's tumors suddenly ceased in 2013, we began to give serious thought to the book.

We would like to thank Professor Lucy Shapiro and Rene's co-advisor, Professor Harley McAdams. They have been instrumental to this book in many ways. Their unwavering support over the years enabled us to persist in our quest for a cure. Critically, Lucy connected us with Dr. Lloyd Old without whom there'd be no book.

We thank Joshua Cook for the numerous iterations of line edits and for copyediting. With great patience and persevering attention to detail, he helped us clarify what we needed to communicate.

We thank our beta readers, Professor Stephen Chee, Tom Tye and Virginia Kalogeraki, for their indispensable feedback.

We owe a debt of gratitude to the numerous medical professionals who went above and beyond their call of duty in caring for Rene. Their dedication to their profession and patients cannot be adequately acknowledged in these short pages. Beyond providing treatment, some sacrificed many hours to educate us on nuances and technical aspects of medicine. Others helped us think through difficult decisions.

Specifically, we'd like to thank the oncology team at Stanford who provided the highest standards of conventional therapy to keep Rene alive. Dr. Michael Kaplan, whose expert hands saved Rene's life not once, but twice. Dr. Charlotte Jacobs and the compassionate nurses at the Stanford chemo ward. Dr. Quynh-Thu Le, who kept Rene safe through radiation and many years of follow-up. Dr. Nancy Fischbein, for helping us to understand head MRIs. Dr. Gerald Berry, for analyzing tumor tissue for evidence of immune cells.

We'd also like to thank Dr. George Demetri of Dana-Farber Cancer Institute for extending compassion to us, analyzing Rene's scans and orienting us in the early, bewildering days of diagnosis.

Instrumental at helping us understand the nature of sarcoma were Rene's physicians at MDA. Dr. Robert Benjamin, whose wealth of experience has enabled us to make very difficult but informed decisions. Dr. Patrick Hwu, Head of Cancer Medicine at MDA, for the countless hours guiding our thinking about immunotherapy, and for making immunotherapy clinical trials a reality for sarcoma patients. Dr. Ehab Hanna, whose experience with sarcoma surgeries proved indispensable in our decision making. We would also like to thank Dr. Padmanee Sharma for her efforts in exploring off-label Yervoy therapy in 2011.

The team at the Ludwig Institute for Cancer Research, New York sacrificed much to make the NY-ESO-1 vaccine a reality. Dr. Linda Pan, for organizing the single patient protocol; Dr. Sacha Gnjatic, for analyzing Rene's blood for immune cells; Dr. Achim Jungbluth, for analyzing Rene's tumor samples. Because of their continued support, we had access to critical treatment-related information that would've been impossible to obtain elsewhere.

We owe a debt of gratitude to the staff of the Palo Alto Medical Foundation (PAMF), Mountain View: Dr. Rosendo So-Rosillo, Lolomi Cardoso, R.N. and Laura Perry, R.N., for making the NY-ESO-1 vaccine a reality.

For many years, Dr. Ravin Agah, our primary physician at PAMF, has supported us in innumerable ways, going far beyond his responsibilities. He stayed by our side through the darkest moments and fought tirelessly with us, providing medical, logistical, strategic and emotional support. Without him, we simply couldn't have sustained our fight. We are truly blessed to have him as a primary physician.

We'd like to thank Dr. Stephen Hoption-Cann and Don MacAdam of MBVax, Canada, for resurrecting Coley's Toxins, providing crucial hope to those of us who see Coley's Toxins as a potential cure with the longest history. Thank you for sacrificing time to field our copious questions as we researched the toxins.

And we thank Dr. Ralph Moss, of the Moss Reports for his research into Coley's Toxins and for bringing awareness of it to cancer patients.

Dr. Vikas Sukhatme of Harvard Medical School first followed our initial treatment with Coley's Toxins, then educated us on key concepts and practical ways to maximize immunotherapy. We are deeply grateful for his kindness.

We thank Dr. Raymond Chang and the staff of the Meridian Medical Group, New York, for making off-label therapies available to cancer patients and for helping us think through the pros and cons of conventional therapies, as well as facilitating the immunotherapy treatments in Germany.

Dr. Axel Rolle of Coswig Specialist Hospital, Germany was kind to us, spending many hours answering our questions in person and over the phone, as we sought to understand the nuances of his laser lung resection technique. We owe him a debt of gratitude.

We are extremely grateful to Dr. Peter Littrup, Dr. Hussein Aoun, Barbara Adam, R.N. of the Karmanos Cancer Center for helping us understand the pros and cons of cryoablation, for providing state-of-the-art medical care, and for advancing the field of cryoablation.

Dr. John Haddad, Maria Iacopelli-Barker, CRNA, Dr. Konstantin Rusin and the anesthesiology team at the Detroit Medical Center took care of us during a dark moment and provided exquisite anesthesiology care, ensuring safe cryoablation of lung tumors during the high-dose omega-3-6 and ketogenic dietary regimens.

We thank Dr. Thomas Nesselhut, Dr. Jan Nesselhut, Dr. Dirk Lorenzen, and the nurses at the Group Practice for Cell Therapy, Germany for enabling us and other patients worldwide to obtain dendritic vaccination and NK cell infusions.

We are deeply indebted to Dr. Jatin Shah of Memorial Sloan-Kettering Cancer Center for taking the time to explain to us what we needed to hear, not what we wanted to hear.

Before the sudden cessation of Rene's tumors, we were preparing to obtain PD-1 off-label. Although we ended up not needing it, we are deeply grateful to Dr. Mark Renneker of UC San Francisco and Dr. Peter Boasberg of The Angeles Clinic in Santa Monica for helping us derive concrete plans to obtain off-label PD-1.

For publishing crucial research on omega-3-6 and documenting patient DH's astonishing success, we are forever grateful to Dr. Ron Pardini at the University of Nevada, Reno. We also thank patient DH for sharing his experience with us.

We'd also like to thank Dr. Jonathan Chung, Dr. Tilman Koelsch and Tamara Greer of the National Jewish Health Department of Radiology in Denver, for their support since 2013 with DWI-MRIs of the lung, and Dr. Juergen Biederer of Heidelberg University Hospital for referring us to Dr. Jonathan Chung.

We'd like to recognize our friends and family who volunteered for the NK cell donation process: Ethan Chan, Matthew Chan, Steve and Grace Fong, David and Dorothea Henry, Pete and Esther Hwang, Brian and Annie Lee, Scott and Megan Liesinger, Annette Lucman, Eddie and Dora Kwan, Monica Schwartz. We will never forget their sacrifice.

Many other friends and family supported us over the marathon years of surviving cancer, blessing us with moral and financial support. Without them, our journey wouldn't have been possible.

Last but not least, we'd like to acknowledge and thank the hundreds of cancer patients and caregivers we've interacted with over the years, who've generously shared with us their wisdom, borne of searing first-hand experience. They've journeyed alongside us over the years, in our common quest to survive, encouraging and admonishing, laughing and crying with us. It is our sincerest hope that this book will, in some way, benefit them and others battling cancer—as much as their shared wisdom has benefited us.

Figure Credits

A. **Chapter 1, Figure 2 (left image):** Courtesy of National Human Genome Research Institute.

B. **Chapter 3, Figure 6:** Reprinted with permission. © 2000 American Society of Clinical Oncology. All rights reserved. Lewis, Jonathan J., et al. "Synovial sarcoma: a multivariate analysis of prognostic factors in 112 patients with primary localized tumors of the extremity." Journal of Clinical Oncology 18.10 (2000): 2087-2094. (Text overlaid on graph for clarity)

C. **Chapter 3, Figure 7:** Reprinted with permission. © 2007 Wiley Periodicals, Inc. Head Neck 2007. All rights reserved. Harb, William J., et al. "Survival in patients with synovial sarcoma of the head and neck: association with tumor location, size, and extension." Head & neck 29.8 (2007): 731-740.

D. **Chapter 3, Figure 8:** Bar chart from the National Cancer Institute's Surveillance, Epidemiology, and End Results (SEER) website (http://seer.cancer.gov/statfacts/html/colorect.html)

E. **Chapter 5, Figures 14:** Reprinted with permission from the Cancer Research Institute

F. **Chapter 5, Figures 15:** By Cancer Research Institute [Public domain], via Wikimedia Commons

G. **Chapter 5, Figures 17:** By Cancer Research Institute (Own work) [CC BY-SA 3.0 (http://creativecommons.org/licenses/by-sa/3.0)], via Wikimedia Commons

H. **Chapter 11, Figures 36 and 37:** Reprinted courtesy of © Copyright 2015 Mohiuddin et al. Mohiuddin M, Park H, Hallmeyer S, et al. (December 18, 2015) High-Dose Radiation as a Dramatic, Immunological Primer in Locally Advanced Melanoma. Cureus 7(12): e417. doi:10.7759/cureus.417

I. **Chapter 15, Figure 43:** Ronald S. Pardini et al., Figures 1 and 2. From Pardini, Ronald S., et al. "Nutritional intervention with omega-3 fatty acids in a case of malignant fibrous histiocytoma of the lungs." Nutrition and cancer52.2 (2005): 121-129. Reprinted by permission of Taylor & Francis Ltd.

J. **Chapter 16, Figures 44 and 45:** Graph concept based on Sharma, Padmanee, and James P. Allison. "Immune checkpoint targeting in cancer therapy: toward combination strategies with curative potential." Cell 161.2 (2015): 205-214.

K. **Tribute to Dr. Lloyd Old, Figure 46:** By Cancer Research Institute (Own work) [CC BY-SA 3.0 (http://creativecommons.org/licenses/by-sa/3.0)], via Wikimedia Commons

Notes

Introduction

1. Nauts, Helen Coley, George A. Fowler, and Frances H. Bogatko. A Review of the Influence of Bacterial Infection and of Bacterial Products "(Coley's Toxins)" on Malignant Tumors in Man A Critical Analysis of 30 Inoperable Cases Treated by Coley's Mixed Toxins, in Which Diagnosis Was Confirmed by Microscopic Examination: Selected for Special Study. Stockh., 1953. 30. Print.

2. In the later half of 2014, PD-1 blocking antibodies, Opdivo, by Bristol-Myers Squibb and Keytruda, by Merck, were approved for metastatic melanoma. Then, during the 2014 American Society of Hematology (ASH) annual meeting, astonishing results of 90% complete remission for high-risk Acute Lymphoblastic Leukemia (ALL) patients using Chimeric Antigen Receptor modified T cells were presented. These patients would have died as chemo was ineffective.

3. Sampson, John H., et al. "Demographics, prognosis, and therapy in 702 patients with brain metastases from malignant melanoma." Journal of neurosurgery 88.1 (1998): 11-20.

4. Mohney, Gillian. "What You Need to Know About Jimmy Carter's Cancer Diagnosis." ABC News. ABC News Network, 20 Apr. 2015. Web. 05 June 2016.

5. Barker, Christopher A., and Michael A. Postow. "Combinations of radiation therapy and immunotherapy for melanoma: a review of clinical outcomes." International Journal of Radiation Oncology* Biology* Physics 88.5 (2014): 986-997

6. Muro, K., et al. "LBA15A phase 1B study of pembrolizumab (PEMBRO; MK-3475) in patients (Pts) with advanced gastric cancer." Annals of Oncology25.suppl 4 (2014): mdu438-15.

7. "Cancer Facts & Figures 2016." American Cancer Society. Web. 30 May 2016.

8. "General Statistics." Fatality Facts. IIHS-HLDI, n.d. Web. 09 June 2016.

9. McCarthy, Edward F. "The toxins of William B. Coley and the treatment of bone and soft-tissue sarcomas." The Iowa orthopaedic journal 26 (2006): 154.

Chapter 1: Pain and Numbness

1. Singer, Samuel, et al. "Synovial sarcoma: prognostic significance of tumor size, margin of resection, and mitotic activity for survival." Journal of Clinical Oncology 14.4 (1996): 1201-1208.

Chapter 2: A Damaged Immune System

1. "What Are the Radiation Risks from CT?" U.S. Food and Drug Administration. Web. 04 Mar. 2016.

2. Giovannucci, Edward. "Insulin, insulin-like growth factors and colon cancer: a review of the evidence." The Journal of nutrition 131.11 (2001): 3109S-3120S.

3. Di Marco, A., M. Gaetani, and B. Scarpinato. "Adriamycin (NSC-123,127): a new antibiotic with antitumor activity." Cancer chemotherapy reports. Part 153.1 (1969): 33.

4. Brouwer, C. A. J., et al. "Long-term cardiac follow-up in survivors of a malignant bone tumour." Annals of oncology 17.10 (2006): 1586-1591.

5. Goodman, Louis S., et al. "Nitrogen mustard therapy: Use of methyl-bis (beta-chloroethyl) amine hydrochloride and tris (beta-chloroethyl) amine hydrochloride for Hodgkin's disease, lymphosarcoma, leukemia and certain allied and miscellaneous disorders." Journal of the American Medical Association 132.3 (1946): 126-132.

6. Kolaczkowska, Elzbieta, and Paul Kubes. "Neutrophil recruitment and function in health and inflammation." Nature Reviews Immunology 13.3 (2013): 159-175.

7. Welte, Karl. "Discovery of G-CSF and early clinical studies." Twenty years of G-CSF. Springer Basel, 2012. 15-24.

Chapter 3: Deciding to Do More

1. Lodish H, Berk A, Zipursky SL, et al. Molecular Cell Biology. 4th edition. New York: W. H. Freeman; 2000. Section 24.1, Tumor Cells and the Onset of Cancer.

2. Lewis, Jonathan J., et al. "Synovial sarcoma: a multivariate analysis of prognostic factors in 112 patients with primary localized tumors of the extremity." Journal of Clinical Oncology 18.10 (2000): 2087-2094.

3. Harb, William J., et al. "Survival in patients with synovial sarcoma of the head and neck: association with tumor location, size, and extension." Head & neck 29.8 (2007): 731-740.

4. In April 2012, Pazopanib (also known as Votrient), a tyrosine kinase inhibitor, was approved for advanced soft tissue sarcoma in patients that failed chemotherapy. FDA news release.

Chapter 4: Exploring Alternative Cures

1. Ji, Hong-Fang, Xue-Juan Li, and Hong-Yu Zhang. "Natural products and drug discovery." EMBO reports 10.3 (2009): 194-200.

2. Stone, Edmund. "An account of the success of the bark of the willow in the cure of agues. In a letter to the Right Honourable George Earl of Macclesfield, President of RS from the Rev. Mr. Edmund Stone, of Chipping-Norton in Oxfordshire." Philosophical Transactions 53 (1763): 195-200.

3. Schrör, Karsten. Acetylsalicylic acid. John Wiley & Sons, 2010.

4. Le Dran H. F. Traité des opérations de chirurgie. Paris: C. Osmont, 1742.

5. Zahl, Per-Henrik, Jan Mæhlen, and H. Gilbert Welch. "The natural history of invasive breast cancers detected by screening mammography." Archives of internal medicine 168.21 (2008): 2311-2316

6. Kolata, G. "Study Suggests Some Cancers May Go Away". The New York Times. November 24, 2008.

7. Challis, G. B., and H. J. Stam. "The spontaneous regression of cancer: a review of cases from 1900 to 1987." Acta Oncologica 29.5 (1990): 545-550.

8. "Helicobacter Pylori and Cancer." National Cancer Institute. Web. 10 Mar. 2016.

9. Cheuk, Wah, et al. "Regression of gastric large B-Cell lymphoma accompanied by a florid lymphoma-like T-cell reaction: immunomodulatory effect of Ganoderma lucidum (Lingzhi)?" International journal of surgical pathology 15.2 (2007): 180-186.

10. Gerson, Max. A Cancer Therapy: Results of Fifty Cases and the Cure of Advanced Cancer by Diet Therapy: A Summary of 30 Years of Clinical Experimentation. Bonita, CA: Gerson Institute, 1990. Print.

11. Levine, Mark, et al. "Vitamin C pharmacokinetics in healthy volunteers: evidence for a recommended dietary allowance." Proceedings of the National Academy of Sciences 93.8 (1996): 3704-3709.

12. Welsh, J. L., et al. "Pharmacological ascorbate with gemcitabine for the control of metastatic and node-positive pancreatic cancer (PACMAN): results from a phase I clinical trial." Cancer chemotherapy and pharmacology 71.3 (2013): 765-775.

13. Papac, Rose J. "Spontaneous regression of cancer." Cancer treatment reviews 22.6 (1996): 395-423.

14. Lokich, Jacob. "Spontaneous regression of metastatic renal cancer: case report and literature review." American journal of clinical oncology 20.4 (1997): 416-418.

15. Beverley, Peter CL. "Primer: making sense of T-cell memory." Nature Clinical Practice Rheumatology 4.1 (2008): 43-49.

16. McCarthy, Edward F. "The toxins of William B. Coley and the treatment of bone and soft-tissue sarcomas." The Iowa orthopaedic journal 26 (2006): 154.

Chapter 5: Coley's Toxins: A 100-Year-Old Immunotherapy

1. Hall, Stephen S. A Commotion in the Blood: Life, Death, and the Immune System. New York: Henry Holt, 1997. 23. Print.

2. Hall, 23.

3. Hall, 24.

4. Hall, 25.

5. Hall, 25.

6. Hall, 26.

7. Hall, 27.

8. Hall, 27.

9. Hall, 27.

10. Hall, 28.

11. Hall, 40.

12. Hall, 40.

13. Hall, 40.

14. Hall, 40.

15. Edgar, Irving I. "Modern Surgery and Lord Lister." Journal of the history of medicine and allied sciences 16.2 (1961): 145-160

16. Hall, Stephen S. A Commotion in the Blood: Life, Death, and the Immune System. New York: Henry Holt, 1997. 41. Print.

17. Hall, 52.

18. Hall, 55.

19. Hall, 56.

20. Hall, 56.

21. McCarthy, Edward F. "The toxins of William B. Coley and the treatment of bone and soft-tissue sarcomas." The Iowa orthopaedic journal 26 (2006): 154.

22. Nauts, Helen Coley, and John R. McLaren. "Coley toxins—the first century." Consensus on Hyperthermia for the 1990s. Springer US, 1990. 483-500.

23. Nauts, Helen Coley, George A. Fowler, and Frances H. Bogatko. A Review of the Influence of Bacterial Infection and of Bacterial Products "(Coley's Toxins)" on Malignant Tumors in Man A Critical Analysis of 30 Inoperable Cases Treated by Coley's Mixed Toxins, in Which Diagnosis Was Confirmed by Microscopic Examination: Selected for Special Study. Stockh., 1953. 29. Print.

24. Nauts, 29.

25. Nauts, 29.

26. Nauts, 29.

27. Nauts, 29.

28. Nauts, 30.

29. Zacharski, L. R., and V. P. Sukhatme. "Coley's toxin revisited: immunotherapy or plasminogen activator therapy of cancer?" Journal of Thrombosis and Haemostasis 3.3 (2005): 424-427.

30. Thomas-Tikhonenko, Andrei, and Christopher A. Hunter. "Infection and cancer: the common vein." Cytokine & growth factor reviews 14.1 (2003): 67-77.

31. Tsung, Kangla, and Jeffrey A. Norton. "Lessons from Coley's toxin." Surgical oncology 15.1 (2006): 25-28.

32. Wiemann, Bernadette, and Charlie O. Starnes. "Coley's toxins, tumor necrosis factor and cancer research: a historical perspective." Pharmacology & therapeutics 64.3 (1994): 529-564.

33. Karbach, Julia, et al. "Phase I clinical trial of mixed bacterial vaccine (Coley's toxins) in patients with NY-ESO-1 expressing cancers: immunological effects and clinical activity." Clinical Cancer Research 18.19 (2012): 5449-5459.

34. Aggarwal, Bharat B. "Nuclear factor-kB: the enemy within." Cancer cell 6.3 (2004): 203-208.

35. Matzinger, Polly. "The danger model: a renewed sense of self." Science 296.5566 (2002): 301-305.

36. Smyth, Mark J., Dale I. Godfrey, and Joseph A. Trapani. "A fresh look at tumor immunosurveillance and immunotherapy." Nature immunology 2.4 (2001): 293-299.

37. van der Graaf, Winette TA, et al. "Pazopanib for metastatic soft-tissue sarcoma (PALETTE): a randomised, double-blind, placebo-controlled phase 3 trial." The Lancet 379.9829 (2012): 1879-1886.

38. Nauts, Helen Coley, George A. Fowler, and Frances H. Bogatko. A Review of the Influence of Bacterial Infection and of Bacterial Products "(Coley's Toxins)" on Malignant Tumors in Man A Critical Analysis of 30 Inoperable Cases Treated by Coley's Mixed Toxins, in Which Diagnosis Was Confirmed by Microscopic Examination: Selected for Special Study. Stockh., 1953. 18-19. Print.

39. "FDA Approval for Bevacizumab." National Cancer Institute. Web. 04 Dec. 2014.

40. Nauts, Helen Coley, and John R. McLaren. "Coley toxins—the first century." Consensus on Hyperthermia for the 1990s. Springer US, 1990. 483-500.

41. Richmond, Phyllis Allen. "American attitudes toward the germ theory of disease (1860–1880)." Journal of the history of medicine and allied sciences 9.4 (1954): 428-454.

42. DeVita, Vincent T., and Edward Chu. "A history of cancer chemotherapy." Cancer research 68.21 (2008): 8643-8653.

43. McCarthy, Edward F. "The toxins of William B. Coley and the treatment of bone and soft-tissue sarcomas." The Iowa orthopaedic journal 26 (2006): 154.

44. Hall, Stephen S. A Commotion in the Blood: Life, Death, and the Immune System. New York: Henry Holt, 1997. 83-89. Print.

45. Hollister, Leo E., et al. "The Kefauver-Harris Amendments of 1962: A Critical Appraisal of The First Five Years." The Journal of clinical pharmacology and the journal of new drugs 8.2 (1968): 69-73.

46. Hess, David J. Can bacteria cause cancer?: Alternative medicine confronts big science. NYU Press, 1997. 15. Print.

47. DiMasi, Joseph A., Ronald W. Hansen, and Henry G. Grabowski. "The price of innovation: new estimates of drug development costs." Journal of health economics 22.2 (2003): 151-185.

48. "Lloyd J. Old, M.D." Cancer Research Institute. Web. 30 May 2016.

49. Axelrod, Rita S., et al. "Effect of the mixed bacterial vaccine on the immune response of patients with non-small cell lung cancer and refractory malignancies." Cancer 61.11 (1988): 2219-2230.

50. Tang, Zhao You, et al. "Preliminary result of mixed bacterial vaccine as adjuvant treatment of hepatocellular carcinoma." Medical oncology and tumor pharmacotherapy 8.1 (1991): 23-28.

51. Kölmel, K. F., et al. "Treatment of advanced malignant melanoma by a pyrogenic bacterial lysate. A pilot study." Oncology Research and Treatment 14.5 (1991): 411-417.

52. "Coley's Toxins for Cancer (Feb/March 2006)." Townsend Letter. Feb. 2006. Web. 29 Mar. 2016.

53. Old, Lloyd J., Donald A. Clarke, and Baruj Benacerraf. "Effect of Bacillus Calmette-Guerin infection on transplanted tumours in the mouse." (1959): 291-292.

54. Karbach, Julia, et al. "Phase I clinical trial of mixed bacterial vaccine (Coley's toxins) in patients with NY-ESO-1 expressing cancers: immunological effects and clinical activity." Clinical Cancer Research 18.19 (2012): 5449-5459.

Chapter 6: Targeting Cancer with T Cells

1. Beverley, Peter CL. "Primer: making sense of T-cell memory." Nature Clinical Practice Rheumatology 4.1 (2008): 43-49.(table 2)

2. Robbins, Paul F., et al. "Tumor regression in patients with metastatic synovial cell sarcoma and melanoma using genetically engineered lymphocytes reactive with NY-ESO-1." Journal of Clinical Oncology 29.7 (2011): 917-924.

3. Mellman, Ira, George Coukos, and Glenn Dranoff. "Cancer immunotherapy comes of age." Nature 480.7378 (2011): 480-489.

4. Bodey, Bodey, et al. "Failure of cancer vaccines: the significant limitations of this approach to immunotherapy." Anticancer research 20.4 (1999): 2665-2676.

5. Gnjatic, Sacha, et al. "NY-ESO-1: Review of an Immunogenic Tumor Antigen." Advances in cancer research 95 (2006): 1-30.

6. "Juno's CAR T and TCR investigational product candidates demonstrate promising outcomes in clinical trials in patients with B-cell cancers." Juno Therapeutics. N.p., 8 Dec. 2014. Web. 03 July 2016.

7. Morgan, Richard A., et al. "Case report of a serious adverse event following the administration of T cells transduced with a chimeric antigen receptor recognizing ERBB2." Molecular Therapy 18.4 (2010): 843-851.

8. June, Carl H. "Adoptive T cell therapy for cancer in the clinic." The Journal of clinical investigation 117.6 (2007): 1466-1476.

9. O'Donnell-Tormey, Jill, and Edward A. McDermott. "The cancer vaccine collaborative: a new model of coordinated discovery." Cancer Immunity Archive 12.1 (2012): 10.

10. Rosenberg, Steven A., Paul Spiess, and Rene Lafreniere. "A new approach to the adoptive immunotherapy of cancer with tumor-infiltrating lymphocytes." Science 233.4770 (1986): 1318-1321.

Chapter 7: How Tumors Evade the Immune System

1. "Treatment at MD Anderson: In Our Patients' Words." Why MD Anderson. Web. 17 Mar. 2016.

2. Winslow, Ron. "How the Promise of Immunotherapy Is Transforming Oncology." WSJ. Wall Street Journal Online, 4 Dec. 2014. Web. 15 Apr. 2016.

3. The Autoimmune Diseases Coordinating Committee. "Progress in Autoimmune Diseases Research." National Institutes of Health, Mar. 2005. Web. 15 Apr. 2016.

4. "FDA Approval for Ipilimumab." National Cancer Institute. 3 Jul. 2011. Web. 22 Apr. 2016.

5. Levy, Robert. "Hope Blossoms." Dana-Farber Cancer Institute. Web. 18 Apr. 2016.

6. Schadendorf, Dirk, et al. "Pooled analysis of long-term survival data from phase II and phase III trials of ipilimumab in unresectable or metastatic melanoma." Journal of clinical oncology (2015): JCO-2014.

7. Topalian, Suzanne L., Charles G. Drake, and Drew M. Pardoll. "Immune checkpoint blockade: a common denominator approach to cancer therapy." Cancer cell 27.4 (2015): 450-461.

8. Kolata, Gina. "Breaking Through Cancer's Shield." The New York Times. The New York Times, 2013. Web. 23 Mar. 2016.

9. "Immunotherapy: How a Former Cop Beat Cancer." Wall Street Journal Online. Web. 12 Dec. 2014. (http://www.wsj.com/video/immunotherapy-how-a-former-cop-beat-cancer/11325F03-9EA6-4B83-A2F9-619856C64ADD.html)

10. "Immunotherapy: How a Former Cop Beat Cancer." Wall Street Journal Online. Web. 12 Dec. 2014. (http://www.wsj.com/video/immunotherapy-how-a-former-cop-beat-cancer/11325F03-9EA6-4B83-A2F9-619856C64ADD.html)

11. Hamid, Omid, et al. "Safety and tumor responses with lambrolizumab (anti–PD-1) in melanoma." New England Journal of Medicine 369.2 (2013): 134-144.

12. Topalian, Suzanne L., et al. "Safety, activity, and immune correlates of anti–PD-1 antibody in cancer." New England Journal of Medicine 366.26 (2012): 2443-2454.

13. Ansell, Stephen M., et al. "PD-1 blockade with nivolumab in relapsed or refractory Hodgkin's lymphoma." New England Journal of Medicine 372.4 (2015): 311-319.

14. Dunn, Gavin P., Lloyd J. Old, and Robert D. Schreiber. "The three Es of cancer immunoediting." Annu. Rev. Immunol. 22 (2004): 329-360.

15. Mellman, Ira, George Coukos, and Glenn Dranoff. "Cancer immunotherapy comes of age." Nature 480.7378 (2011): 480-489.

16. "U.S. Food and Drug Administration." FDA Approves Keytruda for Advanced Melanoma. 4 Sept. 2014. Web. 23 Mar. 2016.

17. "U.S. Food and Drug Administration." FDA Expands Approved Use of Opdivo to Treat Lung Cancer. 4 Mar. 2015. Web. 23 Mar. 2016.

18. Borghaei, Hossein, et al. "Nivolumab versus docetaxel in advanced nonsquamous non-small-cell lung cancer." New England Journal of Medicine 373.17 (2015): 1627-1639.

19. "FDA Expands Approved Use of Opdivo to Treat Lung Cancer." U.S. Food and Drug Administration, 9 Oct. 2015. Web. 11 May 2016.

20. Topalian, Suzanne L., M.D., et al. "Safety, Activity, and Immune Correlates of Anti–PD-1 Antibody in Cancer." The New England Journal of Medicine 366 (2012): 2443-454.

21. Herbst, Roy S., et al. "Pembrolizumab versus docetaxel for previously treated, PD-L1-positive, advanced non-small-cell lung cancer (KEYNOTE-010): a randomised controlled trial." The Lancet (2015)

22. "Cancer of the Lung and Bronchus." Surveillance, Epidemiology, and End Results Program. National Cancer Institute. Web. 22 Apr. 2016.

23. Yamamoto, Ryo, et al. "PD-1–PD-1 ligand interaction contributes to immunosuppressive microenvironment of Hodgkin lymphoma." Blood 111.6 (2008): 3220-3224.

24. Hamid, Omid, et al. "Safety and tumor responses with lambrolizumab (anti–PD-1) in melanoma." New England Journal of Medicine 369.2 (2013): 134-144.

25. Pollack, Andrew. "Approval for Drug That Treats Melanoma." The New York Times. 25 Mar. 2011. Web. 03 June 2016.

26. Constans, M., et al. "Autologous stem cell transplantation for primary refractory Hodgkin's disease: results and clinical variables affecting outcome." Annals of oncology 14.5 (2003): 745-751.

27. Akhtar, S., et al. "Primary refractory Hodgkin's lymphoma: outcome after high-dose chemotherapy and autologous SCT and impact of various prognostic factors on overall and event-free survival. A single institution result of 66 patients." Bone marrow transplantation 40.7 (2007): 651-658.

28. Mink, Scott A., and James O. Armitage. "High-dose therapy in lymphomas: a review of the current status of allogeneic and autologous stem cell transplantation in Hodgkin's disease and non-Hodgkin's lymphoma." The Oncologist 6.3 (2001): 247-256.

29. Ansell, Stephen M., et al. "PD-1 blockade with nivolumab in relapsed or refractory Hodgkin's lymphoma." New England Journal of Medicine 372.4 (2015): 311-319.

30. "Study of Pembrolizumab (MK-3475) as First-Line Monotherapy and Combination Therapy for Treatment of Advanced Gastric or Gastroesophageal Junction Adenocarcinoma (MK-3475-062/KEYNOTE-062)." Clinicaltrials.gov. N.p, 8 July 2015. Web. 18 Apr. 2016.

31. Muro, K., et al. "LBA15A phase 1B study of pembrolizumab (PEMBRO; MK-3475) in patients (Pts) with advanced gastric cancer." Annals of Oncology 25.suppl 4 (2014): mdu438-15.

32. "Management of Glioblastoma in Older Adults." UpToDate.com. 06 Apr. 2016. Web. 17 Apr. 2016.

33. Abelson, Reed. "Drug Sales Bring Huge Profits, And Scrutiny, to Cancer Doctors." The New York Times. 26 Jan. 2003. Web. 17 Apr. 2016.

34. Colla, Carrie H., et al. "Impact of payment reform on chemotherapy at the end of life." Journal of Oncology Practice 8.3S (2012): e6s-e13s.

35. Chen, Kang-Jie, et al. "Selective recruitment of regulatory T cell through CCR6-CCL20 in hepatocellular carcinoma fosters tumor progression and predicts poor prognosis." PloS one 6.9 (2011): e24671.

36. Qureshi, Omar S., et al. "Trans-endocytosis of CD80 and CD86: a molecular basis for the cell-extrinsic function of CTLA-4." Science 332.6029 (2011): 600-603.

37. Le, Dung T., and Elizabeth M. Jaffee. "Regulatory T-cell modulation using cyclophosphamide in vaccine approaches: a current perspective." Cancer research 72.14 (2012): 3439-3444.

38. Walker, Lucy SK. "Treg and CTLA-4: two intertwining pathways to immune tolerance." Journal of autoimmunity 45 (2013): 49-57.

39. Allison, James. "Cytotoxic T-lymphocyte-associated Protein 4 and Cancer Therapy." Blood 126.23 (2015): SCI-7

40. Zou, Weiping, Jedd D. Wolchok, and Lieping Chen. "PD-L1 (B7-H1) and PD-1 pathway blockade for cancer therapy: Mechanisms, response biomarkers, and combinations." Science translational medicine 8.328 (2016): 328rv4-328rv4.

41. Zou, Weiping, Jedd D. Wolchok, and Lieping Chen. "PD-L1 (B7-H1) and PD-1 pathway blockade for cancer therapy: Mechanisms, response biomarkers, and combinations." Science translational medicine 8.328 (2016): 328rv4-328rv4.

Chapter 8: Activating the Immune System with Coley's Toxins

1. James, John T. "A new, evidence-based estimate of patient harms associated with hospital care." Journal of patient safety 9.3 (2013): 122-128.

2. See outlined box on page 126 describing far-infrared heating pads.

3. Cann, SA Hoption, J. P. Van Netten, and C. Van Netten. "Dr William Coley and tumour regression: a place in history or in the future." Postgraduate medical journal 79.938 (2003): 672-680.

4. Brightbill, Hans D., et al. "Host defense mechanisms triggered by microbial lipoproteins through toll-like receptors." Science 285.5428 (1999): 732-736.

5. Netea, Mihai G., Bart Jan Kullberg, and Jos WM Van der Meer. "Circulating cytokines as mediators of fever." Clinical Infectious Diseases 31.Supplement 5 (2000): S178-S184.

6. Ostberg, Julie R., Bradley R. Ertel, and Julie A. Lanphere. "An important role for granulocytes in the thermal regulation of colon tumor growth." Immunological investigations 34.3 (2005): 259-272.

7. Evans, Sharon S., Elizabeth A. Repasky, and Daniel T. Fisher. "Fever and the thermal regulation of immunity: the immune system feels the heat." Nature Reviews Immunology 15.6 (2015): 335-349.

8. Coca, Santiago, et al. "The prognostic significance of intratumoral natural killer cells in patients with colorectal carcinoma." Cancer 79.12 (1997): 2320-2328.

9. Burd, Randy, et al. "Tumor cell apoptosis, lymphocyte recruitment and tumor vascular changes are induced by low temperature, long duration (fever-like) whole body hyperthermia." Journal of cellular physiology 177.1 (1998): 137-147.

10. Multhoff, Gabriele, et al. "Heat shock protein 72 on tumor cells: a recognition structure for natural killer cells." The Journal of Immunology 158.9 (1997): 4341-4350.

11. Bachleitner-Hofmann, Thomas, et al. "Heat shock treatment of tumor lysate-pulsed dendritic cells enhances their capacity to elicit antitumor T cell responses against medullary thyroid carcinoma." The Journal of Clinical Endocrinology & Metabolism 91.11 (2006): 4571-4577.

12. Mackowiak, Philip A. "Brief history of antipyretic therapy." Clinical infectious diseases 31.Supplement 5 (2000): S154-S156.

13. Botting, Regina. "Antipyretic therapy." Front Biosci 9.956 (2004): e66.

14. Minamisawa, Hiroaki, Maj-Lis Smith, and Bo K. Siesjö. "The effect of mild hyperthermia and hypothermia on brain damage following 5, 10, and 15 minutes of forebrain ischemia." Annals of neurology 28.1 (1990): 26-33.

15. Plaisance, Karen I., et al. "Effect of antipyretic therapy on the duration of illness in experimental influenza A, Shigella sonnei, and Rickettsia rickettsii infections." Pharmacotherapy: The Journal of Human Pharmacology and Drug Therapy 20.12 (2000): 1417-1422.

16. Sugimura, Tetsu, et al. "Risks of antipyretics in young children with fever due to infectious disease." Pediatrics International 36.4 (1994): 375-378.

17. Earn, David JD, Paul W. Andrews, and Benjamin M. Bolker. "Population-level effects of suppressing fever." Proceedings of the Royal Society of London B: Biological Sciences 281.1778 (2014): 20132570.

18. Schulman, Carl I., et al. "The effect of antipyretic therapy upon outcomes in critically ill patients: a randomized, prospective study." Surgical infections 6.4 (2005): 369-375.

19. Schulman, 374.

20. Lee, Byung Ho, et al. "Association of body temperature and antipyretic treatments with mortality of critically ill patients with and without sepsis: multi-centered prospective observational study." Critical Care 16.1 (2012): 1-13.

21. Bernard, Gordon R., et al. "The effects of ibuprofen on the physiology and survival of patients with sepsis." New England Journal of Medicine 336.13 (1997): 912-918.

22. Hasday, Jeffrey D., and Allen Garrison. "Antipyretic therapy in patients with sepsis." Clinical infectious diseases 31.Supplement 5 (2000): S234-S241.

23. "What Ever Happened to Coley's Toxins?" Cancer Research Institute. 02 Apr. 2015. Web. 28 Mar. 2016.

24. Nauts, Helen Coley, and John R. McLaren. "Coley toxins—the first century." Consensus on Hyperthermia for the 1990s. Springer US, 1990. 486-486.

Chapter 9: The Violence of the Immune System

1. Rice, Penelope, et al. "Febrile-range hyperthermia augments neutrophil accumulation and enhances lung injury in experimental gram-negative bacterial pneumonia." The Journal of Immunology 174.6 (2005): 3676-3685.

2. Hotchkiss, Richard S., Jerrold H. Levy, and Marcel Levi. "Sepsis-induced disseminated intravascular coagulation, symmetrical peripheral gangrene, and amputations." Critical care medicine 41.10 (2013): e290-e291.

3. Murray, Patrick R., and Henry Masur. "Current Approaches to the Diagnosis of Bacterial and Fungal Bloodstream Infections for the ICU." Critical care medicine 40.12 (2012): 3277.

4. Mayo Clinic Staff. "Sepsis." Symptoms and Causes of Sepsis. 15 Jan. 2016. Web. 03 June 2016.

5. Kumar, Anand, et al. "Duration of hypotension before initiation of effective antimicrobial therapy is the critical determinant of survival in human septic shock." Critical care medicine 34.6 (2006): 1589-1596.

6. Rittirsch, Daniel, Michael A. Flierl, and Peter A. Ward. "Harmful molecular mechanisms in sepsis." Nature Reviews Immunology 8.10 (2008): 776-787.

7. Landesberg, Giora, et al. "Diastolic dysfunction and mortality in severe sepsis and septic shock." European heart journal 33.7 (2012): 895-903.

8. "Sepsis Questions and Answers." Centers for Disease Control and Prevention. Centers for Disease Control and Prevention, 05 Oct. 2015. Web. 01 Apr. 2016.

9. Liu, Vincent, et al. "Hospital deaths in patients with sepsis from 2 independent cohorts." Jama 312.1 (2014): 90-92.

10. "Inpatient Care for Septicemia or Sepsis: A Challenge for Patients and Hospitals." Centers for Disease Control and Prevention. 22 June 2011. Web. 03 June 2016.

11. "Sepsis Fact Sheet." - National Institute of General Medical Sciences. Aug. 2014. Web. 01 Apr. 2016.

12. Carmeli, Yehuda, et al. "Health and economic outcomes of antibiotic resistance in Pseudomonas aeruginosa." Archives of Internal Medicine 159.10 (1999): 1127-1132.

13. Dubos, René J., and Russell W. Schaedler. "Effects of cellular constituents of Mycobacteria on the resistance of mice to heterologous infections: I. Protective effects." The Journal of experimental medicine 106.5 (1957): 703.

14. Howard, J. G., et al. "The effect of Mycobacterium tuberculosis (BCG) infection on the resistance of mice to bacterial endotoxin and Salmonella enteritidis infection." British journal of experimental pathology 40.3 (1959): 281.

15. Personal communication with Heather's husband.

16. FDA. "Chapter 9 Import Operations And Actions." Apr. 2013. Web. 1 Apr. 2016.

17. The Autoimmune Diseases Coordinating Committee. "Progress in Autoimmune Diseases Research." National Institutes of Health, Mar. 2005. Web. 15 Apr. 2016.

18. Hancock, Steven L., I. Ross McDougall, and Louis S. Constine. "Thyroid abnormalities after therapeutic external radiation." International Journal of Radiation Oncology* Biology* Physics 31.5 (1995): 1165-1170.

19. Boasberg, Peter, Omid Hamid, and Steven O'Day. "Ipilimumab: unleashing the power of the immune system through CTLA-4 blockade." Seminars in oncology. Vol. 37. No. 5. WB Saunders, 2010.

20. Borodic, Gary, David M. Hinkle, and Yihong Cia. "Drug-induced graves disease from CTLA-4 receptor suppression." Ophthalmic Plastic & Reconstructive Surgery 27.4 (2011): e87-e88.

21. Benvenga, Salvatore, et al. "Usefulness of l-carnitine, a naturally occurring peripheral antagonist of thyroid hormone action, in iatrogenic hyperthyroidism: a randomized, double-blind, placebo-controlled clinical trial." The Journal of Clinical Endocrinology & Metabolism 86.8 (2001): 3579-3594.

22. Leslie, William D., et al. "A randomized comparison of radioiodine doses in Graves' hyperthyroidism." The Journal of Clinical Endocrinology & Metabolism 88.3 (2003): 978-983.

23. Nakamura, Hirotoshi, et al. "Comparison of methimazole and propylthiouracil in patients with hyperthyroidism caused by Graves' disease." The Journal of Clinical Endocrinology & Metabolism 92.6 (2007): 2157-2162.

24. Blomgren, Henric, et al. "Changes of the blood lymphocyte population following 131 I treatment for nodular goiter." International Journal of Radiation Oncology* Biology* Physics 13.2 (1987): 209-215.

25. Molinaro, Eleonora, et al. "Mild decreases in white blood cell and platelet counts are present one year after radioactive iodine remnant ablation." Thyroid 19.10 (2009): 1035-1041.

26. Tajiri, Junichi, et al. "Antithyroid drug–induced agranulocytosis: the usefulness of routine white blood cell count monitoring." Archives of Internal Medicine 150.3 (1990): 621-624.

27. Törring, Ove, et al. "Graves' hyperthyroidism: treatment with antithyroid drugs, surgery, or radioiodine--a prospective, randomized study. Thyroid Study Group." The Journal of Clinical Endocrinology & Metabolism 81.8 (1996): 2986-2993.

28. Yu, Christine, Inder J. Chopra, and Edward Ha. "A novel melanoma therapy stirs up a storm: ipilimumab-induced thyrotoxicosis." Endocrinology, diabetes & metabolism case reports 2015 (2015).

29. Burch, Henry B., and L. Wartofsky. "Life-threatening thyrotoxicosis. Thyroid storm." Endocrinology and metabolism clinics of North America 22.2 (1993): 263-277.

30. Terris, David J., et al. "American Thyroid Association statement on outpatient thyroidectomy." Thyroid 23.10 (2013): 1193-1202.

31. "MCG Historical Highlights." MCG Historical Highlights. Web. 04 Apr. 2016.

32. Kain, Zeev N., et al. "Attenuation of the Preoperative Stress Response with Midazolam Effects on Postoperative Outcomes." The Journal of the American Society of Anesthesiologists 93.1 (2000): 141-147.

Chapter 10: Waiting for Immunotherapy to Work

1. Demicheli, R., et al. "The effects of surgery on tumor growth: a century of investigations." Annals of Oncology (2008): mdn386.

2. Gil, Ziv, et al. "Analysis of prognostic factors in 146 patients with anterior skull base sarcoma: an international collaborative study." Cancer 110.5 (2007): 1033-1041.

3. Carswell, E. A., et al. "An endotoxin-induced serum factor that causes necrosis of tumors." Proceedings of the National Academy of Sciences 72.9 (1975): 3666-3670.

4. See chapter 5 beginning on page 65

5. Schwartz, Herbert S., and Dan M. Spengler. "Needle tract recurrences after closed biopsy for sarcoma: three cases and review of the literature." Annals of surgical oncology 4.3 (1997): 228-236.

6. Nauts, Helen Coley, and Walker E. Swift. "The treatment of malignant tumors by bacterial toxins as developed by the late William B. Coley, MD, reviewed in the light of modern research." Cancer Res 6 (1946): 205-216.

7. Old, Lloyd J. "Tumor necrosis factor (TNF)." Science (New York, NY) 230.4726 (1985): 630.

8. "FDA Approves Votrient for Advanced Soft Tissue Sarcoma." fda.gov. 26 Apr. 2012. Web. 12 Apr. 2016.

9. "Votrient." Novartisoncology.com. Web. 13 Apr. 2016.

10. McCarthy, Edward F. "The toxins of William B. Coley and the treatment of bone and soft-tissue sarcomas." The Iowa orthopaedic journal 26 (2006): 154.

Chapter 11: Combining Immunotherapy for Better Results

1. Ablin, R. J. "Cryoimmunotherapy." Br Med J 3.5824 (1972): 476-476.

2. Downie, Gordon, and William Krimsky. "Response to spray cryotherapy in a patient with adenocarcinoma in the parietal pleura." Respiration 80.1 (2010): 73-77.

3. Nishida, Hideji, et al. "Cryoimmunology for malignant bone and soft-tissue tumors." International journal of clinical oncology 16.2 (2011): 109-117.

4. Sabel, Michael S. "Cryo-immunology: a review of the literature and proposed mechanisms for stimulatory versus suppressive immune responses." Cryobiology 58.1 (2009): 1-11.

5. Erinjeri, Joseph P., and Timothy WI Clark. "Cryoablation: mechanism of action and devices." Journal of Vascular and Interventional Radiology 21.8 (2010): S187-S191.

6. Chu, Katrina F., and Damian E. Dupuy. "Thermal ablation of tumours: biological mechanisms and advances in therapy." Nature reviews Cancer 14.3 (2014): 199-208.

7. Weber, Sharon M., and Fred T. Lee Jr. "Cryoablation: history, mechanism of action, and guidance modalities." Tumor Ablation. Springer New York, 2005. 250-265.

8. "April 29, 2010 Approval Letter." U.S. Food and Drug Administration. 29 Apr. 2010. Web. 20 Apr. 2016.

9. Ralph Moss, Ph.D. was the cancer journalist we purchased paid reports from in 2009 when we were first interested in studying alternative approaches to treating cancer.

10. Nesselhut T, et al. Marker expression of monocyte-derived dendritic cells in healthy individuals and cancer patients; correlation to clinical response. ASCO 2003; Abstract No. 723.

11. Lesterhuis, W. Joost, et al. "Synergistic effect of CTLA-4 blockade and cancer chemotherapy in the induction of anti-tumor immunity." PloS one 8.4 (2013): e61895.

12. Waitz, Rebecca, et al. "Potent induction of tumor immunity by combining tumor cryoablation with anti–CTLA-4 therapy." Cancer research 72.2 (2012): 430-439.

13. "Pre-Operative, Single-Dose Ipilimumab And/or Cryoablation in Early Stage/Resectable Breast Cancer." ClinicalTrials.gov. 29 Dec. 2011. Web. 20 Apr. 2016.

14. See chapter 7 pages 115-116, "Coley's Toxins and the Fearsome Bodyguards of Tumors."

15. Levy, Moshe Yair, et al. "Cyclophosphamide unmasks an antimetastatic effect of local tumor cryoablation." Journal of Pharmacology and Experimental Therapeutics 330.2 (2009): 596-601.

16. Larkin, James, et al. "Combined nivolumab and ipilimumab or monotherapy in untreated melanoma." New England Journal of Medicine 373.1 (2015): 23-34.

17. Everson, Tilden C., and Warren H. Cole. "Spontaneous regression of cancer: preliminary report." Annals of Surgery 144.3 (1956): 366.

18. Postow, Michael A., et al. "Immunologic correlates of the abscopal effect in a patient with melanoma." New England Journal of Medicine 366.10 (2012): 925-931.

19. "President Carter Shares Cancer Diagnosis." Emory Winship Cancer Institute. N.p., 20 Aug. 2015. Web. 4 June 2016.

20. Mohiuddin, Majid et al. "High-Dose Radiation as a Dramatic, Immunological Primer in Locally Advanced Melanoma." Ed. Alexander Muacevic and John R Adler. Cureus 7.12 (2015): e417. PMC. Web. 22 Apr. 2016.

21. James, John T. "A new, evidence-based estimate of patient harms associated with hospital care." Journal of patient safety 9.3 (2013): 122-128.

22. Makary, Martin A., and Michael Daniel. "Medical error—the third leading cause of death in the US." BMJ 353 (2016): i2139.

Chapter 12: Immunotherapy in Germany

1. Tremblay, Lorraine N., and Arthur S. Slutsky. "Ventilator-induced injury: from barotrauma to biotrauma." Proceedings of the Association of American Physicians 110.6 (1997): 482-488.

2. Chen, Kuan-Yu, et al. "Pneumothorax in the ICU: patient outcomes and prognostic factors." CHEST Journal 122.2 (2002): 678-683.

3. Meisel, S., et al. "Another complication of thoracostomy--perforation of the right atrium." CHEST Journal 98.3 (1990): 772-773.

4. Chan, Lisa, et al. "Complication rates of tube thoracostomy." The American journal of emergency medicine 15.4 (1997): 368-370.

5. Ball, Chad G., et al. "Chest tube complications: how well are we training our residents?." Canadian Journal of Surgery 50.6 (2007): 450.

6. Gammie, James S., et al. "The pigtail catheter for pleural drainage: a less invasive alternative to tube thoracostomy." JSLS 3.1 (1999): 57-61.

7. Kulvatunyou, N., et al. "Randomized clinical trial of pigtail catheter versus chest tube in injured patients with uncomplicated traumatic pneumothorax." British Journal of Surgery 101.2 (2014): 17-22.

8. Thomas, Terry L., and Patricia A. Stewart. "Mortality From Lung Cancer And Respiratory Disease Among Pottery Workers Exposed To Silica And Talc." American journal of epidemiology 125.1 (1987): 35-43.

9. Cramer, Daniel W., et al. "Ovarian cancer and talc: a case-control study." Obstetrical & Gynecological Survey 37.11 (1982): 686.

10. Allen, Marshall. "How Many Die From Medical Mistakes in U.S. Hospitals?" Propublica. org. 19 Sept. 2013. Web. 26 Apr. 2016.

11. Si, Tongguo, Zhi Guo, and Xishan Hao. "Immunologic response to primary cryoablation of high-risk prostate cancer." Cryobiology 57.1 (2008): 66-71.

12. Bundesverfassungsgericht [BVG, German Federal Constitution Court], Beschluss vom 6.12.2005 – 1 BvR 347/98 – BverfGE. pp. 115–25.

13. Lenk, Christian, and Gunnar Duttge. "Ethical and legal framework and regulation for off-label use: European perspective." Therapeutics and clinical risk management 10 (2014): 537.

14. Anassi, Enock, and Uche Anadu Ndefo. "Sipuleucel-T (provenge) injection: the first immunotherapy agent (vaccine) for hormone-refractory prostate cancer." Pharmacy and Therapeutics 36.4 (2011): 197.

15. "Improvement of Dendritic Cell Therapy in Glioblastoma Multiforme WHO 4 by New-castle Disease Virus." ASCO. 2011. Web. 03 May 2016.

16. Chang, Raymond. "Statins for Cancer." Off-label Cancer Treatments. 08 Feb. 2009. Web. 02 May 2016.

17. Bhat, Rauf, and Carsten Watzl. "Serial killing of tumor cells by human natural killer cells–enhancement by therapeutic antibodies." PLoS One 2.3 (2007): e326.

18. Ruggeri, Loredana, et al. "Effectiveness of donor natural killer cell alloreactivity in mis-matched hematopoietic transplants." Science 295.5562 (2002): 2097-2100.

19. Mandelboim, Ofer, et al. "Recognition of haemagglutinins on virus-infected cells by NKp46 activates lysis by human NK cells." Nature 409.6823 (2001): 1055-1060.

20. Zamai, Loris, et al. "NK cells and cancer." The Journal of Immunology 178.7 (2007): 4011-4016.

21. Suck, Garnet, et al. "NK-92: an 'off-the-shelf therapeutic'for adoptive natural killer cell-based cancer immunotherapy." Cancer Immunology, Immunotherapy (2015): 1-8.

22. "NK-92 Clinical Trials." ClinicalTrials.gov, 08 June 2016. Web. 08 June 2016.

23. See chapter 3 pages 41-42.

24. Chen, Pauline W. "When Patients Feel Abandoned by Doctors." The New York Times. The New York Times, 12 Mar. 2009. Web. 01 June 2016.

25. Glantz, Michael J., et al. "Gender disparity in the rate of partner abandonment in patients with serious medical illness." Cancer 115.22 (2009): 5237-5242.

Chapter 13: Taking No Chances: Consolidative Surgery

1. Vitello, Paul. "Lloyd J. Old, Champion of Using Cells to Fight Cancer, Dies at 78." The New York Times. 04 Dec. 2011. Web. 08 May 2016.

2. Personal communication.

3. Personal communication.

4. "Jatin P. Shah, MD, FACS." Memorial Sloan Kettering Cancer Center. Web. 03 May 2016.

5. Malawer, Martin M., and Paul H. Sugarbaker. Musculoskeletal Cancer Surgery: Treatment of Sarcomas and Allied Diseases. Dordrecht: Kluwer Academic, 2001. Print.

6. Jones, Chris. "Roger Ebert: The Essential Man." Esquire. 16 Mar. 2010. Web. 09 May 2016.

7. "Lloyd J. Old, M.D." Cancer Research Institute. Web. 08 May 2016.

8. Millam, Doris. "The history of intravenous therapy." Journal of Infusion Nursing 19.1 (1996): 5-15.

Chapter 14: Injecting Tumors

1. Durani, Piyush, and David Leaper. "Povidone–iodine: use in hand disinfection, skin prepa-ration and antiseptic irrigation." International Wound Journal 5.3 (2008): 376-387.

2. Song, Wenru, and Ronald Levy. "Therapeutic vaccination against murine lymphoma by intratumoral injection of naive dendritic cells." Cancer research 65.13 (2005): 5958-5964.

3. Brody, Joshua D., et al. "In situ vaccination with a TLR9 agonist induces systemic lympho-ma regression: a phase I/II study." Journal of Clinical Oncology 28.28 (2010): 4324-4332.

4. Immune activators are described at the end of chapter 7 (see outlined box on page 119)

5. "CICON15 Report from Day 2." Cancer Research Institute. 17 Sept. 2015. Web. 10 May 2016.

6. Marabelle, Aurélien, et al. "Depleting tumor-specific Tregs at a single site eradicates disseminated tumors." The Journal of clinical investigation 123.6 (2013): 2447-2463.

7. Scott, William. An Indexed System of Veterinary Treatment; a Work on Modern Medical, Surgical, and Biological Therapy. Chicago: Eger, 1922. 603. Print.

8. LoCicero, Joseph, et al. "New applications of the laser in pulmonary surgery: hemostasis and sealing of air leaks." The Annals of thoracic surgery 40.6 (1985): 546-550.

9. Rolle, Axel, and Arpad Pereszlenyi. "Laser resection of lung metastasis." Multimedia Manual of Cardio-Thoracic Surgery 2005.0628 (2005): mmcts-2004.

10. Orr, F. William, Michael R. Buchanan, and Leonard Weiss. Microcirculation in cancer metastasis. CRC Press, 1991. Print.

11. Rolle, Axel, et al. "Is surgery for multiple lung metastases reasonable? A total of 328 consecutive patients with multiple-laser metastasectomies with a new 1318-nm Nd: YAG laser." The Journal of thoracic and cardiovascular surgery131.6 (2006): 1236-1242.

12. Gerner, Peter. "Postthoracotomy pain management problems." Anesthesiology clinics 26.2 (2008): 355-367.

13. Billingsley, Kevin G., et al. "Pulmonary metastases from soft tissue sarcoma: analysis of patterns of disease and postmetastasis survival." Annals of surgery 229.5 (1999): 602.

14. Alonso-Camino, Vanesa, et al. "The profile of tumor antigens which can be targeted by immunotherapy depends upon the tumor's anatomical site." Molecular Therapy 22.11 (2014): 1936-1948.

15. Bang, Hyun J., et al. "Percutaneous cryoablation of metastatic lesions from non–small-cell lung carcinoma: initial survival, local control, and cost observations." Journal of Vascular and Interventional Radiology 23.6 (2012): 761-769.

16. Bucerius, Jan, et al. "Pain is significantly reduced by cryoablation therapy in patients with lateral minithoracotomy." The Annals of thoracic surgery 70.3 (2000): 1100-1104.

17. Callstrom, Matthew R., and J. William Charboneau. "Image-guided palliation of painful metastases using percutaneous ablation." Techniques in vascular and interventional radiology 10.2 (2007): 120-131.

18. Schjeldahl, Peter. "Should Detroit Sell Its Art?" The New Yorker. N.p., 24 July 2013. Web. 12 May 2016.

19. Lu, Pengfei, Valerie M. Weaver, and Zena Werb. "The extracellular matrix: a dynamic niche in cancer progression." The Journal of cell biology 196.4 (2012): 395-406.

20. Hanahan, Douglas, and Lisa M. Coussens. "Accessories to the crime: functions of cells recruited to the tumor microenvironment." Cancer cell 21.3 (2012): 309-322.

21. Whiteside, T. L. "The tumor microenvironment and its role in promoting tumor growth." Oncogene 27.45 (2008): 5904-5912.

22. Rolle, Axel, and Arpad Pereszlenyi. "Laser resection of lung metastasis." Multimedia Manual of Cardio-Thoracic Surgery 2005.0628 (2005): mmcts-2004.

23. Rabinovich, Gabriel A., Dmitry Gabrilovich, and Eduardo M. Sotomayor. "Immunosuppressive strategies that are mediated by tumor cells." Annual review of immunology 25 (2007): 267.

312 | Notes to chapters 14-15

24. Hsieh, Chia-Ling, Ding-Shinn Chen, and Lih-Hwa Hwang. "Tumor-induced immunosuppression: a barrier to immunotherapy of large tumors by cytokine-secreting tumor
vaccine." Human gene therapy 11.5 (2000): 681-692.

Chapter 15: Diet-Based Immunotherapy

1. Fearon, Kenneth C., et al. "Definition of cancer cachexia: effect of weight loss, reduced food
intake, and systemic inflammation on functional status and prognosis." The American
journal of clinical nutrition 83.6 (2006): 1345-1350.

2. Evans, William J., et al. "Cachexia: a new definition." Clinical nutrition 27.6 (2008): 793-
799.

3. Deans, Christopher, and Stephen J. Wigmore. "Systemic inflammation, cachexia and prognosis in patients with cancer." Current Opinion in Clinical Nutrition & Metabolic Care
8.3 (2005): 265-269.

4. Beutler, B., and A. Cerami. "Tumor necrosis, cachexia, shock, and inflammation: a common
mediator." Annual review of biochemistry 57.1 (1988): 505-518.

5. Karin, Michael, Toby Lawrence, and Victor Nizet. "Innate immunity gone awry: linking
microbial infections to chronic inflammation and cancer." Cell 124.4 (2006): 823-835.

6. "Diabetes Latest." Centers for Disease Control and Prevention. Centers for Disease Control and Prevention, 17 June 2014. Web. 17 May 2016.

7. Xu, Haiyan, et al. "Chronic inflammation in fat plays a crucial role in the development of obesi-
ty-related insulin resistance." The Journal of clinical investigation 112.12 (2003): 1821-1830.

8. Donath, Marc Y. "Targeting inflammation in the treatment of type 2 diabetes: time to
start." Nature reviews Drug discovery 13.6 (2014): 465-476.

9. Petersen, Anne Marie W., and Bente Klarlund Pedersen. "The anti-inflammatory effect of
exercise." Journal of applied physiology 98.4 (2005): 1154-1162.

10. Aeberli, Isabelle, et al. "Low to moderate sugar-sweetened beverage consumption impairs glucose and lipid metabolism and promotes inflammation in healthy young men:
a randomized controlled trial." The American journal of clinical nutrition 94.2 (2011):
479-485.

11. Hansson, Göran K. "Inflammation, atherosclerosis, and coronary artery disease." New
England Journal of Medicine 352.16 (2005): 1685-1695.

12. Coussens, Lisa M., and Zena Werb. "Inflammation and cancer." Nature 420.6917 (2002):
860-867.

13. Talmadge, James E., and Dmitry I. Gabrilovich. "History of myeloid-derived suppressor
cells." Nature Reviews Cancer 13.10 (2013): 739-752.

14. Kessenbrock, Kai, Vicki Plaks, and Zena Werb. "Matrix metalloproteinases: regulators of
the tumor microenvironment." Cell 141.1 (2010): 52-67.

15. Talmadge, James E., and Dmitry I. Gabrilovich. "History of myeloid-derived suppressor
cells." Nature Reviews Cancer 13.10 (2013): 739-752.

16. Coussens, Lisa M., and Zena Werb. "Inflammation and cancer." Nature 420.6917 (2002):
860-867.

17. Ramlackhansingh, Anil F., et al. "Inflammation after trauma: microglial activation and
traumatic brain injury." Annals of neurology 70.3 (2011): 374-383.

18. Dreyfuss, Uriel Y., et al. "Ewing's Sarcoma of the hand following recurrent trauma a case report." The Hand 12.3 (1980): 300-303.

19. Coussens, Lisa M., Laurence Zitvogel, and A. Karolina Palucka. "Neutralizing tumor-promoting chronic inflammation: a magic bullet?." Science 339.6117 (2013): 286-291.

20. Anand, Preetha, et al. "Bioavailability of curcumin: problems and promises." Molecular pharmaceutics 4.6 (2007): 807-818.

21. Rothwell, Peter M., et al. "Effect of daily aspirin on long-term risk of death due to cancer: analysis of individual patient data from randomised trials." The Lancet 377.9759 (2011): 31-41.

22. Pardini, Ronald S., et al. "Nutritional intervention with omega-3 Fatty acids in a case of malignant fibrous histiocytoma of the lungs." Nutrition and cancer 52.2 (2005): 121-129.

23. Wu, Gang. "The Nude Mouse Tale: Omega-3 Fats save the Life of a Terminal Cancer Patient." Nevada Agricultural Experiment Station News. N.p., 09 Nov. 2005. Web. 11 June 2016.

24. Kato, Taeko, et al. "Influence of omega-3 fatty acids on the growth of human colon carcinoma in nude mice." Cancer letters 187.1 (2002): 169-177.

25. Pardini, Ronald S., et al. "Nutritional intervention with omega-3 Fatty acids in a case of malignant fibrous histiocytoma of the lungs." Nutrition and cancer 52.2 (2005): 121-125.

26. Personal communication with patient DH

27. Von Schacky, Clemens, Sven Fischer, and Peter C. Weber. "Long-term effects of dietary marine omega-3 fatty acids upon plasma and cellular lipids, platelet function, and eicosanoid formation in humans." Journal of Clinical Investigation 76.4 (1985): 1626.

28. Katan, Martijn B., et al. "Kinetics of the incorporation of dietary fatty acids into serum cholesteryl esters, erythrocyte membranes, and adipose tissue: an 18-month controlled study." Journal of lipid research 38.10 (1997): 2012-2022.

29. Jenski, Laura J., et al. "Omega-3 Fatty Acid Modification of Membrane Structure and Function. I. Dietary Manipulation of Tumor Cell Susceptibility to Cell-and Complement-Mediated Lysis." (1993): 135-146.

30. Kang, Jing X., and Angela Liu. "The role of the tissue omega-6/omega-3 fatty acid ratio in regulating tumor angiogenesis." Cancer and Metastasis Reviews 32.1-2 (2013): 201-210.

31. Barber, M. D., et al. "The effect of an oral nutritional supplement enriched with fish oil on weight-loss in patients with pancreatic cancer." British Journal of Cancer 81.1 (1999): 80.

32. Wigmore, Stephen J., et al. "The effect of polyunsaturated fatty acids on the progress of cachexia in patients with pancreatic cancer." Nutrition 12.1 (1996): S27-S30.

33. Gogos, Charalambos A., et al. "Dietary omega-3 polyunsaturated fatty acids plus vitamin E restore immunodeficiency and prolong survival for severely ill patients with generalized malignancy." Cancer 82.2 (1998): 395-402.

34. Smith, Stephanie. "'He's Going to Be Better than He Was Before'" CNN. Cable News Network, 18 Jan. 2014. Web. 26 May 2016.

35. Talan, Jamie. "Omega-3 Played a Big Role in Healing Coal Miner's Brain." Chicago Tribune. 02 May 2006. Web. 26 May 2016.

36. Berquin, Isabelle M., Iris J. Edwards, and Yong Q. Chen. "Multi-targeted therapy of cancer by omega-3 fatty acids." Cancer letters 269.2 (2008): 363-377.

37. Turk, Harmony F., Rola Barhoumi, and Robert S. Chapkin. "Alteration of EGFR Spatio-temporal Dynamics Suppresses Signal Transduction." Ed. David Holowka. PLoS ONE 7.6 (2012): e39682. PMC. Web. 16 May 2016.

38. Kang, Jing X., and Angela Liu. "The role of the tissue omega-6/omega-3 fatty acid ratio in regulating tumor angiogenesis." Cancer and Metastasis Reviews 32.1-2 (2013): 201-210.

39. Pardini, Ronald S. "Nutritional intervention with omega-3 fatty acids enhances tumor response to anti-neoplastic agents." Chemico-biological interactions 162.2 (2006): 89-105.

40. Ehrlich, Steven. "Omega-6 Fatty Acids." University of Maryland Medical Center. Web. 16 May 2016.

41. "Omega-3 Fatty Acids, Fish Oil, Alpha-linolenic Acid." Omega-3 Fatty Acids, Fish Oil, Alpha-linolenic Acid. 1 Nov. 2013. Web. 26 May 2016.

42. "Nutrition Facts and Analysis for Beef, Top Sirloin, Separable Lean and Fat, Trimmed to 0" Fat, All Grades, Cooked, Broiled [Sirloin Steak, Sirloin Strip]." http://nutritiondata.self.com/facts/beef-products/3586/2

43. Nutrition Facts, Calories in Food, Labels, Nutritional Information and Analysis – NutritionData.com. Self Nutrition Data, n.d. Web. 10 June 2016.

44. Neal, Elizabeth G., et al. "The ketogenic diet for the treatment of childhood epilepsy: a randomised controlled trial." The Lancet Neurology 7.6 (2008): 500-506.

45. See chapter 11, "Vikas Sukhatme, M.D., Sc.D." on page 182.

46. Talmadge, James E., and Dmitry I. Gabrilovich. "History of myeloid-derived suppressor cells." Nature Reviews Cancer 13.10 (2013): 739-752.

47. Talmadge, 739-752.

48. Bayne, Lauren J., et al. "Tumor-derived granulocyte-macrophage colony-stimulating factor regulates myeloid inflammation and T cell immunity in pancreatic cancer." Cancer cell 21.6 (2012): 822-835.

49. Mehta, Hrishikesh M., Michael Malandra, and Seth J. Corey. "G-CSF and GM-CSF in Neutropenia." The Journal of Immunology 195.4 (2015): 1341-1349.

50. Gottfried, Eva, et al. "Tumor-derived lactic acid modulates dendritic cell activation and antigen expression." Blood 107.5 (2006): 2013-2021.

51. Fischer, Bianca, et al. "Acidic pH inhibits non-MHC-restricted killer cell functions." Clinical Immunology 96.3 (2000): 252-263.

52. Husain, Zaheed, et al. "Tumor-derived lactate modifies antitumor immune response: effect on myeloid-derived suppressor cells and NK cells." The Journal of Immunology 191.3 (2013): 1486-1495.

53. Ruskin, David N., Masahito Kawamura Jr, and Susan A. Masino. "Reduced pain and inflammation in juvenile and adult rats fed a ketogenic diet." PLoS One 4.12 (2009): e8349.

54. Bays, Harold E. "Safety considerations with omega-3 fatty acid therapy." The American journal of cardiology 99.6 (2007): S35-S43.

55. Metcalf, Robert G., et al. "Effects of fish-oil supplementation on myocardial fatty acids in humans." The American journal of clinical nutrition 85.5 (2007): 1222-1228.

56. Tsekos, Evangelos, et al. "Perioperative administration of parenteral fish oil supplements in a routine clinical setting improves patient outcome after major abdominal surgery." Clinical Nutrition 23.3 (2004): 325-330.

57. Chen, Bo, et al. "Safety and efficacy of fish oil–enriched parenteral nutrition regimen on postoperative patients undergoing major abdominal surgery a meta-analysis of randomized controlled trials." Journal of Parenteral and Enteral Nutrition 34.4 (2010): 387-394.

58. Berliner, Adam R., and Derek M. Fine. "There's something fishy about this bleeding." NDT plus (2011): sfr046.

59. Berry-Kravis, Elizabeth, et al. "Bruising and the ketogenic diet: Evidence for diet-induced changes in platelet function." Annals of neurology 49.1 (2001): 98-103.

60. The resolution of the CT images was slightly lower than that of diagnostic scans, making precise measurement tricky. Also, Dr. Littrup had spoken with Eddy after the procedure and said the lesion seemed to be a tiny bit smaller.

Chapter 16: Seizing the Cure

1. Chou, Shinn-Huey S., et al. "Cheerio sign." Journal of thoracic imaging 28.1 (2013): W4.

2. "Cancer Facts & Figures 2016." American Cancer Society. Web. 30 May 2016.

3. Grainger, David. Forbes. Forbes Magazine, 29 Jan. 2015. Web. 23 May 2016.

4. Muro, K., et al. "LBA15A phase 1B study of pembrolizumab (PEMBRO; MK-3475) in patients (Pts) with advanced gastric cancer." Annals of Oncology 25.suppl 4 (2014): mdu438-15.

5. "FDA Approves Keytruda for Advanced Melanoma." U.S. Food and Drug Administration. 4 Sept. 2014. Web. 24 May 2016.

6. Levy, Robert. "Hope Blossoms." Dana-Farber Cancer Institute. Web. 18 Apr. 2016.

7. Schadendorf, Dirk, et al. "Pooled analysis of long-term survival data from phase II and phase III trials of ipilimumab in unresectable or metastatic melanoma." Journal of clinical oncology (2015): JCO-2014.

8. "Keytruda, Immune Drug for Deadly Skin Cancer, Shows Long-term Survival." CBSNews. CBS Interactive, 19 May 2016. Web. 21 May 2016.

9. Najjar, Yana G., and James H. Finke. "Clinical perspectives on targeting of myeloid derived suppressor cells in the treatment of cancer." Cancer Immunotherapy & Immuno-monitoring: Mechanism, Treatment, Diagnosis, and Emerging Tools (2014): 52.

10. Lake, Richard A., and Bruce WS Robinson. "Immunotherapy and chemotherapy—a practical partnership." Nature Reviews Cancer 5.5 (2005): 397-405.

11. Danna, Erika A., et al. "Surgical removal of primary tumor reverses tumor-induced immunosuppression despite the presence of metastatic disease." Cancer research 64.6 (2004): 2205-2211.

12. Hsieh, Chia-Ling, Ding-Shinn Chen, and Lih-Hwa Hwang. "Tumor-induced immunosuppression: a barrier to immunotherapy of large tumors by cytokine-secreting tumor vaccine." Human gene therapy 11.5 (2000): 681-692.

13. Graph based on Sharma, Padmanee, and James P. Allison. "Immune checkpoint targeting in cancer therapy: toward combination strategies with curative potential." Cell 161.2 (2015): 205-214.

14. van der Graaf, Winette TA, et al. "Pazopanib for metastatic soft-tissue sarcoma (PALETTE): a randomised, double-blind, placebo-controlled phase 3 trial." The Lancet 379.9829 (2012): 1879-1886.

15. Patel, Vir. "Poliovirus Cancer Treatment by Duke Researchers Receives 'breakthrough' Status from FDA." The Chronicle. 20 May 2016. Web. 23 May 2016.

16. "Partners Online Specialty Consultations." E-consults. Web. 24 May 2016.

17. "UpToDate Subscriptions for Patients and Caregivers." UpToDate. Web. 11 June 2016.

18. "Impacting All Cancers." Cancer Research Institute. Web. 11 June 2016.

19. Google Scholar provides the number of other articles that cite a study.

20. "ClinicalTrials.gov" ClinicalTrials.gov. National Institutes of Health, n.d. Web. 24 May 2016.

21. "Gene-Modified T Cells, Vaccine Therapy, and Nivolumab in Treating Patients With Stage IV or Locally Advanced Solid Tumors Expressing NY-ESO-1 (NYM)." Clinical-Trials.gov. 13 May 2016. Web. 24 May 2016.

22. Wallen, Herschel, et al. "Fludarabine modulates immune response and extends in vivo survival of adoptively transferred CD8 T cells in patients with metastatic melanoma." PloS one 4.3 (2009): e4749.

23. Topalian, Suzanne L., et al. "Survival, durable tumor remission, and long-term safety in patients with advanced melanoma receiving nivolumab." Journal of Clinical Oncology 32.10 (2014): 1020-1030.

24. West, Howard, M.D. "How Is Immunotherapy Administered? (An Immunotherapy Primer for Patients, Pt. 2) | GRACE :: Treatments & Symptom Management." GRACE Treatments Symptom Management. 30 Dec. 2014. Web. 27 May 2016.

25. Vacchelli, Erika, et al. "Trial watch: FDA-approved Toll-like receptor agonists for cancer therapy." Oncoimmunology 1.6 (2012): 894-907.

26. Holmes, E. C., et al. "Intralesional BCG immunotherapy of pulmonary tumors." The Journal of thoracic and cardiovascular surgery 77.3 (1979): 362-368.

27. Marabelle, Aurélien, et al. "Intratumoral immunization: a new paradigm for cancer therapy." Clinical Cancer Research 20.7 (2014): 1747-1756.

28. Vatner, Ralph E., and Silvia C. Formenti. "Myeloid-derived cells in tumors: effects of radiation." Seminars in radiation oncology. Vol. 25. No. 1. WB Saunders, 2015.

29. Rosenberg, Steven A., and Nicholas P. Restifo. "Adoptive cell transfer as personalized immunotherapy for human cancer." Science 348.6230 (2015): 62-68.

30. Marabelle, Aurélien, et al. "Intratumoral immunization: a new paradigm for cancer therapy." Clinical Cancer Research 20.7 (2014): 1747-1756.

A Tribute to Dr. Lloyd Old

1. "Lloyd J. Old, M.D." Cancer Research Institute. Web. 30 May 2016.

2. "FDA-Approved Cancer Immunotherapies and CRI's Impact: Bladder Cancer." Cancer Research Institute. Cancer Research Institute, n.d. Web. 13 June 2016.

3. "Lloyd J. Old, M.D." Cancer Research Institute. Web. 30 May 2016.

Glossary

Abscess: A swollen area of body tissue containing an accumulation of pus.

Abscopal effect: A phenomenon where treating one tumor causes other untreated tumors in the body to shrink—presumably through an immune effect.

Acute inflammation: An immune response to injury (trauma, irritant, pathogen) that aims to eliminate the source of injury, repair the wound and clean out dead tissue. Acute inflammation resolves when these goals are achieved.

Adaptive immune system: The immune system's second line of defense that creates large numbers of specific T cells that can recognize and eradicate a pathogen.

Adjuvant: Stimulants that promote a strong response by the immune system (such as to a cancer vaccine).

Adoptive T cell therapy: An immunotherapy where T cells are isolated from the patient, then manipulated in the laboratory. There are 3 kinds of adoptive T cell therapy: T cell receptor (TCR) , chimeric antigen receptor T cell (CAR-T) and tumor-infiltrating lymphocyte (TIL). The T cells are genetically modified in TCR and CAR-T procedures to home in on a cancer signature. In all three forms, the T cells are multiplied to large numbers, then re-infused into patients.

Adoptive therapy: *See* adoptive T cell therapy

Antibodies: Small proteins that latch on to specific targets (antigens).

Antigen: A substance that can stimulate an immune response, resulting in the creation of T cells and antibodies against it. In this book, antigens mainly refer to protein signatures found on the surface of cells.

Autoimmunity: When the immune system inadvertently attacks the body's own healthy cells and tissues.

Axilla: Armpit.

B cells: An immune cell that produces antibodies.

Bacillus Calmette-Guerin: A live bacterial vaccine for the treatment of superficial bladder cancer.

Benign tumor: An abnormal growth of cells that does not invade or spread to other parts of the body.

Biopsy: A small tissue sample removed from the body for further analysis, usually removed with a needle, or sometimes during surgery.

Bone marrow: The soft, spongy tissue inside some bones in the body, where blood cells are made.

Cachexia: A state of weakness and wasting away seen in many advanced diseases, notably cancer. Strongly associated with inflammation.

Cancer vaccine: A biological preparation injected to prevent or treat cancer. Most often an injection of tumor antigen mixed with immune stimulants (adjuvants) to generate antibodies and T cells against the tumor.

Cancerous tumor: An abnormal growth of cells capable of invading and spreading to other parts of the body.

CAR T cell therapy (Chimeric antigen receptor T-cell therapy): A form of adoptive T cell therapy (*See* adoptive T cell therapy) where special receptors are engineered onto T cells so they can lock onto surface proteins on cancer cells.

Centrifuge: A machine that spins to separate out components based on their different densities.

Chemoradiation: Chemotherapy and radiation therapy.

Chimeric antigen receptor: A receptor protein engineered on the surface of T cells to recognize a certain antigen. When it binds to the antigen, it activates the T cell. The receptor protein is genetically engineered and not found in nature.

Chromosome: A structure of tightly coiled DNA.

Chromosome spread: A test that shows the DNA chromosome composition of a cell, such as a cancer cell.

Chronic inflammation: A state where immune cells are stuck in a constant state of activation and damage the body over time. Can cause or fuel cancer.

Clinical trial: A research study to investigate how well a medical therapy works. Various phases of clinical trials include Phase I (safety), Phase II (effectiveness), Phase III (large scale test of effectiveness against established therapies or placebo).

Coley's Toxins: A cancer immunotherapy (an injection of two dead strains of bacteria) developed in the 1890s by Dr. William Coley

Cryoablation: A treatment to kill tumors with extreme cold. There are various methods of delivering the cold, but in this book, we mainly describe percutaneous cryoablation (where needles are inserted through the skin to reach tumors within the body).

CT scan: A computed tomography (CT) scan, also known as a computerized axial tomography (CAT) scan, is a medical imaging technique that combines many X-ray images to form a three-dimensional internal view of the body.

CTLA-4: A protein found on the surface of T cells, that acts as a brake on the T cells when activated.

Curative surgery: Surgery performed with the intent of curing cancer, achieved by completely removing all tumor(s) and surrounding microscopic disease.

Cytokine storm: The uncontrolled secretion of cytokines in the body, leading to a massive activation of the immune system that can cause internal bleeding, organ failure and death.

Cytokines: Signals (proteins) secreted by immune cells to control the activity of other immune cells.

Dendritic cell: An immune cell that engulfs pathogens, then travels to lymph nodes to activate large numbers of T cells that can recognize and eradicate that pathogen.

Dendritic vaccine: An immunotherapy where dendritic cells are extracted from a patient, pulsed with tumor antigen(s), activated and multiplied in the laboratory, then reinfused into the patient.

DNA: Deoxyribonucleic acid, the hereditary material in humans and almost all other organisms, found in all of our cells. The information encoded in DNA serves as a master program that determines the traits of a cell and its functions.

Doxorubicin: Chemotherapy drug that kills rapidly dividing cells, derived from a natural antibiotic.

Durability of tumor shrinkage: How long the tumor shrinkage lasts.

En bloc surgery: A surgical procedure that aims to remove, in one piece, the entire tumor along with a wide cuff of healthy tissue around it.

Endoscope: A long, flexible medical device with an attached light, used by doctors to examine the insides of the body.

ENT: A physician who specializes in treating problems of the ear, nose and throat.

Erysipelas: An infection caused by the bacteria Streptococcus pyogenes, characterized by a bright, red rash.

FDA: U.S. Food and Drug Administration, the federal agency responsible for protecting public health by regulating and supervising food safety, medical devices and drugs.

First-line treatment: The first set of treatments given to a patient after diagnosis.

G-CSF: Granulocyte colony stimulating factor, a protein normally produced by immune cells to stimulate the release of neutrophils from the bone marrow.

Growth factors: Substances secreted by immune cells in our body to regulate growth and healing of tissues.

Heat-killed bacteria: Dead bacteria that are rendered harmless by heating them up.

HLA type: A genetic blood test to determine the type of immune proteins (including MHC proteins) produced in a person.

Ifosfamide: Chemotherapy drug that kills rapidly dividing cells, derived from mustard gas.

Inflammation: A response by immune cells within the body to heal wounds and eliminate a perceived threat such as an infection.

Infusion: Fluids or medications introduced into body through the vein through intravenous drip.

Innate immune system: The immune system's first line of defense that is always "standing ready" to attack invading pathogens and heal damaged tissues.

Institutional review board: A committee that reviews, approves and monitors research performed on patients.

Interventional radiologist: A physician who specializes in using minimally-invasive, image-guided procedures to diagnose and treat diseases.

Intratumoral immunotherapy : Immunotherapy that involves injecting substances directly into the tumor to generate an immune response at the site of the tumor. Examples are injections of Coley's toxins, CpG, dendritic cells.

Intravenous therapy (IV therapy): An infusion of liquid substances such as medicine directly into the vein.

Ketogenic diet: A very low-carbohydrate, high-fat diet used in medicine to control epilepsy. (Scientific studies have shown that a short course of the ketogenic diet may deplete tumors of MDSCs.)

Keytruda: The brand name for Pembrolizumab, a PD-1 inhibitor antibody, manufactured by Merck. A cancer immunotherapy that prevents the shutdown of T cells.

Killer T cell: A type of T cell capable of directly killing cancer cells by introducing holes on the surface of the target cell and pumping poisons through the holes.

Leukapheresis: A procedure that separates white blood cells from the blood. Blood is extracted from a vein in one arm and filtered for white blood cells. Unused components (red cells, plasma, platelets) are returned into the other arm.

Leukemia: Cancer of the blood cells, usually of white blood cells, but sometimes of red blood cells and platelets.

Lymph nodes: Small structures throughout the lymphatic system that filter out harmful substances and where dendritic cells activate T cells.

Lymphocyte: A type of white blood cell, that includes T cells, B cells and natural killer (NK) cells.

Lytic: The ability to destroy other cells.

Macrophages: An immune cell that eats microbes and sends signals to summon other immune cells.

Major histocompatibility complex: The major histocompatibility complex (MHC) is a set of cell surface proteins essential for the adaptive immune system to recognize foreign molecules.

Malignant tumor: *See* cancerous tumor

Margins: The rim of tissue surrounding a surgically resected tumor. If the edges are free of microscopic tumor, the margins are said to be negative (or "clear"). If tumor is found at the cut edge, margins are said to be positive.

MDSC: *See* myeloid-derived suppressor cell

Medical oncologist: A physician who treats cancer with systemic therapies (such as drugs, hormonal treatment and targeted therapies). Often the main healthcare provider for cancer patients.

Memory T cells: A T cell that encounters a pathogen (or cancer cell) but continues to persist long after the pathogen has been eradicated. Upon re-exposure, it expands to large numbers to quickly eradicate the pathogen.

Metastasis: The spread of cancers cells from a tumor to another part of the body.

MHC: *See* major histocompatibility complex

MHC class I: A cell surface protein that advertises internal proteins within a cell, thus allowing T cells to identify the cell's internal proteins.

Mixed response: The phenomenon where treatment leads to the shrinkage of some tumors but the growth of others.

Molecular fingerprint: A description used in this book for the HLA type.

MRI: Magnetic resonance imaging, a scan that uses a strong magnetic field and radio waves to create a detailed image of the internal organs and tissues within the body.

Myeloid-derived suppressor cell: A fearsome immune cell that assists tumors in many ways, protecting tumors against other immune cells, promoting the growth of tumors, helping them to form blood vessels and to spread around the body.

National Cancer Institute: A U.S. federal agency that conducts its own cancer research and supports cancer research throughout the U.S.

Natural killer cell: An immune cell that identifies and destroys cells that cannot be recognized by T cells (due to the absence of MHC Class I protein).

NCI: *See* National Cancer Institute

Necrosis: Death of cells within a tumor, usually occuring in the center of fast-growing tumors that have outgrown their blood supply.

Neoadjuvant therapy: Treatment given to help shrink a tumor before the main treatment (surgery).

Neupogen: A stimulant comprising G-CSF, given to patients whose immune systems are suppressed by chemotherapy. It works by forcing the bone marrow to produce more neutrophils.

Neurologist: A doctor who diagnoses and treats disorders of the nervous system.

Neutrophil: A type of white blood cell that kills pathogens such as bacteria, viruses and fungi. It is part of the innate immune system.

NK cell: *See* natural killer cell

No evidence of disease (NED): When cancer tests (such as scans) reveal there is no further detectable cancer in the patient's body. Synonymous with remission.

Non-Hodgkin's lymphoma: A cancer where tumors develop from lymphocytes (a type of white blood cell in our body).

NY-ESO-1: An important protein found in many cancers and elicits a strong immune response.

Off-label therapy: When a doctor prescribes a drug or therapy for an unapproved disease indication (in other words, clinical trials have not been run or completed, but the physician has decided the benefits are worth the risks).

Omega-3: An essential fatty acid necessary for human health that comes mainly from fish and algae. Decreases inflammation in the body.

Omega-3-6: An abbreviation for the dietary strategy of eliminating dietary omega-6 fats, while consuming large quantities of omega-3 in the form of fish oil.

Omega-6: An essential fatty acid found abundantly in nuts and seeds, necessary for human health, but is overabundant in the modern western diet, and fuels inflammation in the body.

Opdivo: The brand name for Nivolumab, a PD-1 inhibitor antibody, manufactured by Bristol-Myers Squibb. A cancer immunotherapy that prevents the shutdown of T cells.

Out-of-pocket: Cost of treatment or medications not covered by insurance.

Outpatient clinic: A medical clinic where patients do not stay overnight.

Overall response rate: *See* response rate

Pathologist: A physician or scientist who examines and analyzes tissue samples to diagnose diseases and determine appropriate treatment.

PD-1: A protein found on the surface of T cells, that acts as a shut down switch when activated.

PD-L1: a protein often found on tumors that activates PD-1 on T cells, causing T cells to shut down.

Peptide fragments: Short portions of proteins, made up of amino acids.

Peripherally inserted central catheter: Thin plastic catheter that is inserted into the upper arm vein and threaded all the way to the opening of the heart, used to deliver intravenous medications over a longer period of time.

PET scan: A scan where radioactive sugar is injected into the bloodstream. Due to their fast growth, cancerous cells preferentially take up the radioactive sugar and light up on the scan. PET scans are usually combined with CT scans which provide fine anatomical detail in order to pinpoint the location of high sugar uptake.

PICC line: *See* peripherally inserted central catheter

Pleurodesis : A procedure that fuses the surface of the lung to the chest wall, done to prevent future lung collapse (pneumothorax).

Pneumothorax: The collapse of a lung caused by a leak (hole) in the lung.

Primary tumor: The original or first tumor in the body from which a cancer spreads.

Prognosis: A forecast of the likely outcome of a disease, e.g. whether a cancer patient is likely to survive, or how long the patient may have to live.

Radiation oncologist: A physician who treats cancer with radiation therapy.

Radiologist: A physician who specializes in interpreting scans to diagnose diseases.

Receptor: A protein on the surface of cells that fits specifically with another protein.

Red Death: A common nickname given to the chemo drug doxorubicin. *See* doxorubicin

Response rate: The percentage of patients who show shrinkage or disappearance of tumors after receiving treatment.

Sarcoma: Malignant cancer derived from soft tissue or the bones.

Sepsis: A massive immune response to an infection, which involves the release of an overwhelming amount of inflammatory proteins into the bloodstream that can kill patients.

Single patient protocol: A clinical trial set up for only one patient.

Spontaneous regression: The unexpected improvement of cancer that would otherwise progress.

Spontaneous remission: *See* spontaneous regression

Stem cell: An immature cell that can develop into different kinds of mature cells.

Stomach ulcer: A painful, eroded area in the the lining of the stomach.

Subcutaneous injection: Injection under the skin.

Survival curve: A graph showing the percentage of patients with a specific type of cancer that remain alive over time.

T cell receptor: A protein on the T cell that recognizes a specific antigen (signature). When bound to the antigen it activates the T cell.

T cells: The "soldier cells" of the adaptive immune system, capable of multiplying into very large numbers to attack pathogens and tumors.

Targeted therapy: A newer type of cancer treatment that uses drugs, hormones or other substances to more precisely destroy cancer cells, usually while doing less damage to normal cells compared to chemotherapy.

Tumor: An abnormal growth within the body.

Tumor antigen: A protein signature present in a patient's tumor.

Tumor burden: The amount of cancer in the body, reflected in the number and size of tumors.

Tumor flare: The phenomenon of a tumor appearing larger on scans due to an increase of immune cells attacking the tumor.

Tumor microenvironment: The immune cells, blood vessels and structural scaffolding surrounding the tumor, recruited by the tumor to protect itself and support its growth.

Vaccine: *See* cancer vaccine

Yervoy: The brand name for the drug Ipilimumab, a CTLA-4 inhibitor antibody, manufactured by Bristol-Myers Squibb. A cancer immunotherapy that releases the brakes of the immune system.

Index

Reading Group Guide

During the years of battling cancer, Rene and Eddy are forced to wrestle with difficult choices—decisions such as whether to pursue experimental immunotherapy and how much they were willing to sacrifice in pursuit of an elusive cure. They also encounter sobering issues such as the prevalence of medical mistakes, the overprescription of chemotherapy and the exorbitant pricing of drugs that aren't covered by insurance. They learn the hard way that patients attempting experimental treatments may face opposition from some doctors. Through these experiences, Rene and Eddy discover the value of arming themselves with facts and facing life's difficult decisions head on.

The following questions will stimulate discussion on issues raised in the book.

Discussion Questions

1) Decisions were a major focus of Rene and Eddy's journey.

a) When purchasing a large item such as a car, how do you decide what to buy? What are some considerations you might research? How many dealers do you talk with before buying?

b) What about major medical decisions? How do you decide on the treatment to take? Do you research the doctor's recommendation and compare the pros and cons versus other approaches? Why or why not?

2) Rene and Eddy faced repeated devastating news: being diagnosed with an aggressive cancer with no effective treatments; the recurrence of her jaw tumor despite starting immunotherapy while "cancer free"; a second recurrence of her jaw tumor after "doubling down" on immunotherapy; lung tumors growing in succession every 3 months.

a) How did they react each time when confronted with bad news?

b) What do you think was the most important factor that kept them fighting?

3) Many cancer patients attempt experimental drugs toward the end of their battle—when all conventional therapies are exhausted. By then, most patients are in poor shape, their bodies riddled with tumors and debilitated from treatment side effects. In contrast, Rene and Eddy pursued immunotherapy soon after finishing first-line chemoradiation—when Rene had no visible cancer in her body.

a) What were some reasons why they pursued experimental immunotherapy so early on?

b) What advantages and disadvantages did early action confer?

4) The five-year survival for Rene's cancer was 40 percent with conventional therapy—meaning 60 percent of patients die by year five despite chemoradiation. Two views on cancer survival statistics are presented in chapter 3 (pages 45-46) and chapter 13 (pages 210-211):

View #1: Statistics don't matter to a single patient—one either survives (100% survival) or one dies (0% survival) by the cutoff date.

View #2: Statistics reflect how well the treatment will work. Therefore, they should be scrutinized to decide on treatment options (or whether to treat at all).

a) Why did some of Rene's doctors adopt view #1—that statistics didn't matter in her situation?

b) Recall a situation where a doctor recommended treatment for a difficult disease (to you or someone close). Did statistics matter? Why or why not?

c) In chapter 13 (page 211), Dr. Old recounts the story of a friend who declines chemo in the last stages of cancer. What are some of the factors that might lead someone to come to that decision?

5) Rene and Eddy chose to sacrifice their life savings, careers and prospects of starting a family—all for an uncertain chance of pursuing an elusive cure with experimental therapies. How much one is willing to sacrifice in pursuit of a cure is an intensely personal decision. Put in their situation, what would you be willing to sacrifice and why?

6) Changing one's diet isn't easy. For some cancer patients facing the prospect of death, savoring a favorite food is one of the few pleasures left to enjoy. With food being an important part of Rene's life, she was still able to make drastic dietary changes, adhering to the omega-3-6 and ketogenic diets (chapter 15, pages 254-255).

a) What are some reasons why Rene was able to restrict her diet and forgo her favorite foods?

b) How does Rene's diet-based immunotherapy compare with the other treatments she did in terms of difficulty and side effects?

7) A possible reason why Coley's Toxins faded into obscurity was the difficulty of administering repeat injections over a long period of time. In contrast, a few rapid radiation sessions would often result in dramatic tumor shrinkage (even if the cancer would later return).

a) Discuss the dichotomy between an arduous therapy (Coley's Toxins) that could cure some patients with advanced cancer (like Mrs. Gruver in chapter 5), versus a quick and convenient procedure (radiation) that doesn't cure advanced cancer.

b) Discuss other examples of this dichotomy in other areas of society, where convenience and scalability are prioritized over solutions that require more effort. Discuss the long-term consequences of these choices.

8) In chapter 7 (page 113), Rene recounts the example of her 97-year-old grandmother who was prescribed chemoradiation for localized rectal cancer. In another example (page 112), an equally frail Mark was prescribed chemo even though the risk-benefit didn't justify it. These two examples highlight the over-prescription of expensive drugs that don't necessarily benefit patients. Discuss why this happens and what patients can do to avoid these situations.

9) Medical mistakes are prevalent and a leading cause of death in the U.S. Each year, up to 400,000 preventable deaths occur due to medical mistakes. (Reference on page 304, note #1, chapter 8.)
   a) What medical mishaps did Rene experience?
   b) Have you or someone you know experienced a medical mishap?
   c) What practical steps can you take to minimize medical mistakes?

10) After Rene recovers from sepsis contracted during Coley's Toxins treatment in Mexico, Rene's oncologist gives her a "30-day notice to find another physician" (chapter 9, pages 143-144).
   a) Imagine if this happened to you. How would you feel if your oncologist told you to look for another doctor? How would you respond?
   b) Imagine if you were the oncologist. How would you feel about a patient who contracted sepsis from treatment in Mexico, taking into account that sepsis is often contracted in U.S. hospitals? How would you respond to the patient?

11) Rene and Eddy chose to spend their life savings (amounting to hundreds of thousands) on experimental immunotherapy, extensive medical travel and non-covered procedures such as cryoablation. Discuss some of the financial issues surrounding medical treatment in today's society. For example:
   a) Cutting-edge immunotherapies, such as PD-1 and CAR-T, wouldn't exist without decades' worth of federally funded basic research in immunology—footed by U.S. taxpayers. Should taxpayers be compensated, perhaps with reduced drug pricing that would, in turn, translate to a lowering of insurance premiums? Why or why not?
   b) Non-profit hospitals routinely impose a 400-percent markup on medicines not covered by insurance (such as off-label drugs). Are these markups warranted?

About the Authors

Rene Chee is a biologist who was diagnosed with a rare and aggressive cancer in 2008, while she was a postdoctoral scholar at the Stanford School of Medicine. Her training of more than a decade in the field of biology was applied to the most critical experiment of all, her own survival. She holds an M.S. in biological sciences from Stanford University and a Ph.D. in biology from the University of California, San Diego.

Edward Chee is an electrical and computer engineer by training. When his wife, Rene, was diagnosed with cancer one year after they married, he became versed in cancer biology and medicine by immersing himself in scientific literature and consulting doctors and researchers. Taking on the roles of nurse, advocate and researcher, he has fought tirelessly to help Rene survive dismal odds. He holds an M.S. in electrical engineering from Stanford University.

For more information, visit their website at *CuringCancerBook.com*, where you'll find links to follow them on Facebook and Twitter.

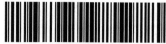

Made in the USA
Lexington, KY
08 October 2016